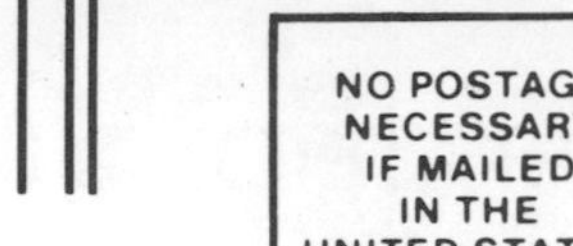

NO POSTAGE
NECESSARY
IF MAILED
IN THE
UNITED STATES

BUSINESS REPLY CARD

FIRST CLASS PERMIT NO. 33107 PHILADELPHIA, PA

POSTAGE WILL BE PAID BY ADDRESSEE

HANLEY & BELFUS, INC.
Medical Publishers
P.O. Box 1377
Philadelphia, PA 19105-9990

NO POSTAGE
NECESSARY
IF MAILED
IN THE
UNITED STATES

BUSINESS REPLY CARD

FIRST CLASS PERMIT NO. 33107 PHILADELPHIA, PA

POSTAGE WILL BE PAID BY ADDRESSEE

HANLEY & BELFUS, INC.
Medical Publishers
P.O. Box 1377
Philadelphia, PA 19105-9990

STATE OF THE ART REVIEWS (STARs)

SUBJECT	FREQUENCY	PRICE (U.S.)	PRICE (Foreign)	PRICE (Single)
☐ CARDIAC SURGERY	Triannual	$88.00	$98.00	$38.00
☐ NEUROSURGERY	Biannual	$75.00	$84.00	$42.00
☐ OCCUPATIONAL MEDICINE	Quarterly	$68.00	$78.00	$29.00
☐ PHYSICAL MED & REHAB (PM&R)	Quarterly	$66.00	$76.00	$28.00
☐ SPINE	Triannual	$78.00	$88.00	$34.00

☐ 1989 subscription ☐ 1988 subscription ☐ Single issue

Check subject title above. Title ____________

I enclose payment: ☐ Check ☐ Visa ☐ MasterCard

Credit Card # ____________ Exp. Date ________

Name ____________

Signature ____________

Title ____________

Street Address ____________

Company/Hospital ____________

City/State/Zip ____________

Send order to:

HANLEY & BELFUS, INC.

210 South 13th Street / Philadelphia, PA 19107 / 215-546-7293

Cardiac Surgery

Cyanotic Congenital Heart Disease

L. Douglas Cowgill, M.D.
Guest Editor

Volume 3/Number 1 February 1989
HANLEY & BELFUS, INC. Philadelphia

STATE OF THE ART REVIEWS

Publisher: HANLEY & BELFUS, INC.
210 South 13th Street
Philadelphia, PA 19107

CARDIAC SURGERY: State of the Art Reviews (ISSN 0887-9850)
February 1989 Volume 3, Number 1 (ISBN 0-932883-88-5)

CARDIAC SURGERY: State of the Art Reviews is published triannually (three times per year) by Hanley & Belfus, Inc., 210 South 13th Street, Philadelphia, Pennsylvania 19107.

POSTMASTER: Send address changes to CARDIAC SURGERY: State of the Art Reviews, Hanley & Belfus, Inc., 210 South 13th Street, Philadelphia, PA 19107.

This issue is Volume 3, Number 1.

The Editor of this publication is Linda C. Belfus.

CONTENTS

Tricuspid atresia is one of the most serious cardiac congenital diseases, occurring when there is absence or imperforation of the tricuspid valve. Embryology, anatomy, classification/variable features, clinical features, diagnostic methods, and treatment are discussed.

The original Fontan procedure and subsequent modifications are described and illustrated. No single form of repair is universally favored or uniformly applicable; however, principles to guide a flexible approach to reconstruction are outlined. The appropriate selection of patients for the Fontan procedure ("the Ten Commandments"), surgical technique, and postoperative are also considered.

The authors advocate aggressive surgical treatment of patients with a univentricular heart in view of the good intermediate results. They suggest that detailed anatomic identification, early intervention to reduce pulmonary vascular occlusive disease in unrestricted pulmonary blood flow, and systemic-pulmonary artery shunts when pulmonic stenosis is present, followed by early surgical repair, can favorably alter the natural history of this disease.

Ebstein's anomaly is diagnosed over a rather wide age range—from neonates to late in life. The wide variation in pathology, hemodynamics, and symptoms as well as surgical treatment and outcome are discussed.

TAPVD is a rare but serious cardiac malformation that usually occurs in isolation. Surgical results have been dramatically improved in the last two decades, largely owing to improved techniques of cardiopulmonary bypass and perioperative management.

Anomalous systemic venous return is an important, sometimes confusing, type of congenital heart disease. It includes the unroofed coronary sinus syndrome and may coexist with other anomalies. Anatomy, classification, diagnosis, treatment, and postoperative results are also addressed.

CONTRIBUTORS

H. Ashraf, M.D., FRCS
Cardiovascular Surgeon, Miami Children's Hospital and Cedars Medical Center, Miami, Florida

David N. Campbell, M.D.
Associate Professor of Surgery, Section of Cardiovascular-Thoracic Surgery, University of Colorado Health Services Center, Denver, Colorado

David R. Clarke, M.D.
Associate Professor of Surgery, University of Colorado Health Services Center; Chief of Cardiothoracic Surgery, University Hospital and The Children's Hospital, Denver, Colorado

Daniel M. Cohen, M.D.
Fellow, Pediatric Cardiovascular Surgery, The Hospital for Sick Children, Toronto, Ontario, Canada

L. Douglas Cowgill, M.D.
Department of Surgery, Dean Clinic, Madison, Wisconsin

Pedro J. del Nido, M.D.
Assistant Professor of Surgery, University of Illinois College of Medicine, Chicago, Illinois

John W.E. Douglas-Jones
Division of Cardiovascular and Thoracic Surgery, Marshfield Clinic, Marshfield, Wisconsin

Robert M. Freedom, M.D., FRCPC, FACC
Professor of Pediatrics and Pathology, and Head, Division of Cardiology, University of Toronto Faculty of Medicine, Toronto, Ontario, Canada

Frank L. Hanley, M.D.
Assistant Professor of Surgery, University of California, San Francisco, School of Medicine, San Francisco, California

John C. Laschinger, M.D.
Chief Resident, Division of Cardiothoracic Surgery, Washington University School of Medicine, St. Louis, Missouri

Sidney Levitsky, M.D.
Professor of Surgery, University of Illinois College of Medicine, Chicago, Illinois

William I. Norwood, M.D., Ph.D.
Professor of Surgery, University of Pennsylvania School of Medicine, Chief of Cardiothoracic Surgery, The Children's Hospital of Philadelphia, Philadelphia, Pennsylvania

Albert D. Pacifico, M.D.
Professor and Director, Division of Cardiothoracic Surgery, University of Alabama at Birmingham, Birmingham, Alabama

John D. Pigott, M.D.
Assistant Professor of Surgery, University of Pennsylvania School of Medicine; Division of Cardiothoracic Surgery, The Children's Hospital of Philadelphia, Philadelphia, Pennsylvania

Stephen Jay Roth, M.D.
Department of Pediatrics, Division of Pediatric Cardiology, Marshfield Clinic, Marshfield, Wisconsin

David C. Sabiston, Jr., M.D.
James B. Duke Professor and Chairman, Department of Surgery, Duke University Medical Center, Durham, North Carolina

S. Subramanian, M.D.
Chairman, Cardiovascular Surgery, Miami Children's Hospital; Chief, Cardiac Surgery, Cedars Medical Center, Miami, Florida

Kevin Turley, M.D.
Associate Professor of Surgery, University of California, San Francisco, School of Medicine, San Francisco, California

Ross Michael Ungerleider, M.D.
Assistant Professor of Surgery, and Chief, Pediatric Cardiac Surgery, Duke University Medical Center, Durham, North Carolina

Edward D. Verrier, M.D., Ph.D.
Associate Professor of Surgery, University of California, San Francisco, School of Medicine, San Francisco, California

Clarence S. Weldon, M.D.
Formerly, Professor of Surgery, and Head, Division of Cardiothoracic Surgery, Washington University School of Medicine, St. Louis, Missouri

William G. Williams, M.D., FRCSC
Associate Professor of Surgery, University of Toronto Faculty of Medicine, Toronto, Ontario, Canada

PUBLISHED ISSUES, 1986–1988

Volume 1, Number 1 — **Coronary Artery Bypass Grafting**
Edited by Jack G. Copeland, M.D.
and Steven Goldman, M.D.
Tucson, Arizona

Volume 1, Number 2 — **Current Heart Valve Prostheses**
Edited by Fred A. Crawford, Jr., M.D.
Charleston, South Carolina

Volume 1, Number 3 — **Surgery of the Aorta**
Edited by L. Douglas Cowgill, M.D.
Marshfield, Wisconsin

Volume 2, Number 1 — **Concomitant Cardiac and Peripheral Vascular Disease**
Edited by Hamner Hannah, III, M.D.
Kansas City, Missouri

Volume 2, Number 2 — **Myocardial Preservation**
Edited by W. Randolph Chitwood, Jr., M.D.
Lexington, Kentucky

Volume 2, Number 3 — **Mediastinal and Sternal Infections**
Edited by Thomas J. Vander Salm, M.D.
Worcester, Massachusetts

Volume 2, Number 4 — **Cardiothoracic Transplantation**
Edited by Robert W. Emery, M.D.
and Marc R. Pritzker, M.D.
Minneapolis, Minnesota

FUTURE ISSUES

Innovations in Congenital Heart Surgery
Edited by Irving Kron, M.D.,
Charlottesville, VA
and Constantine Mavroudis, M.D.,
Louisville, KY

Cardiac Pacing
Edited by Lenox D. Baker, M.D.
Norfolk, Virginia

Thoracic Transplantation: Medical Management and Complications
Edited by Robert W. Emery, M.D.,
Marc R. Pritzker, M.D., and
Frazier F. Eales, M.D.
Minneapolis, Minnesota

Cardiac Arrhythmia Surgery
Edited by James L. Cox, M.D.
St. Louis, Missouri

Subscriptions and single issues available from the publisher—Hanley & Belfus, Inc., Medical Publishers, 210 South 13th Street, Philadelphia, PA 19107 (215) 546-7293.

PREFACE

> Heretofore a "blue baby" with a malformed heart was considered beyond the reach of surgical aid.
>
> Alfred Blalock and Helen Taussig, 1945

Nearly 45 years have passed since Alfred Blalock and Helen Taussig collaborated on the first systemic artery-pulmonary artery shunt, offering hope to children afflicted with certain cyanotic forms of congenital heart disease. When cardiopulmonary bypass became available in the 1950s, the possibility of definitive repair for many lesions arose and accelerated the pace of learning. The atrial switch procedures, developed for the fundamentally abnormal circulation of transposition of the great arteries, illustrated the ingenuity with which congenital heart surgery might be approached. The introduction of the Rashkind procedure was an early model for subsequent therapeutic catheterization techniques. In the 1970s, the right-heart bypass procedure allowed separation of systemic and pulmonary circulations for lesions with hypoplastic right ventricle, univentricular heart, and, more recently, hypoplastic left ventricle. Advances in the last 10 years are too numerous to abbreviate here but include both primary repair and transatrial approach for tetralogy of Fallot, the successful performance of arterial switch for transposition of the great arteries, and percutaneous balloon valvuloplasty for valvular stenosis. Additionally, the remarkable diagnostic information provided by bedside 2-D echocardiography, the utility of prostaglandin E_1 and hypothermia/circulatory arrest in infants, and the tremendous improvements in perioperative circulatory, nursing, and respiratory care have steadily lowered operative mortality for all but the most complex congenital heart lesions.

Congenital heart disease is typically divided into acyanotic and cyanotic lesions. Although the latter constitute a minority of the total, they present some of the most complex and challenging anatomic and physiologic problems. In addition, a mastery of cyanotic lesions is of immense value for approaching all patients with congenital heart disease. With that perspective this issue of **Cardiac Surgery: State of the Art Reviews** addresses the various cyanotic lesions, with special emphasis on recent developments and recommendations.

The review begins with an introductory overview, intended primarily for the less experienced student. Two chapters on topics of general interest for many cyanotic lesions, therapeutic catheterization techniques and extracardiac shunting procedures, are included. Other chapters individually address the various disorders beginning with an authoritative discussion of the most common cyanotic lesion, tetralogy of Fallot. Special consideration is also given transposition of the great arteries and tricuspid atresia. The importance of the Fontan procedure for so many forms of cyanotic congenital heart disease leads to a separate discussion of that procedure. The review concludes with a discussion of an important issue for many of these lesions—homograft valves.

Many individuals deserve special recognition. I am very grateful to all of the contributors for their excellent manuscripts, with special acknowledgment to my mentors in congenital heart disease, David Clarke and David Campbell. I am thankful for the stimulus provided by Alden Harken, and the encouragement and example of Alan Hopeman.

Having recently taken a position at the Dean Clinic, I would also like to recognize my former institution, the Marshfield Clinic and St. Joseph's Hospital, and their superb cardiology, operating room, perfusionist, and nursing staffs. The help of our assistants, particularly Robert Hanlin, is appreciated, as is that of Al Zimmerman and his excellent library staff. The cheerful dedication of Ardell Specht and Linda Wyman, and the immense clerical work provided by JoAnn Strobel are deeply appreciated. Most importantly, the professional example and personal support of my esteemed colleagues, William O. Myers, Jefferson Ray, John Douglas-Jones, Richard Sautter, and the late Ben Lawton have been inspirational.

Finally, words are insufficient to express my gratitude for the patience, support, and vitality of my wife and family.

L. Douglas Cowgill, M.D.
GUEST EDITOR

L. DOUGLAS COWGILL, MD

APPROACH TO THE PATIENT WITH CYANOTIC CONGENITAL HEART DISEASE

From the Department of Surgery
Dean Clinic
Madison, Wisconsin

Reprint requests to:
L. Douglas Cowgill, MD
Department of Surgery
Dean Clinic
1313 Fish Hatchery Rd.
Madison, WI 53715

As a framework for subsequent chapters, an overview of pathophysiology, classification, diagnosis, and management of cyanotic congenital heart disease is presented here. For those conditions, usually rare, not discussed elsewhere, a brief discussion of management will be provided.

PATHOPHYSIOLOGY

Cyanosis comes from the Greek word for blue, "kyanos," and describes a bluish discoloration of skin and mucous membranes due to excessive concentration of reduced hemoglobin in the blood. Normally systemic hemoglobin oxygen saturation is greater than 95%, but may fall to 92% with crying and other physiologic changes. Arterial desaturation is considered to be present when arterial saturation is less than 91%.[1] The typical oxygen-hemoglobin dissociation curve is sigmoid, becoming relatively flat at pO_2 values greater than 60 mm Hg, so that arterial desaturation implies significant reduction of pO_2 below 50-60 mm Hg.

Lundsgaard[2] demonstrated that the recognition of cyanosis was dependent on the absolute concentration of reduced hemoglobin in the blood, rather than the ratio of reduced to oxygenated hemoglobin. Originally authorities thought that at least 5 gm of hemoglobin per 100 cc of circulating blood needed to be desaturated for cyanosis to be apparent.[2,3] This would mean, for a patient with a hemoglobin of 15 gm%, arterial oxygen saturation would have to be 67% or less for cyanosis to be recognized. As cyanosis may be apparent at O_2 saturations between 75–88%, cyanosis may be detectable with 3 gm% of reduced hemoglobin.[4,5] The hemoglobin value is also very important, as a patient with an O_2 saturation of 75% and hemoglobin of 10 will not be cyanotic (2.5 gm desaturated hemoglobin), whereas another with O_2 saturation of 75% but hemoglobin of 16 would be cyanotic (4 gm of desaturated hemoglobin). Other factors, including pH, pCO_2, amount of 2,3 diphosphoglycerate and percent of fetal hemoglobin also affect the cyanotic appearance by their effect on the oxygen-hemoglobin dissociation curve. Factors that shift the oxygen-hemoglobin curve to the left, such as increased levels of fetal hemoglobin, delay the appearance of cyanosis by keeping oxygen bound to hemoglobin at the expense of oxygen delivery to the tissues. Thus the newborn infant with a high concentration of fetal hemoglobin may have a serious reduction in oxygen tension (pO_2 32–34 mm Hg) before cyanosis is apparent.[6] This also implies measurement of oxygen tension is much more discriminatory than measurement of oxygen saturation.

In their classic studies on the causes of cyanosis, Lundsgaard and Van Slyke[7] demonstrated four important factors in the production of cyanosis: (1) the height of hemoglobin, (2) the volume of venous blood shunted into the systemic circulation, (3) the rate of oxygen utilization by peripheral tissues, and (4) the extent of the aeration of blood in the lungs. They also described the clinical and laboratory differentiation between central and peripheral cyanosis. Organs with a substantial flow and small arteriovenous oxygen difference (e.g., tongue and mucous membranes) will not appear cyanotic as early as the peripheral extremities, with a low blood flow and wider arteriovenous oxygen difference (Table 1).[18] Peripheral cyanosis, in which the arterial O_2 saturation is normal, may occur in low flow states (shock, congestive failure, cold environment) when the extremities are cool, tissue oxygen extraction is increased, and the arteriovenous oxygen difference is wide.

Central cyanosis requires reduction of arterial O_2 saturation. Its major causes are cardiac abnormalities (in which cyanosis occurs either from a right-to-left shunt across an atrial septal defect (ASD), ventricular septal defect (VSD), or patent ductus arteriosus (PDA), or because of transposition of the great arteries where the systemic and pulmonary circulations are arranged in parallel) and pulmonary abnormalities. For cardiac lesions with a right-to-left shunt, the degree of arterial desaturation depends largely on the total pulmonary blood flow

TABLE 1. Differential Diagnosis of Cyanosis

Features	Central	Peripheral
Physiologic		
Systemic arterial oxygen saturation	Reduced	Normal
Systemic arteriovenous difference	Normal	Wide
Cardiac output	Normal to high	Low
Clinical		
Intensity	Moderate to severe	Mild
Mucous membranes	Cyanotic	Pink
Temperature of extremities	Warm	Cold, clammy

Reprinted with permission from Pediatr Ann 10:127–132, 1981.

TABLE 2. Differential Diagnosis of Central Cyanosis

Features	Cardiac	Pulmonary	Hematologic
	Intracardiac or great-vessel mixing	Alveolar hypoventilation, ventilation-perfusion imbalance	Methemoglobinemia
Physiologic			
Pulmonary venous pO_2	Normal	Diminished	Normal
Systemic arterial pO_2	Diminished	Diminished	Normal
Systemic arterial pCO_2	Normal	High	Normal
Clinical			
Crying	Cyanosis increases	Cyanosis decreases	Cyanosis unchanged
100% O_2	Cyanosis decreases	Cyanosis usually clears	Cyanosis unchanged

Reprinted with permission from Pediatr Ann 10:127–132, 1981.

or pulmonary-to-systemic flow ratio.[5] The lower the pulmonary flow, the lower the systemic arterial saturation and the worse the cyanosis.

A number of pulmonary abnormalities may cause cyanosis, including primary lung disease, hypoventilation from atelectasis or other cause, extrinsic mechanical interference with lung function, and primary pulmonary hypertension. Because these problems often arise in the newborn infant when serious cardiac causes of cyanosis become evident, their distinction is important (Table 2). The response to breathing 100% oxygen, especially with positive pressure ventilation, is helpful because it should result in $pO_2 > 100$ for most pulmonary problems, while having minimal effect on pure right-to-left shunt. However, serious pulmonary pathology, especially when associated with intrapulmonary right-to-left shunt, may not show a response to 100% oxygen, so this test must be used with an understanding of its limitations.[4,8] A dramatic response to oxygen breathing supports alveolar hypoventilation or ventilation/perfusion mismatch (but does not exclude cyanotic congenital heart disease), whereas lack of any visible response favors a large intracardiac or intrapulmonary right-to-left shunt.

A difficult problem in infancy is the distinction between cyanotic congenital heart disease and persistent pulmonary hypertension (PPH) associated with substantial right-to-left shunt across a patent foramen ovale and/or ductus arteriosus (persistent fetal circulation). Administration of 100% oxygen would not be expected to alter either shunt situation, although initial improvement in pO_2 is occasionally seen with PPH followed by deterioration. Neonates with suspected PPH are often given tolazoline hydrochloride for diagnostic and therapeutic purposes to reduce pulmonary vascular resistance, increase pulmonary blood flow, and reduce right-to-left ductal shunting.[9] However, if tolazoline preferentially reduces systemic over pulmonary vascular resistance, right-to-left ductal shunting may actually increase with worsening of cyanosis. For this reason, close monitoring of systemic blood pressure during tolazoline administration has been recommended to aid interpretation of hemodynamic events.[8,9]

The other type of pulmonary hypertension deserving comment is Eisenmenger's syndrome, in which chronic, severe left-to-right shunt (usually VSD or PDA) causes delayed development of pulmonary hypertension, with reversal of shunt across the defect and production of cyanosis. Other causes of cyanosis include methemoglobinemia, polycythemia, shock, sepsis, hypoglycemia, and central nervous system disease.[4]

Differential cyanosis describes cyanosis confined to the upper or lower extremities, and may be missed unless the extremities are carefully compared. It requires right-to-left ductal shunting, and generally indicates serious cyanotic congenital heart disease. In most cases, the lower extremities will be cyanotic with the upper extremities pink, such as cases of aortic obstruction (coarctation or interrupted arch). A reverse pattern of differential cyanosis, with cyanotic upper extremities and pink lower ones, indicates transposition of the great arteries with patent ductus arteriosus.

The degree of restriction to pulmonary blood flow is central to the understanding of cyanosis pathophysiology. Normally the transition from fetal to adult circulatory patterns begins at birth with the onset of respirations and the exclusion of the low-resistance placental circulation. With lung expansion, oxygenation, and chemical mediators of vasodilatation, pulmonary vascular resistance falls and the foramen ovale and ductus arteriosus close. Once right-to-left shunting is eliminated, normal adult-type circulatory patterns are established, although the decline of pulmonary vascular resistance to normal adult levels may take weeks to months.[10]

In cyanotic patients with elevated pulmonary vascular resistance, pulmonary blood flow is reduced with persistent right-to-left shunting across atrial, ventricular, or ductal defects. Furthermore, the usual increase in oxygen uptake that normally occurs at the start of exercise may fail to occur. This can be measured noninvasively to evaluate the degree to which pulmonary blood flow is constrained in response to exercise.[11]

In addition to the anatomic restriction to pulmonary blood flow, polycythemia (secondary to sustained and profound arterial hypoxemia) increases vascular resistance by increasing viscosity.[12] Generally, the relative blood viscosity rises exponentially with increased hematocrit. In the systemic circulation, the increased blood viscosity may be offset by increase in blood volume and peripheral vasodilatation. Since restriction to pulmonary blood flow prevents expansion of pulmonary blood volume, pulmonary vascular resistance increases relative to systemic vascular resistance, and right-to-left shunting is worsened. Moreover, the low flow, hyperviscosity, and polycythemia cause stasis, which in turn may cause formation of pulmonary and cerebral thrombi when the hematocrit rises above 65%.[13–16]

Considering the severity of desaturation in many forms of cyanotic congenital heart disease, it is sometimes surprising that many patients do as well as they do. This was the finding of Theodore and colleagues,[17] who studied adults with cyanotic congenital heart disease and found the patients capable of moderate exercise and normal brain function despite severe hypoxia. Also surprising in this study was that mitochondrial O_2 utilization was maintained despite profound reduction in pO_2, without compensatory rise in hemoglobin concentration, cardiac output, or oxyhemoglobin dissociation.

CLASSIFICATION

Although cyanotic congenital heart disease is usually classified broadly into two groups, that with decreased and that with increased pulmonary blood flow, a division into three groups is more precise (Table 3).[8] Lesions with diminished

TABLE 3. Classification of Cyanotic Heart Disease

Group I: Diminished Pulmonary Blood Flow
- A. Ventricular septal communication
  1. Tetralogy of Fallot
  2. Variants of tetralogy of Fallot
     - a. Double outlet right ventricle with pulmonary stenosis
     - b. Tetralogy of Fallot and endocardial cushion defect
     - c. Single ventricle and pulmonary stenosis with or without transposition of the great vessels.
     - d. Complete transposition of the great arteries with ventricular septal defect and pulmonary stenosis
     - e. Congenitally corrected transposition of the great arteries with ventricular septal defect and pulmonary stenosis
     - f. Congenital cardiac anomalies associated with asplenia
     - g. Pulmonary atresia with ventricular septal defect
- B. Atrial septal communication
  - a. Pulmonary atresia with intact ventricular septum
  - b. Tricuspid atresia
  - c. Ebstein's anomaly of the tricuspid valve
  - d. Hypoplastic right ventricle
  - e. Uhl's anomaly of the right ventricle
  - f. Tricuspid insufficiency
  - g. Endocardial fibroelastosis of the right ventricle

Group II: Increased Pulmonary Blood Flow
- A. Truncus arteriosus
- B. Single ventricle
- C. Tricuspid atresia
- D. Total anomalous pulmonary venous connection
- E. Transposition of the great vessels with ventricular septal defect or patent ductus arteriosus
- F. Hypoplastic left ventricle

Group III: Simple transposition of the great vessels

Modified from Moller JH, Neal WA: Heart Disease in Infancy. New York, Appleton-Century-Crofts, 1981, p. 365.

pulmonary blood flow (Qp) include tetralogy of Fallot and its variants and pulmonary atresia. The major variables influencing the severity of cyanosis will be the oxygen consumption, oxygen capacity, the ratio of pulmonary to systemic blood flow (Qp/Qs), and the effective pulmonary blood flow (Qep, which is the portion of systemic venous return circulating through the lungs, and will equal Qp in pure right-to-left shunts). The Qp/Qs depends on the severity of obstruction to pulmonary blood flow, but for these disorders will always be less than one. In patients with ventricular-level shunts, the Qp depends upon the relative resistance to systemic and pulmonary blood flow imposed by the systemic arterioles and pulmonary stenosis, respectively. In patients with atrial-level shunts, the flow is more dependent upon the relative ventricular compliances. Since right ventricular filling in these latter conditions is usually severely limited (tricuspid atresia, pulmonary atresia, Ebstein's anomaly), right-to-left shunting is favored.

The second group of cyanotic lesions is characterized by complete intracardiac mixing of systemic with pulmonary blood flow, and includes total anomalous pulmonary venous connection, truncus arteriosus, and single ventricle without pulmonary stenosis. Depending on whether there is obstruction to pulmonary blood flow or pulmonary venous return, Qp/Qs may either be less than or greater than one. These malformities are termed "admixture" lesions, with both a left-to-right and right-to-left shunt. Quite often in these lesions cyanosis may be mild, and the patient may be in congestive failure (Qp/Qs much greater than one) with pulmonary edema.

The third type of cyanotic heart defect is simple transposition of the great arteries. Since the systemic and pulmonary circulations are arranged in parallel, Qp/Qs is not an important determinant of pO_2 or oxygen content. Qep, however, is inversely related to the degree of cyanosis, and is determined by the degree of bidirectional interatrial shunting across a patent foramen ovale. If a VSD or PDA is also present, cyanosis may be mild and congestive failure may occur.

TETRALOGY OF FALLOT

This condition represents approximately 10% of all congenital heart lesions, and is the commonest cyanotic cardiac lesion beyond infancy. The "tetralogy" consists of a large malalignment VSD, right ventricular outflow tract obstruction, overriding aorta, and right ventricular hypertrophy. The right ventricular outflow tract obstruction is usually in the form of infundibular and valvar stenosis. Occasionally supravalvular or branch pulmonary artery stenosis occurs. The caliber of the pulmonary annulus, trunk, and pulmonary arteries reflects the degree of infundibular stenosis. Occasionally the left pulmonary artery is absent. Other conditions including ASD, anomalous left anterior descending from the right coronary artery, and right aortic arch may be present.

The clinical presentation reflects the degree of right ventricular outflow tract obstruction, with most patients symptomatic with cyanosis, clubbing, squatting, dyspnea on exertion, and hypoxia spells. In the minority with pulmonary atresia, presentation will be early in life with life-threatening cyanosis. "Pink" tetralogy indicates mild right ventricular outflow tract obstruction. Precordial exam reveals a local systolic murmur, often with thrill, and a single-component second sound. Electrocardiogram shows right axis deviation (RAD) (+120 to +150 degrees) with right ventricular hypertrophy (RVH). Chest x-ray classically shows boot-shaped heart (concave main pulmonary artery segment with upturned apex from RVH), decreased pulmonary vascular markings, and in 25% right aortic arch. "Pink" tetralogy may be indistinguishable from VSD. The echocardiogram resembles that seen in truncus arteriosus (enlarged arterial vessel overriding thick interventricular septum), but the pulmonary valve and right ventricular outflow tract should be identifiable in patients with tetralogy, unlike those with truncus arteriosus. Catheterization reveals identical oxygen saturation on the right side of the heart, with systemic right ventricular pressure, gradient(s) across the right ventricular outflow tract, and right-to-left shunt across the large VSD.

A different type of tetralogy of Fallot is that with absent pulmonary valve. If pulmonary incompetence is severe with increased pulmonary blood flow, presentation may be early with congestive failure and severe tracheobronchitis. Cyanosis may be absent and infants may be in severe respiratory distress. The second heart sound is single, and a diastolic murmur may be audible. Chest x-ray is usually distinctive, showing mediastinal widening due to aneurysmal dilatation of the central and hilar pulmonary arteries. Unlike typical tetralogy, in severe cases there is considerable cardiomegaly. In addition to the usual principles of tetralogy of Fallot repair (VSD closure, relief of right ventricular outflow tract obstruction), placement of a homograft valve is indicated for patients beyond infancy.[19-22]

About 1% of patients with tetralogy of Fallot have associated complete atrioventricular canal defects. A murmur of mitral insufficiency may be present. A QRS axis of –90° to –150° is a valuable clue, and a typical gooseneck deformity of left ventricular outflow tract will be seen on angiocardiography. Operation entails correction of both the atrioventricular canal as well as tetralogy defects.[23-27]

TRANSPOSITION OF THE GREAT ARTERIES

This condition accounts for some 5-8% of all congenital heart defects, and is the most common cause of cyanosis in the newborn infant. It is more common in males. The aorta arises anteriorly from the right ventricle (to the right of the pulmonary artery in d-transposition, and to the left in the infrequent l-transposition), with the pulmonary artery arising posteriorly from the left ventricle. Defects that permit bidirectional shunting (usually patent foramen ovale) are necessary for survival. A VSD is present in some 40%. Pulmonic stenosis, either valvular or subvalvular, occurs in about 30% of patients with VSD and 5% without VSD.[28]

Clinically, cyanosis is usually present at birth, but can be delayed several weeks with VSD. The patient is usually a large, tachypneic male infant with moderate to severe cyanosis. The S_2 is loud and single. A systolic murmur is present in only about half of patients, usually when VSD or left ventricular outflow tract obstruction is present. Arterial hypoxemia may be severe, and responds minimally to 100% oxygen. If mixing between pulmonary and systemic venous return is inadequate, the pO_2 ranges between 15 and 30 mm Hg, with values less than 20 being ominous. The three characteristic x-ray findings are a narrow superior mediastinum (due to the superimposition of aortic and pulmonary artery shadows), mild cardiomegaly and mild pulmonary plethora. This "egg-on-its-side" appearance is present in approximately 75% of patients. Electrocardiogram shows RAD (+90° to +200°) with RVH within a few days of life. Two-D echocardiography is usually diagnostic, showing the abnormal position of the great vessels, and features of dynamic left ventricular outflow tract obstruction may be detectable (leftward deviation of the ventricular septum, premature closure of the pulmonary valve).[29] Catheterization is performed urgently to substantiate the diagnosis, exclude associated anomalies, and perform Rashkind balloon atrial septostomy.

Natural history leaves 90% of untreated patients dead within 6 months of age. The sickest infants are those without VSD, but they respond best to Rashkind septostomy. Those with VSD or PDA may do better untreated initially, but are more likely to develop congestive heart failure and pulmonary vascular obstructive disease (PVOD) (unless, in the case of VSD, the patient is protected from congestive heart failure by left ventricular outflow tract obstruction).

Special situations include TGA with large VSD, transposition of the great arteries with VSD and left ventricular outflow tract obstruction, and transposition of the great arteries (TGA) with PDA. For TGA with large VSD, repair has been performed by use of an intraventricular tunnel technique, depending upon the relationship of the VSD to the great vessels and tricuspid valve.[30,31] Alternatively an arterial or atrial switch procedure with transatrial VSD closure may be performed. A tunnel technique is also used for transposition of the great arteries with VSD and left ventricular outflow tract obstruction, using a patch to close the VSD so that the left ventricle is in continuity with the aorta, and using a valved conduit for right ventricular–pulmonary artery continuity (Rastelli procedure). This procedure is preferably delayed until 3–5 years of age to allow a reasonably large homograft valve-conduit to be used, using an initial shunt for palliation if necessary to allow growth.[32–35] Patients with TGA and PDA are at increased risk of death, including natural history of untreated disease, following Rashkind procedure, and following operative repair.[36–39] Closure of the ductus (spontaneously or surgically), even when combined with Rashkind septostomy, may result in severe hypoxia and sudden deterioration, with decreased intra-atrial mixing (due to decreased pulmonary venous return) as well as the loss of the ductal shunt being contributory.[37] These patients need to be managed aggressively, preferably with early arterial or atrial switch procedure.[39]

CONGENITALLY CORRECTED TRANSPOSITION

In this condition, not only is the ventriculoarterial relationship discordant, but so also is the atrioventricular relationship. Consequently the two abnormalities result in functional correction, since the right atrium empties through a (bicuspid) mitral valve into the left ventricle which ejects through the pulmonary artery, and the left atrium empties through a tricuspid valve into the right ventricle which then ejects blood out the aorta. The "right" ventricle is located to the left of the "left" ventricle (ventricular inversion). Although this arrangement results in no functional abnormality by itself, associated intracardiac defects are common. A large VSD is present in some 80%, and since pulmonary (valvular or subvalvular) stenosis occurs in about 50%, these patients are quite often cyanotic. Tricuspid regurgitation (systemic ventricle) is frequent, as are conduction abnormalities (arrhythmia/block). The conduction bundle courses superior and on the left side (right ventricle) of the VSD. Presentation depends on associated defects,with cyanosis (VSD and pulmonary stenosis) or congestive heart failure (large VSD) common. Physical examination depends on presence of VSD, pulmonary stenosis, and tricuspid regurgitation. Electrocardiograms may show varying degrees of 1st, 2nd, or 3rd degree heart block. Additionally, a pattern of reversed direction of initial ventricular depolarization may be indicated by the absence of Q-waves in I, V5 and V6, and the presence of Q waves in right precordial leads. Chest x-ray may suggest the l-transposition of the aorta by a straight shadow along the left upper cardiac border. Echocardiography is reasonably accurate, but cardiac catheterization is required for definitive diagnosis.

DOUBLE-OUTLET RIGHT VENTRICLE

This condition comprises less than 1% of all congenital heart disease. The 50% rule is used to distinguish double-outlet right ventricle from tetralogy of Fallot or TGA, with all of one great artery and more than 50% of the other arising from the right ventricle diagnostic of double-outlet right ventricle.[40] Both the aorta and pulmonary artery arise side-by-side from the right ventricle, with their valves at the same level, and there is aortic/mitral valve discontinuity from a subaortic conus in most cases. The only outlet from the left ventricle is a large VSD, which is classified as subaortic, subpulmonary, doubly committed, or uncommitted.[41] The three most common types are subaortic VSD without pulmonary stenosis (Eisenmenger type), with pulmonary stenosis (Fallot type), and subpulmonary VSD (Taussig-Bing type). Other malformations are common, and many patients are inoperable. Clinical presentation varies considerably depending on the location of VSD, presence of pulmonic stenosis, and associated anomalies, with congestive failure the rule for the Eisenmenger type, and cyanosis for the Fallot and Taussig-Bing types. Chest x-rays will show decreased pulmonary vascularity for the Fallot type, but increased for the Taussig-Bing variety. The latter also reveals a pulmonary artery O_2 saturation greater than aortic. Echocardiography may be helpful for diagnosis (extreme overriding of the aorta, aortic/mitral valve discontinuity), but cardiac catheterization is necessary for accurate diagnosis.

Much rarer than double-outlet right ventricle is double-outlet left ventricle. Common associated anomalies are subaortic VSD, pulmonary stenosis, Ebstein's malformation of the tricuspid valve, hypoplastic right ventricle, and atrioventricular discordance. Congestive failure is present unless pulmonary stenosis (which is frequent) results in cyanosis from diminished pulmonary blood flow. Complete repair usually entails use of an external valved conduit in patients with associated pulmonary or subpulmonary stenosis.[40,42,43]

SINGLE VENTRICLE (UNIVENTRICULAR HEART)

This condition represents less than 1% of all congenital heart disease. In this entity, the ventricular chamber receives both the mitral and tricuspid valves. The great vessels are transposed in about 80% of patients, roughly equally divided between l-and d-transposition. The ventricular chamber is LV-type in 80% (recognized by its smooth trabecular pattern), RV-type in most of the remainder, and rarely a true common ventricle with normal right ventricular and left ventricular components but absent septum. A rudimentary infundibular (outlet) chamber is present in the first two types, giving rise to one of the great arteries. This rudimentary chamber is anterosuperior (usually on the left [l-loop], but often on the right [d-loop]) when the main chamber is left ventricular type , and posteroinferior when the main chamber is of right ventricular type. In the majority with transposition, the aorta arises from the outlet chamber and the pulmonary artery from the main chamber. Aortic stenosis is generally present with d-transposition, while pulmonary stenosis is present in about half of patients with l-transposition. Asplenia or polysplenia syndrome occurs commonly. Anatomic variations are numerous, with the most common subtype (about half) being LV-type main chamber and left-sided (subaortic) anterosuperior outlet chamber.

Clinical presentation varies considerably. About one-third of patients have no pulmonary stenosis, and present similar to those with large VSD with congestive heart failure, distinguishable because common mixing in the single ventricle also produces mild cyanosis (resembling TGA with VSD or truncus arteriosus). The majority of patients with pulmonary stenosis present with cyanosis, usually after infancy, and the clinical picture resembles that of tetralogy of Fallot. Electrocardiogram may show one of four patterns: (1) RVH, (2) LVH, (3) similar RS, rS, or QR complexes across most or all precordial leads, or (4) a pattern of corrected transposition. Chest x-ray shows variable heart size and pulmonary vascularity depending on pulmonary stenosis, but may have a narrow waist due to transposition. Echocardiography may be diagnostic by absence of posterior (inlet) septum between the two atrioventricular valves, and no ventricular septal echo in the usual position. Cardiac catheterization is definitive.

PULMONARY ATRESIA WITH INTACT VENTRICULAR SEPTUM

This condition represents approximately 1% of all types of congenital heart disease. It usually presents in the first 24 hours with intense cyanosis, decreased pulmonary vascularity, and cardiomegaly, with 50% of untreated patients dead within the first month. The pulmonary valve is replaced by an imperforate membrane, and by definition there is no VSD. In approximately 85% of patients the right ventricle is hypoplastic, whereas in the remainder it is large and thin-walled. The tricuspid valve is always abnormal; in the former it tends to be small and stenotic, and in the latter larger and incompetent. A combination of tricuspid stenosis and regurgitation is common and Ebstein's anomaly may occur. A right ventricular assessment by a tripartite classification is useful, with some right ventricles having an absent trabecular portion, some having an absent infundibular and trabecular portion (with only an inlet portion present), and some having a tripartite ventricle with inlet, trabecular, and infundibular portions.[44,45] Fistulous communications between the hypertensive right ventricle and coronary artery (myocardial sinusoids) occur in up to 40%, being common in hypoplastic hypertensive right ventricle without tricuspid regurgitation and rare in dilated right ventricles with tricuspid regurgitation. They are associated with coronary artery sclerosis and myocardial ischemia. For survival an atrial and ductal communication are necessary, and both Rashkind procedure and prostaglandin therapy have been used to maintain necessary shunts. Clinically, cyanosis is usually early and intense and progresses to metabolic acidosis. Hepatomegaly may be present. Murmurs are variable, depending upon ductal flow and tricuspid regurgitation. Electrocardiogram is variable depending upon right ventricular size, but unlike tricuspid atresia (also having hypoplastic right ventricle), left axis deviation (LAD) is rare. Chest x-ray may resemble that of tricuspid atresia, with cardiomegaly from right atrial and left ventricular enlargement, decreased pulmonary vascular markings, and a concave main pulmonary artery segment. Echocardiography demonstrates right ventricular size, a pulmonary valve is not seen, and the presence of a tricuspid valve distinguishes this from tricuspid atresia. Cardiac catheterization provides precise information regarding right ventricular size, pressure (usually suprasystemic), presence of sinusoids, and length of atretic infundibulum.

TRICUSPID ATRESIA

Tricuspid atresia represents 3% of all congenital heart defects. Three associated findings are always present: (1) interatrial communication, (2) hypertrophied left ventricle, and (3) hypoplastic or absent right ventricle. Transposition of the great arteries (usually "d") is present in 30%. The interatrial communication, usually patent foramen ovale, is rarely restrictive. Classification is made according to presence of transposition and degree of pulmonary stenosis, with the most common type, normally related arteries with pulmonary stenosis, accounting for over 50% of all types of tricuspid atresia. The great majority of patients with normally related arteries (85%) have restricted blood flow and present with cyanosis. Conversely, most patients with d-transposition have unrestricted blood flow and present with congestive heart failure. Cyanosis is present at birth in 50% of patients, and 80% of untreated patients cyanotic in the first 30 days of life will be dead by 6 months. A heart murmur from the VSD is usually present, and its absence is a poor prognostic sign suggesting pulmonary atresia. Symptoms of right heart failure (hepatomegaly, distended neck veins, peripheral edema, etc.) suggest a restrictive patent foramen ovale. Electrocardiogram may be very helpful, as LAD is present in over 80% with normally related arteries, and in a cyanotic patient strongly suggests tricuspid atresia. Left ventricular hypertrophy is virtually always present. Chest x-ray is variable according to amount of pulmonary blood flow and relationship of great arteries, but will most often show concave pulmonary artery segment, diminished pulmonary blood flow, and flattening of the right heart border. Echocardiography reveals a minute right ventricle, large left ventricle, and absent tricuspid valve echo. Cineangiography shows the typical sequence of opacification of the heart chambers and a non-opacified area cast by the right ventricle.

EBSTEIN'S ANOMALY

Ebstein's anomaly constitutes less than 1% of all congenital heart defects. Its cardinal feature is the downward displacement of the septal and posterior leaflets of the tricuspid valve into the right ventricle at the junction of the inlet and trabecular portions. Although the anterior leaflet is not usually displaced, it is abnormally attached and quite large. The downward displacement of the tricuspid valve divides the right ventricle into two parts, a thin-walled inlet, "atrialized portion" above the leaflets, and the functional right ventricle composed of the trabecular and infundibular portions. An interatrial communication is present in 80% of patients. Symptoms may result variably from tricuspid insufficiency, functional or anatomic tricuspid valve/right ventricular obstruction, paradoxical disadvantageous systolic and diastolic motion of the atrialized portion of the right ventricle, right-to-left interatrial shunt, and arrhythmias, including Wolff-Parkinson-White. Most patients present with cyanosis, with or without congestive heart failure, and diagnosis may be suggested when cyanosis spontaneously improves due to falling pulmonary vascular resistance and decreased left-to-right shunt. This improvement is usually only transitory, however. A precordial murmur is usually audible, and the second heart sound is widely split. Hepatomegaly is usually present. Electrocardiogram is variable, commonly showing right atrial hypertrophy, right bundle branch block and, in 20%, Wolff-Parkinson-White. Chest x-ray may show extreme cardiomegaly due to massive right atrial enlargement, with diminished pulmonary vascularity. Echocardiography shows the displaced septal leaflet, large anterior leaflet, delayed tricuspid valve closure, and two-part right ventricle. Cardiac catheterization usually reveals a normal right ventricular systolic pressure, a large "a" wave and "v" wave with normal or moderately elevated right atrial pressure, and right-to-left interatrial shunt. Right ventriculography is usually diagnostic, and quantitates the degree of tricuspid regurgitation.

ISOLATED HYPOPLASTIC RIGHT VENTRICLE

This is a very rare condition with strong familial tendency. Unlike tricuspid atresia and pulmonary atresia with IVS, this form of right ventricular hypoplasia is associated with structurally normal valves. There may be fibroelastosis of the endocardium. Clinically patients are cyanotic, usually as newborns, with atrial level right-to-left shunt. Hepatomegaly may be present. There may or may not be a murmur. Electrocardiogram may resemble that of pulmonary atresia. Chest x-ray may resemble that of tricuspid atresia (decreased pulmonary blood flow, prominent right heart border, and concave pulmonary artery segment), and echocardiography is helpful. Catheterization demonstrates normal right ventricular and pulmonary artery pressures, patent valves, a small right ventricle, and atrial right-to-left shunt. Balloon septostomy and systemic-pulmonary artery shunt may be necessary for cyanotic infants.[46–48]

UHL'S ANOMALY OF THE HEART

Uhl's anomaly (parchment right ventricle) is a rare condition characterized by partial or complete absence of right ventricular myocardium and replacement by fibroelastic and adipose tissue in the presence of a normal tricuspid valve. Under 40 cases have been described in the world's literature, with antemortem diagnosis being rare. Clinical presentation is variable, including right heart failure, cyanosis (with associated ASD), and ventricular arrhythmia. Chest x-ray shows considerable cardiomegaly with variable pulmonary vasculature. Electrocardiogram may show generalized low voltage QRS complexes, with or without evidence of P pulmonale. Recently 2-D echocardiography has been very useful, demonstrating paradoxical systolic motion of the ventricular septum and aneurysmal ballooning of the thin anterolateral, apical, and free walls of the right ventricle.[49,50] Angiocardiography may show a normally located tricuspid valve, enormous dilatation of the right ventricle with very scant trabeculae, delayed pulmonary filling, and, in some individuals with ASD, right-to-left shunt.[51] Surgical efforts have been infrequent, including systemic-pulmonary artery shunts, proposal for Fontan repair, and intracardiac repair.[49]

TRICUSPID INSUFFICIENCY

This may occur either as a primary or secondary diagnosis. The primary form is rare, due either to a dysplastic valve or papillary muscle dysfunction (secondary to anoxia or metabolic abnormality), and, in the latter instance, occurs as a reversible lesion in neonates.[52–54] The neonate presents with cyanosis, congestive failure, and a greatly enlarged heart. Hypoxic newborn events and depletion of glycogen stores have been implicated in causing the transitory but severe papillary muscle dysfunction.[55] Symptoms usually occur in the first week of life, often the first day, and begin with cyanosis (with or without congestive heart failure). A murmur along the lower left sternal border is heard. The most common electrocardiographic finding is right atrial enlargement. Chest x-ray resembles Ebstein's, with massive cardiomegaly due to right heart enlargement and diminished pulmonary vascularity. Echocardiography may distinguish this from tricuspid atresia, Ebstein's anomaly, or pulmonary atresia with IVS, but cardiac catheterization is diagnostic. Right ventricular pressure is usually elevated but not to systemic levels, and a right-to-left shunt, patent valves, and tricuspid regurgitation are demonstrated. Intensive medical management (digitalis, diuretics, vasopressor infusion, and correction of acidosis and hypoglycemia) may salvage some critically ill neonates, especially if they can be sustained until pulmonary vascular resistance normally declines and lessens tricuspid regurgitation.[53,54] Tricuspid valve repair or replacement may be necessary in older children.[52]

TOTAL ANOMALOUS PULMONARY VENOUS RETURN

This condition represents approximately 1% of all congenital heart disease, and occurs in two clinical forms: with and without pulmonary venous obstruction. The former group has severe cyanosis and a dismal prognosis when untreated. The latter group has milder cyanosis and slower deterioration, but still two-thirds of untreated patients are dead by one year. There is no pulmonary venous connection to the left atrium, and four types of drainage to the systemic circulation are recognized: supracardiac (50%), intracardiac (20%), infracardiac (20%) and mixed (10%). The infracardiac type drains subdiaphragmatically to the portal vein, one of its tributaries, or a hepatic vein, and is the most common type associated with pulmonary venous obstruction. An interarterial communication is always present for survival, with a bidirectional shunt. The left side of the heart is small, and total anomalous pulmonary venous return (TAPVR) is distinguishable from other admixture lesions by notably lacking left atrial enlargement. Coexistence of other anomalies is common, especially asplenia.

TAPVR without pulmonary venous obstruction hemodynamically resembles large ASD, with the volume of left-to-right shunt determined by the relative ventricular compliances. Unlike ASD, however, obligatory right-to-left shunt produces cyanosis, usually mild, and development of early PVOD is not uncommon. Patients present with congestive heart failure, failure to thrive, and mild cyanosis. A precordial murmur is audible and the second sound is usually widely split and fixed. Electrocardiogram demonstrates RAD and RVH. Chest x-ray shows cardiomegaly (right-sided), increased pulmonary vascularity, and may show a "snowman" appearance with the supracardiac type. Echocardiography demonstrates an enlarged right heart, normal or small left atrium, and may show an echo-free space posterior to the left atrium. Cardiac catheterization is diagnostic and demonstrates the site of pulmonary venous connection. Because of complete right atrial mixing, oxygen saturation is identical (as expected) in all four cardiac chambers in about half of patients, whereas the remainder may show pulmonary artery saturation greater than aortic due to streaming.

TAPVR with obstruction most often occurs in males. Cyanosis is intense, with saturations as low as 20%, since the pulmonary venous obstruction promotes right-to-left interarterial shunting. In addition to cyanosis, patients are tachypneic and have great difficulty with feeding. A murmur is often absent. The second heart sound is often single and loud. Rales and hepatomegaly are common. Electrocardiogram shows RAD and RVH. Chest x-ray shows a normal-sized heart with pulmonary edema resembling pneumonia or hyaline membrane disease. Cardiac catheterization demonstrates a large right-to-left shunt with severe arterial desaturation, with pulmonary hypertension which often exceeds systemic pressures in infants. Angiography demonstrates the site of obstruction. Most untreated patients die within 1–3 months.

TRUNCUS ARTERIOSUS

This represents less than 1% of all congenital heart lesions. Only a single arterial vessel leaves the heart through a single truncal valve that usually has three, less often four cusps (infrequently, two or five). The truncus overrides the ventricular septum, which has a superior, anterior septal defect, and receives the entire output from both ventricles. The valve may be insufficient, especially with time, and occasionally stenotic. The origin of the pulmonary arteries from the truncus is variable. Most often a short pulmonary trunk arises on the left, posterior aspect of the truncus just above the truncal valve, and this in turn gives rise to the left and right pulmonary arteries. Less often the left and right pulmonary arteries arise separately from the truncus, either in proximity or distant from one another. Stenosis of their origins occurs occasionally. Patients whose pulmonary blood supply arises from bronchial arteries from the descending aorta are better classified as tetralogy of Fallot with pulmonary atresia.

Other common anomalies are a right aortic arch and coronary artery abnormalities.

Hemodynamics and clinical presentation depend on the relative resistance to pulmonary and systemic blood flow. Usually congestive heart failure develops early in lie, becomes very severe, and may lead to early PVOD. Cyanosis is present in 50–75% of patients but is most often mild. Pulses are bounding, and there is a wide pulse pressure due to pulmonary artery runoff. A loud precordial murmur is present. The second sound is single and loud, and a diastolic murmur may be heard with truncal valve insufficiency. Electrocardiogram most often shows normal QRS axis with biventricular hypertrophy. Chest x-ray demonstrates cardiomegaly (biventricular plus left atrial enlargement) and increased pulmonary vascularity, which may resemble that of TGA, except the upper mediastinum is wide due to the truncus. A right aortic arch may also be noted. Echocardiography resembles that of tetralogy of Fallot with an enlarged arterial vessel overriding the ventricular septum, usually distinguishable by the absence of a pulmonary valve in truncus arteriosus. Cardiac catheterization demonstrates the anatomy, degree of stenosis or incompetence of the truncal valve, systemic right ventricular and pulmonary artery pressures (unless the latter has separate stenosis), arterial desaturation, and wide pulse pressure (> 40 mm Hg). Most untreated patients die of congestive failure within 6–12 months.

HYPOPLASTIC LEFT HEART

This condition is characterized by aortic valve atresia, a hypoplastic ascending aorta, mitral atresia or hypoplasia, an intact ventricular septum, and severe left ventricular hypoplasia. The left ventricle is small, slit-like, with a thick wall. Heart size, however, is large, from marked right ventricular hypertrophy and dilatation. Pulmonary artery is large, and a large patent ductus arteriosus is obligatory to sustain life, with massive right to left shunt and retrograde flow in the arch and ascending aorta. An interatrial communication allows pulmonary venous return to enter the right atrium. Any fall in pulmonary vascular resistance or ductal constriction worsens systemic blood flow and causes deterioration. Clinically neonates may appear normal at birth, but rapid deterioration is the rule with death usually within a week of birth. Cyanosis may be mild, with aortic saturation as high as 85–90% which improves with 100% O_2. Tachypnea and tachycardia develop within hours of birth, and congestive failure becomes very severe. Poor perfusion and mottled skin portend death, but cyanosis may still not be severe. A murmur is variable. The second sound is loud and single. Electrocardiogram shows RAD and RVH, usually with no left ventricular forces. Chest x-ray shows cardiomegaly and pulmonary plethora. Two-dimensional echocardiography is usually diagnostic, showing a large right ventricle and tricuspid valve, and hypoplastic left ventricle.

Preductal aortic coarctation presenting in a critically ill neonate with right-to-left ductal shunting, as well as interrupted aortic arch, may produce cyanosis. These lesions should especially be considered when there is disparity between upper and lower extremity pulses and/or differential cyanosis. Echocardiography may be diagnostic, but cardiac catheterization is preferred for operative management.[56,57]

ANOMALOUS SYSTEMIC VENOUS RETURN

These lesions are rare causes of cyanosis, and then only when anomalous return is to the left (rather than right) atrium. Anomalous left superior vena cava to the left atrium is the most common in this group to produce cyanosis, but anomalous inferior vena cava to the left atrium (either direct or functionally across a low ASD) or hemiazygous continuation to the left atrium may also rarely cause cyanosis. Associated anomalies are frequent. The presence of cyanosis in the absence of RVH is suggestive. In addition to the usual mild cyanosis, patients may present with cerebrovascular accident or brain abscess. Echocardiography may be diagnostic.[58]

ASPLENIA

Patients with asplenia usually present in infancy with intense cyanosis, normal heart size, and diminished pulmonary blood flow. Cardiac anomalies are complex, and include obstructed total anomalous pulmonary return with pulmonary stenosis and VSD. Despite the complexity, the basic pathology is obstruction to pulmonary blood flow with right-to-left ventricular-level shunt. Patients with asplenia usually have right atriopulmonary isomerism (bilateral right-type atria, bronchi and pulmonary arteries). The presence of asplenia may be suggested on chest x-ray by the abnormal situs (ambiguus), while presence of Howell-Jolly bodies on peripheral blood smear is diagnostic. Asplenia usually carries a poor prognosis.[59,60]

PULMONARY ARTERIOVENOUS FISTULA

This is not a cardiac lesion and is mentioned only for completeness. It is usually a congenital disorder in which a variable number of pulmonary arteries connect, without the interposition of pulmonary capillary bed, to a variable number of pulmonary veins. Tortuous, dilated sacciform aneurysmal sacs form, which may be confined to one lobe or may be more diffuse. About 60% have Osler-Weber-Rendu syndrome, and some patients have coexistent congenital heart disease. Hemodynamically, most patients have normal pulmonary blood flow and pressure, with systemic arterial desaturation between 50–85%. Polycythemia usually occurs from hypoxemia. Clinically most patients are cyanotic, and exercise intolerance is common. Neurologic problems, including brain abscess, occur in about 25% of patients. Hemoptysis is quite common, as is clubbing. Pulse is normal and a faint murmur may be heard in about half of patients over the chest wall. Chest x-ray shows a normal-sized heart (except with large fistula). Rounded parenchymal lung opacities occur in about 50% of individuals in one or both lung fields, occasionally with strand-like opacities due to afferent and efferent vessels. Fluoroscopy may show a pulsatile mass. Angiocardiography is diagnostic. Diagnosis is suggested by a relatively asymptomatic, cyanotic patient with normal heart size, heart sounds and electrocardiogram, and by telangiectatic lesions. Symptomatic patients (exercise intolerance, rupture with hemoptysis or hemorrhage, brain abscess, endocarditis, etc.) should be operated on, with conservative resection whenever possible.[61]

SEQUELAE

Clubbing. Hypertrophic osteoarthropathy, or clubbing, is a widening and thickening of the ends of the fingers and toes with convex nails. It usually occurs 6–12 months after the onset of cyanosis,[5] and gradually disappears once the underlying defect causing cyanosis is corrected. Although most commonly due to cyanotic, congenital heart disease, it may also be caused by pulmonary disease, cirrhosis, and subacute bacterial endocarditis.[5]

Erythrocytosis. Diminished arterial oxygen saturation stimulates production of renal erythropoietin, which in turn stimulates increased bone marrow production of red blood cells. The response becomes counterproductive, however, at hematocrit values above 65–70% due to increased blood viscosity, tendency for thrombosis, and so on. In the face of iron deficiency, a situation of relative anemia may occur, where the hemoglobin level is elevated compared to normal but not optimally for the level of arterial desaturation.[62] This inadequate elevation of hemoglobin may occur even though, deceptively, red cell counts are increased due to erythropoietin.[16]

Hypercyanotic Spells. Known by a variety of names, including "tet" spells and hypoxic spells, these occur in the first year of life (peak incidence 2–4 months). They are associated with tetralogy of Fallot, but may occur in any condition with right ventricular outflow tract obstruction. The degree of resting cyanosis does not appear to be a critical factor. They usually occur in the morning (after defecation, crying, or feeding), and are characterized clinically by (1) a paroxysm of hyperpnea (rapid and deep respirations), (2) irritability and prolonged cry, (3) increasing cyanosis, and (4) decreased intensity of the heart murmur. This may lead to limpness, loss of consciousness, seizure, cerebrovascular accident, and occasionally death.[28]

The pathophysiology of these spells is not precisely understood, but factors that increase right-to-left shunting and lessen pulmonary blood flow (thus loss of heart murmur) are critical. The two most favored hypotheses are infundibular spasm, precipitated by an acute increase in catecholamine,[63] and any stimulus producing hyperpnea (which increases systemic venous return and, in turn, increases the right-to-left shunt).[28,64]

Squatting. Squatting is virtually diagnostic of tetralogy of Fallot, and occurs more commonly in children after they begin to walk. It may be apparent in infants as they lie with their knees drawn up against their chests. This position appears to be beneficial for two reasons: (1) it increases systemic vascular resistance, which increases left-to-right shunt, and (2) it reduces systemic venous return of desaturated blood to the heart, which lowers right-to-left shunt.[65]

Cerebrovascular Accidents. Hemiplegia or lesser deficit occurs occasionally in association with cyanotic congenital heart disease, and can be due to thrombosis (hyperviscosity), anoxia ("tet" spell), or paradoxical emboli. It occurs most commonly in infants and children under 2 years of age, and considerable recovery may occur.[66] Patients with relative anemia and excessive erythrocytosis are particularly susceptible, especially with dehydration, "tet" spells, or surgery (shunt procedures). Brain abscess should be excluded.

Brain Abscess. At least 1–2%[5] and possibly substantially more[67] patients with cyanotic congenital heart disease develop brain abscess. It is most common with tetralogy of Fallot, usually in those over 2 years of age, but may occur with any defect producing right-to-left shunt.[5] The exact mechanism is unknown, but favored ones include infected paradoxical emboli from the venous side which ordinarily would be filtered in the lungs, and anoxic cerebral infarction that becomes infected during a bacteremic episode. Alpha-streptococcus is the most common organism.[5] Symptoms include headache, drowsiness, vomiting, seizures, and focal neurologic signs, with or without fever. CT scan is usually diagnostic.

Coagulation Problems. Impairment of coagulation in patients with polycythemia and cyanotic congenital heart disease has long been recognized.[68–74] Many factors appear to be important, including prolongation of prothrombin time and activated partial thromboplastin times, elevation of fibrin degradation products, decreased levels of factors V, VIII, and fibrinogen, and evidence of fibrinolysis. Thrombocytopenia has also been associated with cyanotic heart disease,[73,74–76] and in conjunction with other abnormalities low-grade chronic disseminated intravascular coagulation has been reported.[71,73,75,77] Impaired platelet function has also been reported.[78,79]

Hyperuricemia. Due to increased red cell production, hyperuricemia, gout, and uric acid nephropathy may be seen in adolescents and adults with longstanding cyanotic congenital heart disease.[80] Impaired urate excretion has also been recognized as partially causative of the hyperuricemia.[81]

DIAGNOSIS

The approach to diagnosis of cyanotic heart disease should be systematic, with the usual initial emphasis on history and physical examination. Echocardiography notwithstanding, a thorough knowledge of the lesions capable of producing cyanosis, their symptoms and signs, and the extraordinarily important information provided by a plain chest x-ray and electrocardiogram are of immense value.[82–84] The characteristic boot-shaped heart of tetralogy of Fallot, egg-shaped heart of TGA, and "snowman" appearance of supracardiac TAPVR are examples of nearly diagnostic chest x-rays, while the giant P waves of Ebstein's suggest that disorder.

A helpful table comparing the electrocardiogram with pulmonary vascularity is provided here for review (Fig. 1). Patients with right ventricular hypertrophy, right axis deviation or normal axis, and pulmonary plethora most likely have transposition of the great arteries, total anomalous pulmonary venous return or double-outlet right ventricle, while those with pulmonary oligemia most likely have tetralogy of Fallot or pulmonary atresia. If the QRS axis is normal with either no ventricular hypertrophy, bilateral ventricular hypertrophy or left ventricular hypertrophy, the five possibilities are transposition of the great arteries, pulmonary atresia, double-outlet right ventricle, truncus arteriosus and tricuspid atresia. Finally, in the small group with left axis deviation and left ventricular hypertrophy, tricuspid atresia is the diagnosis with pulmonary oligemia, and either tricuspid atresia or TGA with pulmonary plethora.[82,83]

Without diminishing in any way the importance of the above systematic approach to diagnosis, it is fair to say that echocardiography, particularly two-dimensional, real-time echocardiography, has revolutionized the diagnosis of cyanotic congenital heart disease.[84–86] This can help to differentiate what might otherwise be a difficult problem clinically, cyanotic congenital heart disease from persistent fetal circulation, with approximately 75% sensitivity and up to 100% specificity.[84] In addition, the various causes of cyanotic congenital heart disease may be differentiated with varying but generally reliable accuracy, as discussed above and very thoroughly elsewhere.[85] Magnetic resonance imaging may also prove helpful in evaluating various cyanotic heart lesions.[877]

Finally, although systemic-pulmonary artery shunts, Norwood procedures and other repairs have been performed recently based upon clinical presentation and real-time 2-D echocardiography,[88,91] cardiac catheterization and cine angiography are generally necessary for surgical treatment, with the additional potential to perform therapeutic maneuvers such as balloon septostomy.

MANAGEMENT

Management of patients with cyanotic congenital heart disease depends upon definitive diagnosis and clinical presentation, which will be discussed at

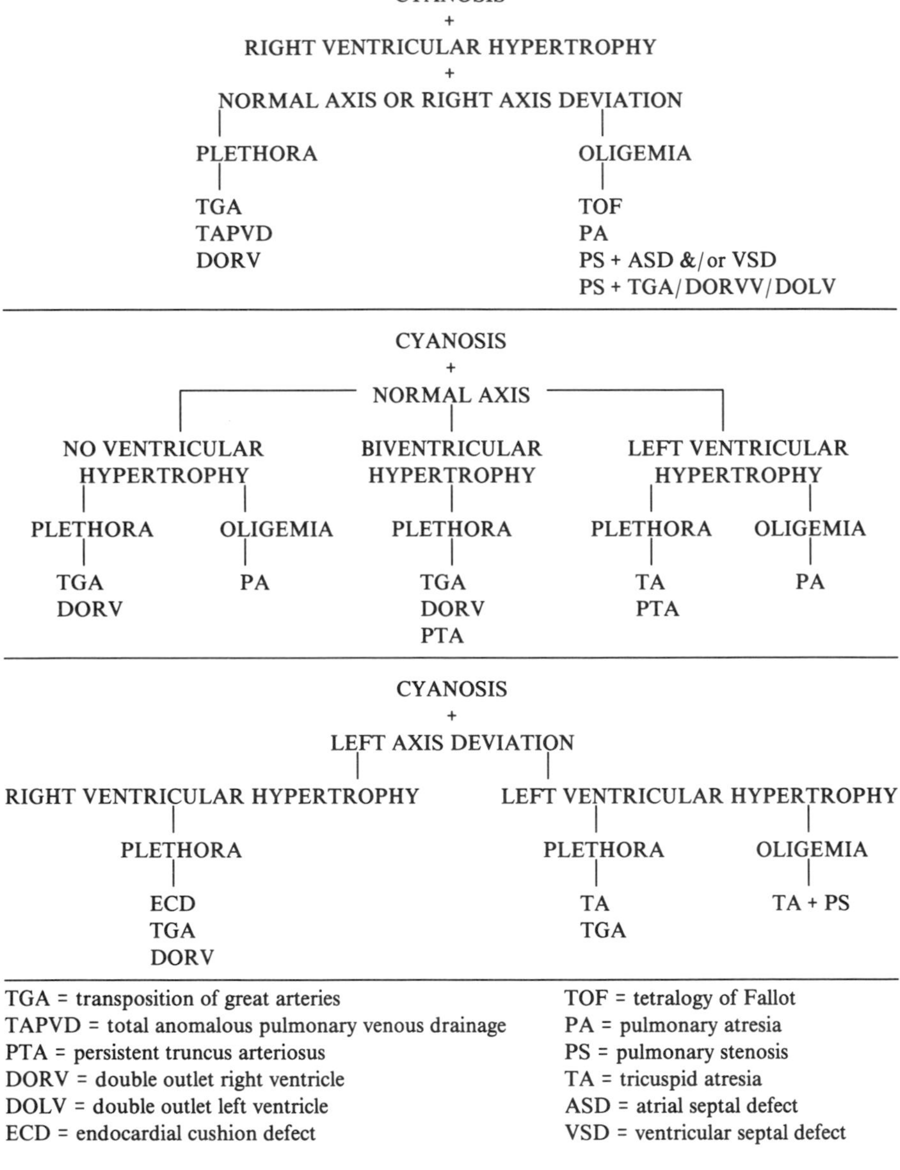

FIGURE 1. Correlation of electrocardiographic and roentgenographic findings in cyanotic congenital heart disease. (From Elliott LP, Scheibler GL: A roentgenologic-electrocardiographic approach to cyanotic forms of heart disease. Pediatr Clin North Am 18:1133–1161, 1971; and Yip WCL, Tay JSH: A practical diagnostic approach to cyanotic heart disease. Singapore Med J 24:189, 1983, with permission.)

length in the following chapters. Certain general principles will be focused on here, which apply broadly to cyanotic patients irrespective of diagnosis.

Should prostaglandin E_1 infusion, for example, be begun in cyanotic infants, especially those critically ill, prior to definitive diagnosis? Newborn infants with congenital heart defects producing severe or complete obstruction to right ventricular outflow depend on a patent ductus arteriosus to provide adequate pulmonary blood flow. Ductal patency is also vital in patients with critical preductal coarctation or interruption of the aortic arch to allow lower body perfusion via right-to-left ductal shunting. Danford and colleagues[92] found that early prostaglandin infusion was indicated in cyanotic term infants with a murmur or poor pulses, regardless of how ill they appeared, and in any critically ill newborn infant who had either cyanosis or poor pulses. Prostaglandin E_1 is infused continuously at a dosage of 0.05–0.1 μg/kg/min. Acyanotic patients with normal pulses should not be treated prior to definitive diagnosis. Other principles of management in this important and difficult subset are immediate administration of 100% oxygen and assisted ventilation (for both diagnostic and therapeutic purposes), appropriate correction of hypotension, anemia, bradycardia, metabolic acidosis, hypoglycemia and hypocalcemia, and preparation for early transfer to a tertiary care nursery.[93] Early bedside real-time echocardiography should then be performed promptly, followed by cardiac catheterization when indicated where, for example, balloon atrial septostomy may stabilize a critically hypoxemic patient with transposition of the great arteries.

The hemoglobin value is an important consideration in cyanotic patients, and can be too low or too high. Based upon the level of arterial saturation, there is an optimal level of hemoglobin at which adequate oxygen is delivered to the tissues. If iron stores are inadequate, compensatory polycythemia does not occur and this relative anemia may cause decreased exercise tolerance and increase the susceptibility to hypercyanotic spells. Consequently, periodic evaluation of the hemoglobin, hematocrit, and red cell indices is indicated with institution of iron therapy at the first sign of relative or actual anemia.[14,94] For more seriously ill patients, the rapid correction of relative anemia by partial exchange transfusion has been shown to have significant hemodynamic benefit, not only by increasing O_2 carrying capacity but also by elevating systemic vascular resistance and thus decreasing right-to-left shunting.[95] Conversely, when the hematocrit reaches 65–70%, the polycythemia becomes counterproductive due to the marked increase in yield shear stress and viscosity of blood, with symptoms as discussed above. In this setting erythrophoresis (not phlebotomy) is recommended,[5] removing 20–30 ml aliquots of blood and replacing with equal volume of colloid. Reducing the hematocrit by more than 10% or to less than 55% is not recommended.[5] A rising hematocrit also suggests worsening hypoxemia, and is a common indication for corrective surgery.

Urgent management is required for patients suffering hypercyanotic spells. The underlying problem is acute pulmonary oligemia, and therapy is directed at its correction. The patient should be placed in the knee-chest position. Oxygen should be administered, although it is usually of little avail by itself. Morphine sulfate (0.1 mg/kg) is given intravenously, which breaks the hyperpnea and sedates the infant, decreasing oxygen utilization. Acidosis and anemia, if present, are corrected. A major development in the treatment of hypercyanotic spells has been the utilization of propranolol, whose beta-adrenergic blockade decreases the right-to-left shunting, although the mechanism is not precisely understood.[96,97] The dosage is 0.1 mg/kg by slow intravenous route with EKG monitoring, and can be given subsequently orally (1–4 mg/kg/d tid or qid) as a preventive measure for further attacks. If these measures fail, methoxamine (35 mg/100 cc) is infused at a rate to increase systolic blood pressure (and increase left-to-right shunt) approximately 30 mg Hg. Occasionally general anesthesia may be necessary to break the spell.[5] Finally surgery, corrective or palliative, should be seriously considered in any patient presenting with hypercyanotic spells.

The management of other sequelae of cyanotic congenital heart disease underlines the importance of timely surgical correction. Clubbing, for example, will gradually disappear in most cases following surgical correction, as will hyperuricemia (which is treated with allopurinol, with or without other uricosuric agents, and discontinuation of thiazides for uric acid levels > 10 mg%, gout, or uric acid nephropathy). The primary treatment modality for cerebrovascular accidents is prevention by correction of relative anemia, excessive polycythemia, and dehydration, prevention of spells, and, again, timely surgical correction. The management of brain abscesses includes a high index of suspicion in cyanotic patients with headaches, vomiting, lethargy, seizures, fever, or focal neurological signs. Aggressive antibiotic therapy and neurosurgical consultation are critical. Again, timely surgical correction may be preventative.[98,99] Morbidity and mortality appear to be inversely related to the oxygen saturation levels.[99] Endocarditis is an additional concern in most of the defects that produce cyanotic congenital heart disease, before and after surgery, and consequently meticulous oral hygiene and appropriate antibiotic prophylaxis for dental, gastrointestinal, or genitourinary procedures are warranted.

Counselling regarding pregnancy can be problematic, with general discouragement unless the patient has had satisfactory surgical repair with reasonable biventricular function. The added blood volume and cardiac workload increases any tendency to congestive failure, and the increased thromboembolic state may result in pulmonary or cerebral thromboemboli. Additionally the runoff into the placental circulation lowers systemic vascular resistance, increasing right-to-left shunting and worsening cyanosis. The material mortality rate is approximately 4% for cyanotic tetralogy of Fallot, much higher for tricuspid atresia,[100] and up to 60% for Eisenmenger's syndrome from VSD.[101] Fetal mortality in unoperated patients is over 50%.[102,103]

Patients with satisfactory repairs for tetralogy of Fallot generally have no increased incidence of problems with pregnancy, but should be followed closely by a cardiologist in the third trimeseter, particularly if pulmonary insufficiency or residual VSD is present.[104] If intracardiac revision is necessary, it should be accomplished prior to pregnancy.[105] Antibiotic prophylaxis for endocarditis should be used at the beginning of labor and for three days post partum.[104]

Not enough information exists regarding the safety of pregnancy for those with Fontan, Senning or Mustard repairs, but in the absence of good biventricular and valvular function, caution would certainly seem appropriate. Regarding contraceptives, diaphragms, spermicidal gels, or condoms are optimal (when sterilization is not desired), as intrauterine devices carry some risk of bacteremia and excessive vaginal bleeding. Oral contraceptives, especially estrogenic, carry a high risk of thromboembolism in a cyanotic, polycythemic patient.

The coagulation abnormalities of cyanotic heart disease, as noted, are multiple and complex. The most common management technique to restore coagulation parameters has been phlebotomy (more recently erythrophoresis).[5,75,106,107] Preoperative heparin therapy has been advocated for evidence of consumptive coagulopathy.[71,75,77] During open heart procedures, sufficient hemodilution appears to be helpful to reduce bleeding episodes. Milam and coworkers[108] found that cyanotic patients whose hemoglobin was lowered to less than 10 gm% had 45% less bleeding, and used 54% fewer blood components than patients whose hemodilution by conventional techniques left hemoglobins above 10 gm%. No significant problems were noted as a result of this excessive (by traditional standards) hemodilution, and postoperative coagulation tests were only slightly more abnormal than in noncyanotic postoperative patients.

The surgical management of individual cyanotic lesions will be discussed elsewhere. Some of the issues critical to the proper management of cyanotic lesions are the appropriate timing of intervention, the one-stage versus two-stage repair of tetralogy of Fallot, atrial versus arterial switch procedures for transposition of the great arteries, and the appropriate selection of patients for Fontan repair. Regarding timing, the tendency to delay surgery for an older, "stronger" patient must be weighed against: (1) the various risks of cyanotic sequelae detailed above, (2) the development of PVOD in cyanotic lesions with increased pulmonary blood flow such as truncus arteriosus,[109] and (3) the development of ventricular dysfunction from chronic volume overload in patients treated initially with palliative shunts.[110,111]

Several complex and rare causes of cyanosis will be discussed briefly here. The asplenia syndrome has been discussed above, including its association with total anomalous pulmonary venous return. Systemic-pulmonary shunts usually have poor results in these patients, especially when the total anomalous pulmonary venous return is obstructed, as congestive heart failure will then be exacerbated if the obstructed venous drainage is not relieved.[112,113] Evidence of a median liver on standard chest x-ray or bilateral "right" bronchograms should suggest right isomerism. Unfortunately, 2-D echocardiography does not diagnose total anomalous pulmonary venous return with situs ambiguus as accurately as with situs solitus or inversus;[114] consequently pulmonary angiography is usually necessary (a prolonged capillary phase with "ground-glass" lung fields, atypical for restricted pulmonary blood flow, suggests obstructed pulmonary venous return).[112]

Because of difficulties in diagnosing obstructed total anomalous pulmonary venous return in complex cyanotic heart disease, and its critically important therapeutic implications, Freedom and associates[115] introduced the "prostaglandin challenge." This dilates the ductus arteriosus and unmasks obstructed total anomalous pulmonary venous return at catheterization, and is strongly endorsed by others as well.[112,113] Di Donato and associates[112] noted a 54% mortality in operated patients with asplenia syndrome (receiving either shunts alone or a combination of shunt plus repair of total anomalous pulmonary venous return), and found the presence of obstructed pulmonary venous return was the major risk factor for surgery. Likewise, De Leon and associates[113] noted very poor survival in complex cyanotic patients with obstructed total anomalous pulmonary venous return treated with shunts alone. They recommend aggressive preoperative diagnostic efforts, including prostaglandin challenge, and repair of total anomalous pulmonary venous return either before or in conjunction with systemic-pulmonary artery shunt for optimal results.

Patients with polysplenia often have interrupted inferior vena cava with azygous continuation. In the setting of complex cyanotic heart disease, superior vena cava-pulmonary artery shunt ("total cavopulmonary shunt") has been used in conjunction with intracardiac defect repair to isolate systemic and pulmonary venous circulations.[116,117] Another technical advance has been the application of the Fontan procedure to patients with anomalous systemic and pulmonary

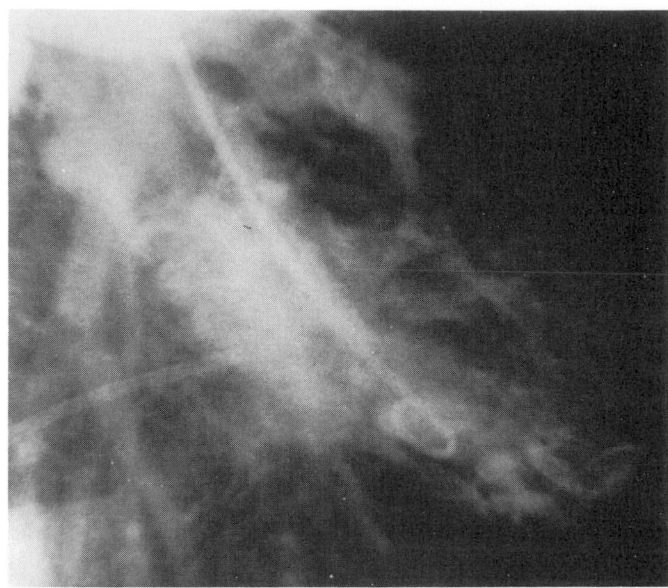

FIGURE 2. Right ventriculogram of 50-year-old patient with tetralogy of Fallot, presenting with severe cyanosis, erythrocytosis, and exercise intolerance. The severe infundibular stenosis is apparent as well as filling of the overriding aorta across the large ventricular septal defect. This patient is now in NYHA Class I two years following closure of the ventricular septal defect and right ventricular outflow tract reconstruction.

venous connections. Originally, these patients were excluded according to Choussat's and Fontan's criteria.[118] Recently Vargas and associates[119] reported 82.3% survival in 17 patients given atriopulmonary anastomosis and correction of anomalous systemic and/or pulmonary venous return. They recommend careful preoperative diagnosis and individualized operative planning to provide unobstructed venous pathways. In the case of anomalous left superior vena cava, they preferred extracardiac exclusion via end-to-side left cavopulmonary shunt (modified Glenn shunt) over complex intra-atrial baffles that may obstruct venous return.

Patients with Eisenmenger's syndrome present a special challenge. According to Wood's series,[120] the average age of death was 33 for aorticopulmonary defect and ventricular septal defect and 36 for atrial septal defect. Hemoptysis (which may be due to pulmonary infarction, pulmonary thrombosis, or rupture of pulmonary artery plexiform lesions) is rare before age 20 but increases to 100% of patients by age 40. Angina pectoris occurs not infrequently in older patients. Sudden death, presumably due to rhythm disturbances, occurred in 14% of Wood's patients,[120] and 41% and 47% of deaths were sudden in two more recent reports.[121,122] The management of patients with Eisenmenger's syndrome is primarily medical, with utilization of the principles already outlined for treatment of polycythemia, relative anemia, hyperuricemia, and so forth. The value of careful erythrophoresis (up to 10% decrease in blood hematocrit) was demonstrated by Rosenthal and coworkers,[123,124] who noted a 38% increase in systemic blood flow and 20% increase in systemic oxygen transport. Pregnancy and oral contraceptives should be avoided, as should high altitude and flying without special precautions.[125] Prompt conversion of atrial arrhythmias, digoxin, and diuretics are all indicated for treatment of congestive heart failure. There is no definitive effective treatment for hemoptysis. Because no vasodilator is specific for the pulmonary vasculature, they may be counterproductive by lowering systemic venous return and increasing right-to-left shunting, and consequently are contraindicated in Eisenmenger's syndrome. In the past, surgery was also contraindicated when pulmonary hypertension was fixed, except in patients with transposition of the great arteries with VSD or PDA who might benefit from palliative intra-atrial baffle.[126] More recently, heart-lung transplantation may be a promising alternative in carefully selected patients.[127] An excellent review of the entire Eisenmenger syndrome is recommended for more detailed discussion.[128]

One final consideration is cyanotic congenital heart disease presenting in adults. Lesions such as transposition of the great arteries, truncus arteriosus, and total anomalous pulmonary venous return rarely survive untreated into adulthood. On the other hand, lesions with diminished pulmonary blood flow, notably tetralogy of Fallot, may allow prolonged life untreated (rarely beyond 60 years of age) if right ventricular outflow tract obstruction is not severe and shunting is balanced. Natural history studies indicate that 20% of untreated patients with tetralogy of Fallot will live beyond 15 years, and 3–5% beyond age 25.[129-131] The predominant cause of late death is approximately evenly distributed among: (1) hypercyanotic spells, (2) cerebrovascular accident or brain abscess, (3) infective endocarditis, and (4) pneumonia and congestive heart failure.[130,131] These patients should be considered for surgical repair, with results of primary repair comparable to those obtained in children (Fig. 2).[132-135] Operative mortality has ranged from 0%[134] to 11%.[133] According to Garson and colleagues[104] in their excellent review of this subject, the major exception to offering primary intracardiac repair to adults with tetralogy of Fallot would be the patient with extremely hypoplastic pulmonary arteries.

REFERENCES

1. Nadas AS, Fyler DF: Pediatric Cardiology. Philadelphia, W.B. Saunders Co., 1972.
2. Lundsgaard C: Studies on cyanosis, I and II. J Exp Med 30:259, 1919.
3. Blalock A, Taussig HB: The surgical treatment of malformations of the heart. JAMA 128:189, 1945.
4. Lees MH: Cyanosis of the newborn infant. J Pediatr 77:484, 1970.
5. Rao PS: Pathophysiologic consequences of cyanotic congenital heart disease. Indian J Pediatr 50:479, 1983.
6. Klaus M, Meyer BP: Oxygen therapy for the newborn. Pediatr Clin North Am 13:731, 1966.
7. Lundsgaard C, Van Slyke DD: Cyanosis. Medical Monographs, Vol. 2. Baltimore, Williams and Wilkins Co., 1923.
8. Yabek SM: Neonatal cyanosis. Reappraised of response to 100% oxygen breathing. Am J Dis Child 138:880, 1984.
9. Goetzman BW, Sunshine P, Johnson JD, et al: Neonatal hypoxia and pulmonary vasospasm: Response to tolazoline. J Pediatr 89:617, 1976.
10. Rheuban KS: The infant with congenital heart disease: Guidelines for care in the first year of life. Clin Perinatol 11:199, 1984.
11. Sietsema KE, Cooper DM, Perloff JK, et al: Dynamics of oxygen uptake during exercise in adults with cyanotic congenital heart disease. Circulation 73:1137, 1986.
12. Nihill MR, McNamara DG, Vick RL: The effects of increased blood viscosity on pulmonary vascular resistance. Am Heart J 92:65, 1976.
13. Wells R: Hyperviscosity syndromes. N Engl J Med 283:183, 1970.
14. Rudolph AJ, Nadas AS, Borges WH: Hematologic adjustments to cyanotic congenital heart disease. Pediatrics 11:454, 1953.

15. Murray JF, Gold P, Johnson BL: The circulatory effects of hematocrit variations in normovolemic and hypervolemic dogs. J Clin Invest 42:1150, 1963.
16. Kontras SB, Bodenbender JG, Craenen J, Hosier DM: Hyperviscosity in congenital heart disease. J Pediatr 76:214, 1970.
17. Theodore J, Robin ED, Burke CM, et al: Impact of profound reductions of PaO_2 on O_2 transport and utilization in congenital heart disease. Chest 87:293, 1985.
18. Levin AR: Management of the cyanotic newborn. Pediatr Ann 10:16, 1981.
19. Miller RA, Lev M, Paul MH: Congenital absence of the pulmonary valve. The clinical syndrome of tetralogy of Fallot with pulmonary regurgitation. Circulation 26:266, 1962.
20. Weldon CS, Rowe RD, Gott VL: Clinical experience with the use of aortic valve homografts for reconstruction of the pulmonary artery, pulmonary valve, and outflow portion of the right ventricle. Circulation 35(Suppl II):11–267, 1967.
21. Macartney F, Miller GAH: Congenital absence of the pulmonary valve. Br Heart J 32:483, 1970.
22. Arensman FW, Francis PD, Helmsworth JA, et al: Early medical and surgical intervention for tetralogy of Fallot with absence of pulmonic valve. J Thorac Cardiovasc Surg 84:430, 1982.
23. d'Allaines C, Colvez L, Fevre C, et al: A rare congenital cardiopathy: Association of tetralogy of Fallot and complete A-V canal. Arch Mal Coeur 62:996, 1969.
24. Tandon R, Moller JH, Edwards JE: Tetralogy of Fallot associated with persistent common atrioventricular canal (endocardial cushion defect). Br Heart J 36:197, 1974.
25. Bharati S, Kirklin JW, McAllister HA, et al: The surgical anatomy of common atrioventricular orifice associated with tetralogy of Fallot, double outlet right ventricle and complete regular transposition. Circulation 61:1142, 1980.
26. Binet JP, Losay J, Hvass U: Tetralogy of Fallot with type C compete atrioventricular canal. J Thorac Cardiovasc Surg 79:761, 1980.
27. Pacifico AD, Kirklin JW, Bargeron LM Jr: Repair of complete atrioventricular canal associated with tetralogy of Fallor or double-outlet right ventricle: Report of 10 patients. Ann Thorac Surg 29:351, 1980.
28. Park MK: Pediatric Cardiology for Practitioners. Chicago, Year Book Medical Publishers, 1984.
29. Aziz KU, Paul MH, Muster AJ: Echocardiographic assessment of left ventricular outflow tract in d-transposition of the great arteries. Am J Cardiol 41:543, 1978.
30. McGoon DC: Intraventricular repair of transposition of the great arteries. J Thorac Cardiovasc Surg 64:430, 1972.
31. Cooley DA, Angelini P, Leachman RD, et al: Intraventricular repair of transposition complexes with ventricular septal defect. J Thorac Cardiovasc Surg 3:461, 1976.
32. Rastelli GC, Wallace RB, Ongley PA: Complete repair of transposition of the great arteries with pulmonary stenosis. A review and report of a case corrected by using a new surgical technique. Circulation 39:83, 1969.
33. Sansa M, Tonkin IL, Bargeron LM Jr, et al: Left ventricular outflow tract obstruction in transposition of the great arteries: An angiographic study of 74 cases. Am J Cardiol 44:88, 1979.
34. Van Gils FA, Moulaert AJ, Oppenheimer-Dekker A, et al: Transposition of the great arteries with ventricular septal defect and pulmonary stenosis. Br Heart J 40:494, 1978.
35. Moulton AL, de Leval MR, Macartney FJ, et al: Rastelli procedure for transposition of the great arteries, ventricular septal defect, and left ventricular outflow tract obstruction. Br Heart J 45:20, 1981.
36. Plauth WH Jr, Nadas AS, Bernhard WF, et al: Changing hemodynamics in patients with transposition of the great arteries. Circulation 42:131, 1970.
37. Waldman JD, Paul MH, Newfield EA, et al: Transposition of the great arteries with intact ventricular septum and patent ductus arteriosus. Am J Cardiol 39:232, 1977.
38. Earle GF, Sade RM, Riopel DA: Banding of patent ductus arteriosus for palliation of cyanotic congenital heart disease. Am Heart J 108:173, 1984.
39. Kirklin JW, Barratt-Boyes BG: Complete transposition of the great arteries. In Kirklin JW, Barratt-Boyes (eds): Cardiac Surgery. New York, John Wiley & Sons, 1986.
40. Pacifico AD, Kirklin JW, Bargeron LM: Complex congenital malformations: Surgical treatment of double-outlet right ventricle and double-outlet left ventricle. In Kirklin JW (ed): Advances in Cardiovascular Surgery. London, New York, Grune & Stratton, 1973.
41. Lev M, Bharati S, Meny CCL, et al: A concept of double outlet right ventricle. J Thorac Cardiovasc Surg 64:271, 1972.
42. Brandt PWT, Calder AL, Barratt-Boyes BG, et al: Double-outlet left ventricle, morphology, cineangiographic diagnosis and surgery treatment. Am J Cardiol 38:897, 1976.
43. Anderson R, Galbraith R, Gibson R, et al: Double outlet left ventricle. Br Heart J 36:554, 1974.

44. Goor DA, Lilleihei CW: Congenital Malformations of the Heart. New York, Grune & Stratton, 1975.
45. Bull C, de Leval M, Mercanti C, et al: Pulmonary atresia and intact ventricular septum: A revised classification. Circulation 66:266, 1982.
46. Raghib C, Amplatz K, Moller JH, et al: Hypoplasia of right ventricle and of tricuspid valve. Am Heart J 70:806, 1965.
47. Sackner MA, Robinson MJ, Jamison WL, et al: Isolated right ventricular hypoplasia with atrial septal defect or patent foramen ovale. Circulation 24:1388, 1961.
48. Freedom RM, Moes CAF: The hypoplastic right heart complex. Semin in Roentgenol 20:169, 1985.
49. Child JS, Perloff JK, Francoz R, et al: Uhl's anomaly (parchment right ventricle): clinical, echocardiographic, radionuclear, hemodynamic and angiocardiographic features in 2 patients. Am J Cardiol 53:635, 1984.
50. Ribeiro PA, Shapiro LM, Foale RA, et al: Echocardiographic features of right ventricular dilated cardiomyopathy and Uhl's anomaly. Eur Heart J 8:65, 1987.
51. Kaul U, Arora R, Rani S: Uhl's anomaly with rudimentary pulmonary valve leaflets: A clinical, hemodynamic, angiographic and pathologic study. Am Heart J 100:673, 1980.
52. Pasque M, Williams WG, Coles JG, et al: Tricuspid valve replacement in children. Ann Thorac Surg 44:164, 1987.
53. Boncek RJ Jr, Graham TP Jr, Morgan JP, et al: Spontaneous resolution of massive congenital tricuspid insufficiency. Circulation 54:795, 1976.
54. Bucciarelli RL, Nelson RM, Egan EA II, et al: Transient tricuspid insufficiency of the newborn: A form of myocardial dysfunction in stressed newborns. Pediatrics 59:330, 1977.
55. Nelson RM, Bucciarelli RL, Eitzman DV, et al: Serum creatine phosphokinase MB fraction in newborns with transient tricuspid insufficiency. N Engl J Med 298:146, 1978.
56. Cowgill LD: Coarctation of the aorta. In Cowgill LD (ed): Surgery of the Aorta, Philadelphia, Hanley & Belfus, Inc. 1987.
57. Douglas-Jones JWE: Aortic arch anomalies. In Cowgill LD (ed): Surgery of the Aorta, Philadelphia, Hanley & Belfus, Inc., 1987.
58. Huhta JC, Smallhorn JF, Macartney FJ, et al: Cross-sectional echocardiographic diagnosis of systemic venous return. Br Heart J 48:388, 1982.
59. Stanger P, Rudolph AM, Edwards JE: Cardiac malpositions. Circulation 56:159, 1977.
60. Moller JH, Neal WA: Heart Disease in Infancy. Norwalk, CT, Appleton-Century-Crofts, 1981.
61. Jimenez MQ, Guillen FA: Arterioverous fistulas. In Adams FH, Emmanouilides GC (eds): Heart Disease in Infants, Children and Adolescents. Baltimore, Williams and Wilkins, 1983.
62. Rudolph AM, Nadas AS, Borges WH: Hematologic adjustments to cyanotic congenital heart disease. Pediatrics 11:454, 1953.
63. Rao PS, Linde LM, Liebman J, Perrin E: Functional closure of physiologically advantageous ventricular septal dcfects: Observations in three cases with tricuspid atresia. Am J Dis Child 127:36, 1974.
64. Guntheroth WG, Morgan BC, Mullins GL: Physiologic studies of paroxysmal hyperpnea in cyanotic congenital heart disease. Circulation 31:70, 1965.
65. Guntheroth WG, Morgan BC, Mullins GL, et al: Venous return with knee-chest position and squatting in tetralogy of Fallot. Am Heart J 75:313, 1968.
66. Garson A Jr, Gillette PC, McNamara DG: Propranolol: The preferred palliation of tetralogy of Fallot. Am J Cardiol 47:1098, 1981.
67. Quaegebeur J, Kirklin JW, Pacifico AD, et al: Surgical experience with unroofed coronary sinus. Ann Thorac Surg 27:418, 1979.
68. Hartmann RC: A hemorrhagic disorder occurring in patients with cyanotic congenital heart disease. Johns Hopkins Med J 91:49, 1955.
69. Burrow L, Watson DG, Bell WN: Blood coagulation studies in children with congenital heart disease. Am Heart J 70:747, 1965.
70. Kontras SB, Sirak HD, Newton WA Jr: Hematologic abnormalities in children with congenital heart disease. JAMA 195:99, 1966.
71. Dennis LH, Stewart JL, Conrad ME: A consumption coagulation defect in congenital cyanotic heart disease and its treatment with heparin. J Pediatr 71:407, 1967.
72. Brodsky I, Gill DN, Lusch CJ: Fibrinolysis in congenital heart disease. Preoperative treatment with ϵ-aminocaproic acid. Am J Clin Pathol 51:51, 1969.
73. Ekert H, Gilchrist GS, Stanton R, Hammond D: Hemostasis in cyanotic congenital heart disease. J Pediatr 76:221, 1970.

74. Wedemeyer AL, Edson JR, Krivit W: Coagulation in cyanotic heart disease. Am J Dis Child 124:656, 1972.
75. Ihenacho HNC, Breeze GR, Fletcher DJ, Stuart J: Consumption coagulopathy in congenital heart disease. Lancet 1:231, 1973.
76. Paul MH, Currimbhoy Z, Miller RA, Schulman I: Thrombocytopenia in cyanotic congenital heart disease. Am J Dis Child 102:597, 1961.
77. Patil AS, Sarup DM, Mehta S: Consumption coagulopathy in a child with congenital cyanotic heart disease and its treatment with heparin. Indian J Pediatr 42:17, 1975.
78. Bhargava M, Sanyal SK, Thapar MK, et al: Impairment of platelet adhesiveness and platelet factor 3 activity in cyanotic congenital heart disease. Acta Haematol 55:216, 1976.
79. Goldschmidt B: Platelet functions in children with congenital heart disease. Acta Paediatr Scand 63:271, 1974.
80. Somerville J: Gout in cyanotic congenital heart disease. Br Heart J 23:31, 1961.
81. Mace SE, Newman AJ, Liebman J: Impairment of urate excretion in patients with cardiac disease. Am J Dis Child 138:1067, 1984.
82. Elliott LP, Schiebler GL: A roentgenologic-electrocardiographic approach to cyanotic forms of heart disease. Pediatr Clin North Am 18:1133, 1971.
83. Yip WCL, Tay JSH: A practical diagnostic approach to cyanotic heart disease. Singapore Med J 24:189, 1983.
84. Linday LA, Ehlers KH, O'Loughlin JE, et al: Noninvasive diagnosis of persistent fetal circulation versus congenital cardiovascular defects. Am J Cardiol 52:847, 1983.
85. Kelley MJ, Jaffe CC, Shoum SM, et al: A radiographic and echocardiographic approach to cyanotic congenital heart disease. Radiol Clin North Am 18:411, 1980.
86. Unger FM, Cavanaugh DJ, Johnson GF, et al: Radiologic and real time echocardiographic evaluation of the cyanotic newborn. Radiographics 6:603, 1986.
87. Chrispin A, Small P, Rutter N, et al: Transectional echo planar imaging of the heart in cyanotic congenital heart disease. Pediatr Radiol 16:293, 1986.
88. Gutgesell HP, Huhta JC, Cohen MH, et al: Two-dimensional echocardiographic assessment of pulmonary artery and aortic arch anatomy in cyanotic infants. J Am Coll Cardiol 4:1242, 1984.
89. Ueda K, Nojima K, Saito A, et al: Modified Blalock-Taussig shunt operation without cardiac catheterization: Two-dimensional echocardiographic preoperative assessment in cyanotic infants. Am J Cardiol 54:1296, 1984.
90. Bush SE, Huhta JC, Vick W III, et al: Hypoplastic left heart syndrome: Is echocardiography accurate enough to guide surgical palliation? J Am Coll Cardiol 7:610, 1986.
91. Jonas RA, Lang P, Hansen D, et al: First-stage palliation of hypoplastic left heart syndrome. J Thorac Cardiovasc Surg 92:6, 1986.
92. Danford DA, Gutgesell HP, McNamara DG: Application of information theory to decision analysis in potentially prostaglandin-responsive neonates. J Am Coll Cardiol 8:1125, 1986.
93. Stevenson DK, Bentiz WE: A practical approach to diagnosis and immediate care of the cyanotic neonate. Stabilization and preparation for transfer to level III nursery. Clin Pediatr 26:325, 1987.
94. Taussig HB: Tetralogy of Fallot: Especially the care of cyanotic infant and child. Pediatrics 1:307, 1948.
95. Beeckman RH, Tuuri DT: Acute hemodynamic effects of increasing hemoglobin concentration in children with a right to left ventricular shunt and relative anemia. J Am Coll Cardiol 5:357, 1985.
96. Ponce Fe, Williams LC, Webb HM, et al: Propranolol palliation of tetralogy of Fallot: Experience with long-term drug treatment in pediatric patients. Pediatrics 52:100, 1973.
97. Cummings GR: Propranolol in tetralogy of Fallot. Circulation 41:13, 1970.
98. Taussig HB, Crocetti A, Eshaghpour E, et al: Long-term observations on the Blalock-Taussig operation. III. Common complications. Johns Hopkins Med J 129:274, 1971.
99. Fishbein CA, Rosenthal A, Fischer EG, et al: Risk factors for brain abscess in patients with congenital heart disease. Am J Cardiol 34:97, 1974.
100. Morera JA, Strong WB: Sexuality, conception, and pregnancy in patients with cyanotic congenital heart disease. In Rao PS (ed): Tricuspid Atresia, New York, Futura Publishing Co., 1982.
101. Gleicher N, Midwall J, Hochberger D, et al: Eisenmenger's syndrome and pregnancy. Obstet Gynecol Surg 34:721, 1979.
102. Perloff JK: Pregnancy and cardiovascular disease. In Braunwald E (ed): Heart Disease. Philadelphia, W.B. Saunders Co., 1980.

103. Whittemore R, Hobbins JC, Engle MA: Pregnancy and its outcome in women with and without surgical treatment of congenital heart disease. Am J Cardiol 50:641, 1982.
104. Garson A, McNamara DG, Cooley DA: Tetralogy of Fallot. In Roberts WD (ed): Adult Congenital Heart Disease. Philadelphia, F.A. Davis Co., 1987.
105. Nissenkorn A, Friedman S, Schonfield A, et al: Fetomaternal outcome in pregnancies after total correction of the tetralogy of Fallot. J Am Coll Cardiol 15:40, 1985.
106. Jackson DP: Hemorrhagic diathesis in patients with cyanotic congenital heart disease. Preoperative management. Ann NY Acad Sci 115:235, 1964.
107. Wedemeyer AL, Lewis JH: Improvement in hemostasis following phlebotomy in cyanotic patients with heart disease. J Pediatr 83:46, 1973.
108. Milam JD, Austin SF, Nihill MR, et al: Use of sufficient hemodilution to prevent coagulation following surgical correction of cyanotic heart disease. J Thorac Cardiovasc Surg 89:623, 1985.
109. Friedman WF, Heiferman MF: Clinical problems of postoperative pulmonary vascular disease. Am J Cardiol 50:631, 1982.
110. Graham TP Jr: Ventricular performance in adults after operation for congenital heart disease. Am J Cardiol 50:612, 1982.
111. Mietus-Snyder M, Lang P, Mayer JE, et al: Childhood systemic-pulmonary shunts: subsequent suitability for Fontan operation. Circulation 76(Suppl III):III-39, 1987.
112. Di Donato R, di Carlo D, Squitieri C, et al: Palliation of cardiac malformations associated with right isomerism (asplenia syndrome) in infancy. Ann Thorac Surg 44:35, 1987.
113. De Leon SY, Gidding SS, Ilbawi MN, et al: Surgical management of infants with complex cardiac anomalies associated with reduced pulmonary blood flow and total anomalous pulmonary venous drainage. Ann Thorac Surg 43:207, 1987.
114. Huhta JC, Gutgesell HP, Nihill MR: Cross-sectional echocardiographic diagnosis of total anomalous pulmonary venous connection. Br Heart J 53:525, 1985.
115. Freedom RM, Olley PM, Coceani F, et al: The prostaglandin challenge: Test to unmask obstructed total pulmonary venous connections in asplenia syndrome. Br Heart J 40:91, 1978.
116. Matsuda H, Kawashima Y, Hirose H, et al: Evaluation of total cavopulmonary shunt operation for single ventricle with common atrioventricular valve and left isomerism. Am J Cardiol 58:180, 1986.
117. Kawauchi M, Asano K, Shindo G, et al: Total cavopulmonary shunt with replacement of common atrioventricular valve for an infant with single atrium and single ventricle. Ann Thorac Surg 40:192, 1985.
118. Choussat A, Fontan F, Besse P, et al: Selection criteria for Fontan procedure. In Anderson RH, Shinebourne EA (eds): Pediatric Cardiology. Edinburgh, Churchill Livingstone, 1978.
119. Vargas FJ, Mayer JE Jr, Jonas RA, et al: Anomalous systemic and pulmonary venous connections in conjunction with atriopulmonary anastomosis (Fontan-Kreutzer). J Thorac Cardiovasc Surg 93:523, 1987.
120. Wood P: The Eisenmenger syndrome of pulmonary hypertension with reversed central shunt. Br Med J 2:701–709, 755–762, 1958.
121. Clarkson PM, Frye RL, DuShane JW, et al: Prognosis for patients with ventricular septal defect and severe pulmonary vascular obstructive disease. Circulation 38:129, 1968.
122. Young D, Marks H: Fate of the patient with the Eisenmenger syndrome. Am J Cardiol 28:659, 1971.
123. Rosenthal A, Nathan DG, Marty AT, et al: Acute hemodynamic effects of red cell volume reduction in polycythemia of cyanotic congenital heart disease. Circulation 42:297, 1970.
124. Rosenthal A, Fyler DC: General principles in the treatment of congential heart disease. In Gellis S, Kagan BM (eds): Current Pediatric Therapy, 7th ed. Philadelphia, W.B. Saunders, 1976.
125. Liebman J, Lucas R, Moss A, et al: Airline travel for children with chronic pulmonary disease. Pediatrics 57:408, 1976.
126. Lindesmith CG, Stiles QR, Tucker BL, et al: The Mustard operation as a palliative procedure. J Thorac Cardiovasc Surg 63:75, 1972.
127. Reitz BA, Wallwork JL, Hunt SA, et al: Heart-lung transplantation. Successful therapy for pulmonary vascular disease. N Engl J Med 306:577, 1982.
128. Graham TP Jr: The Eisenmenger syndrome. In Roberts WC (ed): Adult Congenital Heart Disease. Philadelphia, F.A. Davis, 1987.
129. Abbott M: Atlas of Congenital Cardiac Disease. New York, American Heart Association, 1936.
130. Bowie EA: Longevity in tetralogy and trilogy of Fallot. Discussion of patients and presentation of two further cases. Am Heart J 62:125, 1961.

131. Campbell M: Natural history of cyanotic malformations and comparisons of all common cardiac malformations. Br Heart J 34:31, 1972.
132. Trimble AS, Morce JE, Froggatt MB, et al: Total intracardiac repair of the adult cyanotic tetralogy of Fallot. Can Med Assoc J 103:911, 1970.
133. Bender HW, Haller JA, Brawley RK, et al: Experience in repair of tetralogy of Fallot malformations in adults. Ann Thorac Surg 2:508, 1971.
134. Beach PM, Bowman FO, Kaiser GA, et al: Total correction of tetralogy of Fallot in adolescents and adults. Circulation 43(Suppl 1):37, 1971.
135. Hu DC, Seward JB, Fuga FJ, et al: Total correction of tetralogy of Fallot at age 40 years and older: long term follow-up. J Am Coll Cardiol 5:40, 1985.

STEPHEN JAY ROTH, MD

THERAPEUTIC CATHETERIZATION TECHNIQUES IN CYANOTIC HEART DISEASE

From the Department of Pediatrics
Division of Pediatric Cardiology
Marshfield Clinic
Marshfield, Wisconsin

Reprint requests to:
Stephen Jay Roth, MD
Department of Pediatrics
Division of Pediatric Cardiology
Marshfield Clinic
1000 North Oak Avenue
Marshfield, WI 54449-5777

Over the past several years, therapeutic catheterization techniques in congenital heart disease have unleashed the potential for palliative and curative procedures to the pediatric cardiologist. Lesions traditionally treated by surgery and those not readily amenable to surgery, such as distal areas of pulmonary artery stenosis and pulmonary arteriovenous malformations, can be treated by transcatheter techniques. The advantages of transcatheter therapy include shorter hospitalization, rare need for blood transfusion, lower cost, and absence of scarring.

This chapter reviews techniques of therapeutic catheterization in cyanotic heart disease. Historically, the first transcatheter interventional procedure was the cannulation of the brachial artery for attempted phlebotomy in a patient nearly dead from cholera.[10] Subsequently, Bleichroeder, Unger and Loeb[5] described their pioneering efforts of right heart catheterization upon animals and Bleichroeder.

Although there is a single case report of attempted relief of pulmonary valve stenosis by Rubeo-Alvarez and Limon-Lason[43] in 1950, the advent of modern interventional catheterization techniques in congenital heart disease was the development of the balloon atrial septostomy by Rashkind and Miller[39] in 1966. Initially used in infants for palliation of dextro-transposition of the great arteries (d-TGA), the spectrum of cyanotic congenital heart disease palliated by this technique has dramatically increased as surgical corrective approaches have developed.

CARDIAC SURGERY: State of the Art Reviews—Vol. 3, No. 1, February 1989
Philadelphia, Hanley & Belfus, Inc.

With age, the foramen ovale becomes smaller and the atrial septum thicker, which precludes successful balloon atrial septostomy. Park[33] developed the blade atrial septostomy catheter, which allows access to the left atrium (pulmonary venous atrium) in older infants and children. Mullins[31] increased the applicability of this technique by coordinating it with transseptal left atrial catheterization, which allows access to the left atrium when the atrial septum is, essentially, imperforate.

Conventional treatment of right ventricular obstructive disease consists of either bypassing or opening the obstruction or improving oxygenation by the creation of a systemic to pulmonary artery anastomosis. Traditionally, until a few years ago, techniques to accomplish a valvotomy required a thoracotomy to allow for surgical access with inflow occlusion or cardiopulmonary bypass with all the attendant risks.

Gruntzig[21] pioneered catheter balloon dilatation of coronary arteries in 1978 and suggested guidelines for catheter balloon dilatation. Subsequently, based upon the surgical approach of the Brock pulmonary valvotomy, Kan[23] developed the technique of static catheter balloon dilatation. This has been attempted with other cardiovascular structures such as aortic valve stenosis, coarctation of the aorta, pulmonary artery stenosis, conduit stenosis, pulmonary vein stenosis, aortico-pulmonary shunt stenosis, and, in animals, pulmonary artery band.

At the other end of the spectrum is the work being done to close various sites of cardiac and extracardiac communication. Temporary balloon catheter occlusion of atrial septal defects has been used to judge the adequacy of the right ventricle in forms of the hypoplastic right heart syndrome. Transcatheter delivery of metallic coils, tissue "glues," small particles (Gelfoam, etc.), and detachable balloons, in addition to umbrella devices, has had varying degrees of success.

A newer modality is the laser catheter, initially used to dissolve intravascular plaque, and more recently employed in the fulgaration of ventricular tachycardia and, in animal models, to open stenotic valves.

ATRIAL SEPTOSTOMY

The Rashkind balloon atrial septostomy revolutionized the treatment of cyanotic congenital heart disease. Initially this was performed with a double lumen catheter, but biplane fluoroscopy obviated the need for the pressure port, and, more recently, many advocate balloon atrial septostomy under echocardiographic visualization.[26,45]

In general, in congenital heart disease, although high-resolution, echo-Doppler has replaced "routine" diagnostic catheterization, there has been a marked increase in the number of therapeutic cardiac catheterizations. In d-TGA, surgical correction of anatomy uncomplicated by pulmonary stenosis or a complex ventricular septal defect is often performed in the first week of life. With modern (color) Doppler-echocardiography, the anatomy and physiology can be determined noninvasively, and, following septostomy, the adequacy of the created atrial septal defect can be ascertained accurately.

The technique of balloon atrial septostomy is well known. Whether by echocardiography or fluoroscopy, the balloon atrial septostomy catheter is advanced from the femoral vein, preferably the right, or umbilical vein, across the patent foramen ovale to the left atrium. Although compliant, the balloon will stretch from 12–17 mm in diameter with the usual inflation volume of 1.5–4 cc of contrast diluted with saline. Further inflation results in balloon rupture, which can also occur during the septostomy. For this reason, the balloon is de-aired prior to insertion into the vein. The catheter tip is positioned in the left upper pulmonary vein or posteriorly in the left atrium to ensure it is not in the left atrial appendage or a juxtaposed right atrial appendage. Slow inflation will allow the balloon to be milked from the pulmonary vein or left atrial appendage, and, subsequently, the catheter is slowly withdrawn until resistance is felt, indicating engagement of the atrial septum. The catheter is then rapidly tugged backward to tear, rather than stretch, the atrial septum (septum primum). Often this pulls the balloon back into the inferior vena cava, temporarily occluding it. As the balloon is deflated, it is positioned in the mid right atrium to avoid further obstruction. If the maximum appropriate balloon volume is used initially, then only one pullback need be performed. Other prefer graded balloon volume increases, but this approach may stretch the atrial septum more than tear it. The size of the created defect can be judged by determining the inflation volume that allows the balloon to be pulled through the defect without resistance or measured by echocardiography.

The morbidity and mortality of balloon atrial septostomy are less than 5%.[34] Complications include supraventricular tachycardia, femoral and iliac vein thromboses from the large sheath required, femoral vein and inferior vena cave laceration, infection, and cardiac rupture and tamponade.

With any "new" technique, a comparison of the morbidity and mortality with the accepted standard is necessary. In the case of the balloon septostomy, this is difficult because it virtually has replaced the Blalock-Hanlon atrial septectomy. Over the past two decades, those infants subjected to a the Blalock-Hanlon atrial septectomy were often those in whom a balloon atrial septostomy was unsuccessful or who had otherwise more complicated and tenuous anatomy. From a physiological perspective, the Blalock-Hanlon atrial septectomy can afford for better mixing, as the right pulmonary veins straddle the posterior defect. Sinus node dysfunction has been reported not uncommonly.

Recent hospital morbidity and mortality data for the Blalock-Hanlon atrial septectomy are sparse. Prior to the technique of balloon atrial septostomy, surgical mortality for atrial septectomy was approximately 30%, and is probably the same for an open septectomy, typically performed under inflow occlusion. Currently, surgical mortality of 5–10% is quoted.[25,34] Similar data are reported for the Blalock-Hanlon atrial septectomy performed for palliation of left atrioventricular valve atresia, typically as part of more complex anatomy, such as single ventricle. In those instances, often it is combined with another procedure, such as a pulmonary artery band or systemic to pulmonary artery shunt. Some authors[6,35] recommend proceeding with definitive reparative surgery should the balloon atrial septostomy not be efficacious in simple d-TGA.

In older infants and children, the atrial septum is usually quite thick and essentially imperforate. Under these conditions, the standard catheter balloon atrial septostomy has been shown simply to stretch the foramen ovale. Cardiac rupture can occur, as the intraatrial groove[4] may be the weakest or thinnest structure. A transseptal left atrial catheterization can be performed to position a long (Mullins) sheath within the left atrium through which a Park blade septostomy catheter is manipulated.

The Park blade septostomy catheter is a 65-cm long, 6F, relatively stiff catheter with the lumen containing a stiff controlling wire to allow for blade exposure. The distal end is angled and terminates in a 3.5-cm, thin, stainless steel tube with a 2.5-cm longitudinal slit. Recessed within this tube is a hinged blade that can be extended through the slit to position the cutting blade perpendicular to the catheter shaft. The blade extension is controlled by the stiff wire running through the catheter shaft. The distal end of the wire is connected to the hinging mechanism of the blade, and the proximal end extends through adjustment and locking collars for operator use. Additionally, a proximal side port is used for pressure measurement.

The wire is locked with the blade fully recessed within the distal stainless steel tube, which prevents exposure of the blade during positioning. Whether via a transseptal sheath or directly across the foramen ovale, the catheter is rotated within the left atrium to orient the shallowly angulated tip anteriorly, inferiorly, and leftward. Next, the blade is extended by advancing the wire. The catheter is pulled back slowly. Engagement of the atrial septum can be felt as can the loss of resistance once the blade has cut through the atrial septum and the catheter has been drawn into the right atrium. At this point, the blade is retracted.

Across the new septal tear, a balloon atrial septostomy catheter can be advanced and pulled back in the standard fashion, or a static balloon dilatation catheter can be advanced, positioned, and inflated. If by hemodynamic assessment, angiography, or echocardiography the septostomy is judged inadequate, transseptal left atrial catheterization can be performed at another site and the process repeated or a larger dilatation balloon can be used.

Park[32] reported on a collaborative study by five institutions of blade septostomy in 52 patients over a a 4-year period (1977–1981). Seventy-four percent of the patients with a diagnosis of d-TGA, 60% of the total group, demonstrated improvement based upon criteria relating to the residual atrial pressure gradient and systemic saturation. Five complications occurred in the total group and included one death in a 12-year-old secondary to a lacerated left atrial posterior wall. The right ventricular outflow tract was perforated in a 3-month-old with d-TGA and surgically repaired, at which time a Blalock-Hanlon atrial septectomy was performed. This patient also suffered a central nervous system insult as did three other children.

DILATATION TECHNIQUES

Catheter balloon dilatation for pulmonary valve stenosis was the first intracardiac transcatheter "curative" procedure and remains the most successful with the fewest complications. The roots of this technique are from the early surgical transventricular blunt approach of Brock.[19] Surgical pulmonary valvotomy by Dodrill[11] in 1952 was the first procedure to employ mechanical assistance, as the patient's right lung was ventilated, while right heart bypass allowed for a controlled, unhurried, open pulmonary valvotomy.

The history of transcatheter balloon dilatation begins with the efforts of Dotter and Judkins,[12] who performed studies in 1964 using a lower extremity artery. This was followed in 1976 by Gruntzig,[21] who used a coronary artery. In 1979, in an infant with pulmonary valve stenosis and tricuspid insufficiency, Semb[44] positioned a floating balloon catheter in the main pulmonary artery distal to the pulmonary valve, inflated the balloon with carbon dioxide, and pulled it back in a fashion similar to that for a Rashkind balloon atrial septostomy. The procedure was successful and the infant improved afterward. Kan and White[23] were the first to use a static, fluid-filled balloon catheter positioned across the pulmonary valve to obtain a controlled angioplasty (initially in a bulldog with hereditary pulmonary valve stenosis).

PULMONARY STENOSIS

Anatomy of Pulmonary Valve

To prevent undue trauma to the pulmonary apparatus, dilatation proceeded in a cautious fashion using balloons of diameter smaller than the pulmonary annulus. Although there were initial concerns about the ability to tolerate longstanding pulmonary insufficiency, as the more recent literature was reviewed, it became apparent that pulmonary insufficiency was well tolerated. Gikonyo (Edwards)[18] examined pathology specimens of stenotic pulmonary valves classifying them as domed, unicommissural, bicuspid, tricuspid, hypoplastic annulus, and dysplastic. The salient features of these valves are increased thickness typically due to excessive myxomatous tissue, absence of a normal fibrous annulus, and obstruction by the bulky leaflet of the dysplastic valve along with hypoplasia of the supravalvar and subvalvar regions. In the normal pulmonary valve, the three leaflets originate independently from the annulus without commissural fusion. They correlated these findings with those following open valvotomy and catheter balloon dilatation.

Since the raphe tend to be the thickest portions of the valve, blunt dilatation, whether by a solid sound or static balloon catheter, tears the thinner midportion of the valve leaflet. If the tear is long enough to relieve the obstruction, which probably requires a tear extending from the orifice to the wall, then the leaflet will be flail. Their examination of the dysplastic valve identified three open commissures preoperatively, and indicated that the obstruction occurs from the bulky mass of the leaflets within the (narrow) annulus. It is unlikely that catheter balloon dilatation will be efficacious. Additionally, since the annulus is structurally very abnormal, excessive balloon diameter could result in annulus rupture.

Pulmonary Valve Catheter Balloon Dilatation

Kan,[23,30,49] Perry (Lock),[36] and others[13,24,29,37,38] have developed guidelines concerning balloon size and techniques of dilatation in general. Based upon their experience, they confirm the impressions of postoperative surgical patients that mild pulmonary insufficiency is well tolerated. Catheter balloon dilatation is virtually the procedure of choice for pulmonary valve stenosis, with a prevalence of approximately 8% of congenital heart disease. Patients with pulmonary valve gradients greater than 40 mm Hg and, in several centers, infants with critical pulmonary stenosis are candidates for catheter balloon dilatation.

The basic procedure involves several dilator, sheath, guidewire, and catheter exchanges in order to firmly anchor a relatively thick, flexible guidewire in a distal pulmonary artery. Typically, the guidewire is positioned in the left pulmonary artery, which originates as a straighter branch of the main pulmonary artery than the right. Anchoring the guidewire allows the large, relatively stiff angioplasty catheter to be manipulated across the right ventricular outflow tract and pulmonary valve. The balloon dilatation catheter is considerably stiffer than the diagnostic catheters and, without guidance over a large diameter guidewire, would be difficult to manipulate to the pulmonary artery and could perforate the pre-and postdilatation structures. The guidewire allows the catheter to be atraumatically repositioned should it recoil during dilatation and, with the balloon partially deflated, to be advanced to the left pulmonary artery to restore the cardiac output following the dilatation.

An accurate gradient is estimated by echo-Doppler techniques and confirmed at catheterization, at which time the diameter of the pulmonary annulus is measured. Starting with the smaller sheath used for the catheterization, in the right or left femoral vein, an endhole catheter is positioned to end in a distal branch of the left pulmonary artery. Guidewire, catheter, and sheath exchanges are made up to an .035 inch guidewire and 9F or 10F sheath. The balloon dilatation catheter is advanced over the guidewire and the balloon positioned with the midpoint centered at the pulmonary valve. The balloon position is checked by a low-pressure test inflation to determine the location of the waist. Some advocate positioning a diagnostic catheter within the right ventricle to measure pressure during inflation, administration of oxygen to prevent reflex pulmonary vasoconstriction, lidocaine to mitigate against ventricular dysrhythmias, and atropine to prevent reflex bradycardia.

The pulmonary valve requires less intraballoon dilation pressure, 3 to 4 atm, than the aortic valve. A balloon diameter 20–40% greater than that of the pulmonary annulus is safe and yields a better long-term result than the smaller balloons. A double balloon approach is required for a pulmonary annulus larger than 20 mm, as 25 mm is the largest balloon catheter manufactured. For this approach, one catheter from each femoral vein is advanced in a similar fashion to a single catheter approach, with the sum of the two balloon diameters equal to that of the diameter desired.

Two operators are necessary. One must hold the catheter in the previously determined, hemodynamically stable position and the other must inflate the balloon with dilute contrast and hold the inflation pressure for several seconds. This is repeated 2 or 3 times. With the more stenotic valves, a definite pop can be felt when the valve is successfully dilated. Some advocate de-airing the balloon in vitro, and backfilling with carbon dioxide and contrast. However, this unwraps the balloon and makes it virtually impossible to advance in the relatively smaller sheaths or difficult to pass percutaneously directly over a guidewire. In many clinical situations, the balloon can be safely de-aired in the IVC.

The inflation is viewed, and often recorded, fluoroscopically to verify loss of the waist. Subsequently the catheter is withdrawn while the guidewire is left in place. A hemodynamic catheter is advanced to measure a pullback gradient. There are risks of perforation if a catheter is advanced across a freshly dilated site without the use of a previously placed guidewire. Follow-up cineangiograms are often taken in the right ventricle.

For the past two decades, the surgical results, as discussed by Kirklin,[25] have been excellent. He tabulated hospital mortality for more than 500 patients from several centers. Excluding infants less than 1 month of age, the hospital mortality is approximately 4% with a morbidity of 5–10%. This percentage is not significantly affected by type of procedure, including Brock closed transventricular valvotomy, cardiopulmonary bypass, profound hypothermia with circulatory arrest and limited cardiopulmonary bypass, or mild hypothermia and inflow occlusion, or the periods 1960–1966 or 1967–1979.

The hospital mortality for newborns is quite variable, ranging from 20–50%. This group probably includes several patients with severe right ventricular hypoplasia and sicker neonates before the advent of prostaglandin therapy, and reflects the previous lack of understanding of the need for aortico-pulmonary shunts. Overall, the spectrum of pulmonary stenosis in the neonate is broad, including valvar, annular, and infundibular stenosis, and tricuspid and right ventricular hypoplasia. A coexistent patent ductus arteriosus, elevated pulmonary resistance, and lung disease make the interpretation of the data in this age group quite difficult. An additional reflection of this is demonstrated by the long-term survival and reoperation rate in the neonate compared with older patients. The data are limited, but 2% late mortality and 10–20% significant residual pulmonary stenosis, mainly infundibular, are approximate for non-neonates. For the neonate, 10% late mortality and 30–50% (increasing with time since operation) residual stenosis are common.

It is difficult to extract comparative data for the pulmonary valve catheter balloon dilatation as fewer have been performed (including infrequent neonates), the follow-up interval is shorter, and the stenosis recurrences have decreased with the use of relatively larger diameter balloons. Furthermore, many of the dilatations have been performed in isolated pulmonary valve stenosis without significant infundibular stenosis. In these limited situations, using oversized balloons, there tends to be a gradual dimunition of the transvalvar gradient over time following catheter balloon dilatation of pulmonary valve stenosis. Typically, residual gradients of 20–30% of baseline occur. The dysplastic pulmonary valve is not successfully dilated by catheter balloon dilatation or surgery. The procedure also appears to be successful in patients with restenosis following the traditional surgical approaches. Complications are infrequent, including bundle branch block, vein thrombosis, ventricular tachycardia, and bradycardia. No deaths have been reported.

Catheter Balloon Dilatation of Other Structures

There are isolated reports of catheter balloon dilatation of right ventricular to pulmonary artery conduits, Blalock-Taussig anastomosis, and peripheral pulmonary stenosis. Lloyd et al.,[27] Waldman et al.,[47] and others[36] describe the varied experiences with conduit bioprosthetic valve dilatation. The valves were glutaraldehyde-fixed porcine heterografts and irradiated homografts, 20–21 mm, and had been implanted 4–14 years previously. Some of the patients had preexisting pulmonary insufficiency, and others had none. Pulmonary insufficiency tended to increase following dilatation. If the pulmonary resistance is normal, this may not be of clinical significance. Questions were raised concerning the role that intimal peel might play in the stenosis and whether dislodgment could occur. Waldman reports that the porcine valve function was somewhat preserved and Lloyd indicated that the valve appeared unchanged angiographically. The latter group experienced balloon rupture. Balloon size was no greater than that of the valve. More distal stenotic areas were uncovered that could also be dilated. In others' experience with stenotic calcified porcine valves, the most common finding is calcification of one commissure, and dilatation cracks the valve along that calcified commissure. The procedure was successful in less than half the patients. Complications in this limited number of patients were rare. Despite the low success rate, the data suggest that the procedure offers some relief and can delay the need for conduit replacement.

Transcatheter dilatation of stenotic modified Blalock-Taussig anastomosis using coronary artery and small balloon dilatation catheters has been attempted infrequently.[13,23,24,29,30,36,37,38,49] Access is a problem, especially for shunts ipsilateral to the aortic arch. Although there can be an intimal rind in the Gor-Tex graft, the obstruction is most often at the suture line. The results are not good and some have encountered problems with shunt occlusion from procedure-induced thrombosis, possibly aided by dislodged intimal peel.

Efforts with catheter balloon dilatation of peripheral pulmonary stenosis have been much less successful than in pulmonary valve stenosis. Possibly the development of a catheter delivered vascular stent will make this a viable procedure. Catheter balloon dilatation of peripheral pulmonary stenoses, both native and at the site of anastomosis of a systemic shunt, is successful in approximately half the attempts. Frequently, regions of more distal obstruction are noted which require dilatation after the proximal site has healed. Compared with valve dilatation, the balloon diameters are relatively large at 2–4 times that of the narrow region but less than twice that of the uninvolved pulmonary artery. Morphological studies indicate that success requires intimal and medial tears, and long-term follow-up demonstrates little restenosis.

Many of these sites are not amenable to open thoracotomy either because of the distal location or the need for more exposure than is attainable with the anticipated primary surgery. Additionally, in children who have undergone one or two palliative procedures and possibly a definitive operation, transcatheter therapy has beneficial psychological results and eliminates the need for tedious and risky reoperation in a scarred operative field. It is important to recognize these factors in the interpretation of the complication rate of the transcatheter approach, which exceeds that for transcatheter dilation of pulmonary valve stenosis but is quite low in the few reported cases, and has a much lower success rate.[13,24,30,36,37,38,49] Pulmonary artery rupture with or without balloon rupture, hemoptysis, pulmonary artery thrombosis and aneurysm formation, and death have been reported.

There are isolated reports of dilatation of atrial baffle obstruction in postoperative d-TGA both at the baffle–atrial septum junction and superior vena cava–baffle junction. The results are encouraging, but not enough long-term data have been collected.

Catheter Balloon Dilatation of the Patent Ductus Arteriosus

Lund et al.[28] reported dilatation of the patent ductus arteriosus (PDA) in piglets using a retrograde catheterization approach. Morphologic studies demonstrated damage to the internal elastic lamina, medial hemorrhage, and intact adventitia. Very oversized balloons resulted in rupture. They kept inflation for a long interval, 5 minutes, which clinically is not possible when the pulmonary blood flow is totally patent ductus arteriosus dependent. Corwin et al.[7] tried this approach as palliation just prior to taking the infant to surgery. They used a 5F Berman angiographic catheter advanced prograde with the balloon inflated with air in an infant with an interrupted aortic arch and ventricular septal defect. Suarez de Lezo et al.[9] reported that in vitro PDA dilatation resulted in intima and media damage. Using a static, fluid-filled balloon catheter advanced from the main pulmonary artery, they successfully dilated a PDA in an infant with the hypoplastic left heart syndrome who later died. Microscopic examination revealed findings similar to the in vitro work and focal adventitial hemorrhage. More experimental work needs to be done in this area, as, if permanent dilation of the PDA can be performed, fewer infants may require shunts.

TRANSCATHETER CLOSURE TECHNIQUES

Transcatheter delivery of metallic coils, plastic spheres, tissue "glues," small particles (Gelfoam, etc.), and detachable balloons, in addition to umbrella devices, have had varying degrees of success. Currently, Gianturco coils and balloons are used to close pulmonary arteriovenous malformations, aortic collateral vessels, and residual Blalock-Taussig anastomoses. Typically, the first two lesions are not readily amenable to open surgical technique.

Metallic Coils

Each method has its own proponents. The structure to be occluded should be at least 2 cm long and, ideally, less than 1 cm in diameter.[13] For coil embolization, it is preferable for the vessel to taper at its distal end. The Gianturco coils were developed for use in cerebral vessels. Compared with the detachable balloons, the delivery technique is simpler. Packed, thrombogenic, Dacron-coated coils are placed in a 5F or 6F endhole catheter. The catheter is positioned in the structure to be occluded and the coils extruded from the catheter lumen expanding to 3–8 mm (maximum 15 mm). On the other hand, once in position, the expanded coil is extremely difficult to remove and elicits a greater inflammatory response than balloons. Additionally, the coil itself does not occlude the structure, rather it presents the surface for thrombosis and subsequent occlusion, a process that can take several days. In some instances, a large coil is placed first followed by smaller coils. In regions of high flow, downstream migration is not unlikely. These features tend to limit the applicability of coils to pulmonary arteriovenous malformations with a single small feeder artery, aorticopulmonary collateral vessels, and stenotic Blalock-Taussig anastomoses.[16,46]

Lock[36] reported on Gianturco coil emoblization of 52 vessels in 38 patients. Twenty-five of 38 aortico-pulmonary collateral vessels (major underlying diagnosis was tetralogy of Fallot) were successfully occluded, with an additional nine with near total occlusion. Four of the nine Blalock-Taussig anastomoses were totally occluded, with an additional three with near total occlusion. In one patient, a successful attempt was made to reduce the flow through a Blalock-Taussig anastomosis in a patient with a complex lesion, but subsequent hemolysis, presumably coil induced, necessitated an additional procedure. An example of the potential of these procedures is the gratifying result in a patient with pulmonary atresia and intact ventricular septum with a Blalock-Taussig anastomosis. The right ventricle grew to adequate size following right ventricular outflow tract reconstruction, and the atrial septal defect underwent spontaneous closure. (In the future, transcatheter umbrella closure techniques for atrial septal defects may become more widely available.) Coil occlusion of the shunt eliminated the need for further surgery.

Balloons

Although the detachable balloon catheter delivery system is stiffer and somewhat more complicated than that for coils, there are several advantages to the balloons. More precise positioning can be accomplished, the efficacy of occlusion can be tested by angiography prior to balloon release, and the delivery catheter can be manipulated through more angulated channels. In areas of high flow, a more proximal balloon catheter can be used to decrease the flow while the detachable balloon is positioned and inflated. Once released, the balloon mechanically should completely occlude the vessel. Approximately 10 days are required for complete thrombosis to occur.

There are two types of detachable balloons. One is constructed of semipermeable silicone, delivered via a catheter, inflated with an isotonic saline-contrast solution, and detached. A self-closing valve prevents deflation. Since this is a semipermeable balloon, fluid shifts occur between the blood stream and the balloon interior which, along with the inherent balloon weakness, can result in premature deflation prior to complete thrombosis and/or downstream migration. This balloon can be used to occlude structures no larger than 9 mm.[24]

For larger structures, latex balloons that are filled with two reactive monomeric solutions that rapidly solidify can be used. This technique is more complicated, as the balloon is hand tied to the catheter immediately prior to use. Once positioned, a trial fluid inflation is made to test efficacy of occlusion. If successful, the balloon is deflated, reinflated with the permanent solution, and detached. In areas of high flow, if a more proximal partial occlusion balloon catheter is not used, premature detachment with distal embolization can occur. A marker of premature detachment is the change in shape of the balloon to a teardrop. When this is observed, the balloon can be deflated and repositioned or a second gas-filled balloon catheter can be positioned upstream to temporarily reduce the flow.

The delivery technique involves carefully positioning a 9F introducer catheter through which a 2F catheter with a deflated balloon attached is manipulated. The silicone mini-balloons are 2 mm when collapsed and inflate to 8–12 mm. A smaller 4-mm balloon can be delivered through a 5F catheter. A half dozen case reports exist of attempted balloon occlusion of Blalock-Taussig anastomoses.[18,30,40,41] Complications are infrequent and mild. Balloon embolization to the lung apparently occludes a minor branch artery of little significance.

Closure Techniques in Pulmonary Arteriovenous Malformations

Pulmonary arteriovenous malformations occur in 7–15% of individuals with hereditary hemorrhagic telangiectasia (HHT). There is 10% mortality secondary to hemoptysis and paradoxical embolization, with brain abscess and stroke. Pulmonary arteriovenous malformations tend to occur in the lung bases, perhaps because the lung bases have a relatively high pulmonary blood flow, in HHT as well as late postoperatively in patients with a Glenn anastomosis.[1,20,48] Embolization with particulate matter is relatively contraindicated because of the possibility of systemic embolization. Balloon and coil therapy have been successfully applied without serious complications. Surgery mortality is reportedly approximately 5%. Over time, smaller pulmonary arteriovenous malformations enlarge. Therefore, the recurrence of hypoxemia is exacerbated by the deficiency of lung tissue following earlier surgical resection. The feeder artery distal to branches perfusing the lung normally can be selectively embolized with the transcatheter approach.

Temporary Occlusion Procedures

Diagnostic floating carbon dioxide filled balloon catheters can be used to temporarily occlude structures. In the hypoplastic right heart syndrome there may be enough growth of the right ventricle and tricuspid valve following initial right ventricular outflow reconstruction to support the total pulmonary blood flow. Since a balloon atrial septostomy often has been performed in the newborn period, a test of the adequacy of the right heart can be performed during routine cardiac catheterization by advancing a balloon angiographic catheter (holes proximal to the balloon) across the atrial septal defect to the left atrium.[2,8] With the balloon inflated, often the catheter can be pulled back until the balloon occludes the atrial septal defect. Right atrial pressures are measured as is the systemic oxygenation, which should increase. Currently, a child subsequently would undergo surgical closure of an atrial septal defect. Although not germane to this chapter, catheter-delivered umbrella devices to close atrial septal defects are in investigational stages.

The persistent left superior vena cava can create a problem at the time of open heart surgery. An extra venous cannula is required that can obstruct the surgical field. At the time of diagnostic cardiac catheterization, a balloon wedge catheter can be positioned within this vessel.[15] With the balloon inflated to occlude the vessel, the distal caval pressure is measured. If the pressure does not rise 10 mm Hg after 10 minutes of occlusion, signifying adequate collateral vessels or an innominate vein, then the vessel can be safely ligated at surgery without concern for the development of hydrocephalous or facial swelling.

Laser Catheter

The predominant work with laser catheters has been in the peripheral vascular field. The three lasers used are the carbon dioxide, argon, and neodymium-yttrium aluminum garnet (Nd-YAG). Each produces light at a different wavelength. The action of lasers is tissue vaporization by photochemical changes and heat. Three distinct zones of tissue damage are observed.[3] Argon light was used to create in vitro aortic and mitral valve commissurotomies[17] and to debride calcified aortic valves in vitro.[22] Reimenschneider[42] described the relief of valvar pulmonary and aortic stenosis and dysplastic pulmonary valve stenosis in vitro (as well as coarctation of the aorta) and the creation of an atrial septal defect in an anesthetized dog model.

SUMMARY

The new and rapidly expanding field of interventional catheterization techniques in cyanotic heart disease was reviewed. Similar procedures have been applied to other forms of heart disease, acyanotic and both congenital and acquired. These are exciting techniques that, for the first time, allow "curative" procedures to be performed at cardiac catheterization. Additionally, the benefits to the patient are substantial when compared with the standard surgical approaches. In the majority of these transcatheter procedures, the morbidity and mortality are lower than those of traditional surgery, repairs not accessible surgically can be performed, intrathoracic scarring is reduced thereby decreasing the difficulties in subsequent definitive (re)operation, the length of hospitalization is significantly shortened, and the overall cost is significantly lessened. In children, there is a significant psychological benefit of reduced hospitalization stay and reduced superficial scarring.

Currently, transcatheter techniques have only begun to be utilized. With the development of new catheters and delivery systems, use of new materials for occlusion devices, and energy sources for opening structures, the breadth of applications of these techniques should increase profoundly.

REFERENCES

1. Barth KH, White RI Jr, Kaufman SL, Terry PB, et al: Embolotherapy of pulmonary arteriovenous malformations with detachable balloons. Radiology 142:599, 1982.
2. Bass JL, Fuhrman BP, Lock JE: Balloon occlusion of atrial septal defect to assess right ventricular capability in hypoplastic right heart syndrome. Circulation 68:1081, 1983.
3. Bjork VO, Sternlieb JJ: Prospects for laser application in cardiac operations. Cardiovasc Clin 17:415–420, 1987.
4. Blanchard WB, Knauf DG, Victoria BE: Interatrial groove tear: An unusual complication of balloon atrial septostomy. Pediatr Cardiol 4:149, 1983.
5. Bleichroeder F, Unges E, Loeb W: Intraarterielle therapy. Klin Wochenschr 49:1502, 1912.
6. Cohen DJ, Chopra PS: The Blalock-Hanlon operation: An anachronism? Ann Thorac Surg 44:407, 1987.

7. Corwin RD, Singh AK, Karlson KE: Balloon dilatation of ductus arteriosus in a newborn with interrupted aortic arch and ventricular septal defect. Am Heart J 102:446–447, 1981.
8. Cotter L, Pusey CD, Miller GAH: Extreme right ventricular hypoplasia after relief of severe pulmonary stenosis. Use of balloon catheter occlusion of atrial septal defect in assessing right ventricular function. Br Heart J 44:469, 1980.
9. De Lezo JS, Lopez-Rubio F, Guzman J, Galan A, et al: Percutaneous transluminal angioplasty of stenotic ductus arteriosus. Cathet Cardiovasc Diag 11:493, 1985.
10. Dieffenbach JF: Physiologisch-chirurgisch beobachtigen die cholera-kraken. Cholera Arch 1:86, 1832.
11. Dodrill FD, Hill E, Gerisch RA, et al: Pulmonary valvuloplasty under direct vision using mechanical heart for a complete by-pass of the right heart in a patient with congenital pulmonary stenosis. J Thorac Surg 26:584, 1953.
12. Dotter CT, Judkins MP: Transluminal treatment of arteriosclerotic obstruction: Description of a new technic and a preliminary report of its application. Circulation 30:654, 1964.
13. Fellows KE Jr: Therapeutic catheter procedures in congenital heart disease: Current status and future prospects. Cardiovasc Intervent Radiol 7:170, 1984.
14. Florentine M, Wolfe RR, White RI Jr: Balloon embolization to occlude a Blalock-Taussig shunt. J Am Coll Cardiol 3:200, 1984.
15. Freed MD, Rosenthal a, Bernhard WF: Balloon occlusion of a persistent left superior vena cava in the preoperative evaluation of systemic venous return. J Thorac Surg 65, 1973.
16. Fuhrman BP, Bass JL, Castaneda-Zuniga W, Amplatz K, et al: Coil embolization of congenital thoracic vascular anomalies in infants and children. Circulation 70:285, 1984.
17. Gessman LJ, Reno CW, Chang KS, MacMillan RM, et al: Feasibility of laser catheter valvulotomy for aortic and mitral stenosis. Am J Cardiol 54, 1984.
18. Gikonyo BM, Lucas RV, Edwards JE: Anatomic features of congenital pulmonary valvar stenosis. Pediatr Cardiol 8:109, 1987.
19. Glenn WWL: The evolution of the treatment of isolated pulmonary valve stenosis. Yale J Biol Med 60:471, 1987.
20. Gomes AS, Benson L, George B, Laks H: Management of pulmonary arteriovenous fistulas after superior vena cava-right pulmonary artery (Glenn) anastomosis. J Thorac Cardiovasc Surg 87:636, 1984.
21. Gruntzig AR: Die perkutane rekanalisation chronischer, arterieller verschlusse (dotter-princip) met einem doppelumigen dilatations-katheter. Fortschr Rontgen Str 124:80, 1976.
22. Isner JM, Michlewitz H, Clarke RH, Donaldson RF, et al: Laser-assisted debridement of aortic valve calcium. Am Heart J 109:448, 1985.
23. Kan J, White RI, Mitchell SE, Gardner TJ: Percutaneous balloon valvulotomy: A new method for treating congenital pulmonary valve stenosis. N Engl J Med 307:540, 1982.
24. Kaufman SL: Intrathoracic interventional vascular techniques in congenital cardiovascular disease. J Thorac Imag 2:1, 1987.
25. Kirklin JW, Barratt-Boyes BG: Cardiac Surgery: Morphology, Diagnostic Criteria, Natural History, Techniques, Results and Indications. New York, John Wiley & Sons, 1986.
26. Lau KC, Mok CK, Lo RNS, Leung MP, et al: Balloon atrial septostomy under two dimensional echocardiographic control. Pediatr Cardiol 8:35, 1987.
27. Lloyd TR, Marvin WJ Jr, Mahoney LT, Lauer RM: Balloon dilation valvuloplasty of bioprosthetic valves in extracardiac conduits. Am Heart J 114:268, 1987.
28. Lund G, Cragg A, Rysavy J, Castaneda F: Patency of the ductus arteriosus after balloon dilatation: An experimental study. Circulation 68:621, 1983.
29. McKay RG: Balloon valvuloplasty for treating pulmonic, mitral and aortic valve stenosis. Am J Cardiol 61:102G, 1988.
30. Mitchell SE, Kan JS, White RI Jr: Interventional techniques in congenital heart disease. Semin Roentgenol 20:290, 1985.
31. Mullins CE: Transseptal left heart catheterization: Experience with a new technique in 520 pediatric and adult patients. Pediatr Cardiol 4:239, 1983.
32. Park SC, Neches WH, Mullins CE, Girod DA, et al: Blade atrial septostomy: Collaborative study. Circulation 66:258, 1982.
33. Park SC, Zuberbuhler Jr, Neches WH, Lenox CC, et al: A new atrial septostomy technique. Cath Cardiovasc Diagn 1:195, 1975.
34. Paul M: Moss' Heart Disease in Infants, Children and Adolescents, 3rd ed. In Adams FH, Emmanouilides GG (eds). Baltimore, Williams and Wilkins, 1983.
35. Perry LW, Ruckman RN, Galioto FM Jr, Shapiro SR, et al: Echocardiographically assisted balloon atrial septostomy. Pediatrics 70:402, 1982.

36. Perry SB, Keane JF, Lock JE: Interventional catheterization in pediatric congenital and acquired heart disease AJC. A symposium: Intervent Cardiol 61:109G–115G, 1987.
37. Rashkind WJ: Interventional cardiac catheterization in congenital heart disease. Cardiovasc Clin 15:303–316, 1985.
38. Rashkind WJ: Interventional cardiac catheterization in congenital heart disease. Int J Cardiol 7:1, 1985.
39. Rashkind WJ, Miller WW: Creation of an atrial septal defect without thoracotomy: A palliative approach to complete transposition of the great vessels. JAMA 196:991, 1966.
40. Reidy JF, Baker E, Tynan M: Transcatheter occlusion of a Blalock-Taussig shunt with a detachable balloon in a child. Br Heart J 50:101, 1983.
41. Reidy JF, Jones ODH, Tynan MJ, Baker EJ, et al: Embolisation procedures in congenital heart disease. Br Heart J 54:184, 1985.
42. Riemenschneider TA, Lee G, Ikeda RM, Bommer WJ, et al: Laser irradiation of congenital heart disease: Potential for palliation and correction of intracardiac and intravascular defects. Am Heart J 106:1389, 1983.
43. Rubeo-Alvarez V, Limon-Lason: Treatment of pulmonary valvular stenosis and tricuspid stenosis with a modified cardiac catheter. Washington, D.C., Proc First Nat Conf Cardiovasc Dis. 1950.
44. Semb BKH, Tjonneland S, Stake G, et al: "Balloon valvulotomy" of congenital pulmonary valve stenosis with bicuspid valve insufficiency. Cardiovasc Radiol 2:239, 1979.
45. Steeg CN, Bierman FZ, Hordof AJ, Hayes CJ, et al: "Bedside" balloon septostomy in infants with transposition of the great arteries: New concepts using two-dimensional echocardiographic techniques. J Pediatr 107:944, 1985.
46. Szarnicki R, Krebber HJ, Wack J: Wire coil embolizations of systemic-pulmonary collaterals following surgical correction of pulmonary atresia. J Thorac Cardiovasc Surg 81:124, 1981.
47. Waldman JD, Schoen FJ, Kirkpatrick SE, Mathewson JW, et al: Balloon dilatation of porcine bioprosthetic valves in the pulmonary position. Circulation 76:109, 1987.
48. White RI Jr, Mitchell SE, Barth KH, Kaufman SL, et al: Angioarchitecture of pulmonary arteriovenous malformations: An important consideration before embolotherapy. AJR 140:681, 1983.
49. White RI Jr, Mitchell SE, Kan J: Interventional procedures in congenital heart disease. Cardiovasc Intervent Radiol 9:286, 1986.

L. DOUGLAS COWGILL, MD

SHUNTING PROCEDURES FOR CYANOTIC HEART DISEASE

From the Department of Surgery
Dean Clinic
Madison, Wisconsin

Reprint requests to:
L. Douglas Cowgill, MD
Department of Surgery
Dean Clinic
1313 Fish Hatchery Rd.
Madison, WI 53715

Once the most effective treatment for many cyanotic heart conditions, systemic pulmonary artery shunts (SPAS) are used with less frequency now due to increased emphasis on primary repair. Nevertheless, shunts continue to have a major role in selected patients with pulmonary oligemia, especially those in the first year of life.

The ideal shunt should (1) reliably increase pulmonary blood flow, (2) be relatively simple to construct, (3) have few early or late complications, (4) provide bilateral pulmonary artery blood flow, (5) facilitate pulmonary artery growth, and (6) be simple to take down. This chapter will discuss the various extracardiac shunting operations, with emphasis on patency rates and complications.

SUBCLAVIAN ARTERY-PULMONARY ARTERY SHUNT (BLALOCK-TAUSSIG SHUNT)

The era of surgical treatment for cyanotic heart disease began in 1945 with Blalock and Taussig's report of three patients with tetralogy of Fallot who were shunted.[1] Until then, "a 'blue baby' with a malformed heart was considered beyond the reach of surgical aid."[1] Their understanding of cyanotic heart disease was aided by Lundsgaard and Van Slyke, who demonstrated that there were four factors important in the production of cyanosis: the height of hemoglobin, the volume of the venous blood shunted into the systemic circulation, the rate of utilization of oxygen by peripheral tissues, and the extent of aeration of blood in the

TABLE 1. Studies on Arterial Blood (Case 2)

Dates	Arterial Oxygen Content, Volumes per Cent	Arterial Oxygen Capacity, Volumes per Cent	Arterial Oxygen Saturation per Cent	Arterial CO_2 Content, Volumes per Cent
2/1/45	11.7	32.3	36.3	34.9
2/3/45	Innominate artery anastomosed to left pulmonary artery			
2/12/45	20.3	27.5	73.8	37.8
3/1/45	19.8	23.9	82.8	37.2

Reprinted with permission from JAMA 128:189–202, 1945.

lungs.[2] Taussig recognized that the volume of blood reaching the lungs must be especially important by considering two entities, single ventricle and truncus arteriosus.[1] In both of these, cyanosis occurred only when pulmonary blood flow was restricted anatomically, and she reasoned it could be corrected by increasing pulmonary blood flow. Blalock, working independently with the construction of various shunts in dogs, had proven systemic vessels could be divided and anastomosed to pulmonary arteries experimentally.[1] The collaboration of Taussig and Blalock dramatically changed the fate of many blue babies. All three of their initial patients survived surgery. They noted that the shunts led to "a decline in the red cell count, in the hemoglobin, and in the hematocrit reading; an increase in the oxygen content of the arterial blood; a fall in the oxygen capacity; and most importantly, a decided rise in the oxygen saturation of the arterial blood" (Tables 1 and 2).

Interestingly, in none of the three patients was the "classic Blalock-Taussig shunt" performed, that is, the end of the subclavian artery on the side opposite the aortic arch to the side of the pulmonary artery. Instead, one received a left subclavian-left pulmonary artery shunt with a left aortic arch, and the other two had innominate artery to pulmonary artery shunts. In no case did arm or cerebral ischemia occur. Subsequently, to avoid the kinking that occurred when the subclavian on the side of the arch was used, Blalock recommended using the subclavian on the side opposite the arch (i.e., the subclavian arising from the innominate artery) (Fig. 1).[3] The flexibility Blalock demonstrated when performing shunts is nevertheless instructive.

One further appreciates the Blalock-Taussig shunt by noting that it is still the "standard" by which all other shunts are compared. It has many of the

TABLE 2. Studies on Arterial Blood (Case 3)

Dates	Arterial Oxygen Content, Volumes per Cent	Arterial Oxygen Capacity, Volumes per Cent	Arterial Oxygen Saturation per Cent	Arterial CO_2 Content, Volumes per Cent	Comment
2/8/45	7.3	31.2	23.4	27.5	Patient struggling
2/9/45	10.7	30.2	35.5	29.3	Patient quiet
2/10/45	Innominate artery anastomosed to right pulmonary artery				
2/19/45	17.7	22.2	79.7	37.4	Patient crying
3/6/45	17.7	21.1	83.8	35.2	Patient quiet

Reprinted with permission from JAMA 128:189–202, 1945.

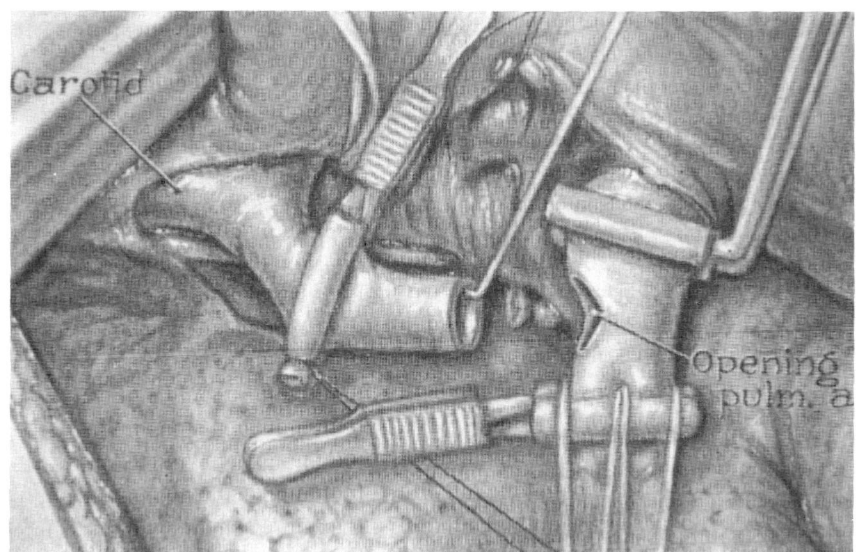

FIGURE 1. The Blalock-Taussig shunt. (Reprinted with permission from Surg Gynecol Obstet 87:385–409, 1948.)

features of an ideal shunt in that it reliably corrects cyanosis; has a low incidence of congestive failure, pulmonary hypertension, and pulmonary artery distortion; has a proven ability to facilitate growth of hypoplastic pulmonary arteries; and is simple to take down. Significant ipsilateral arm ischemia is very uncommon, though arm growth is sometimes poorer than normal, but phrenic nerve injury is a hazard. The Blalock-Taussig shunt does require relatively long dissection time when compared to "central" or "modified" shunts, and originally was less applicable in infants with small subclavian arteries. In 1971 Taussig and associates reported the results of shunts in approximately 1000 patients; they noted that the younger the patient at the time of initial shunt, the shorter the duration of improvement.[4]

The Blalock-Taussig shunt is the procedure of choice for many groups, even in infancy.[5–13] Operative mortality has steadily declined, from as high as 47% in neonates in 1975[6] to less than 10% more recently.[19] The very low incidences of congestive failure (due to the naturally limited size of the subclavian artery) and pulmonary artery distortion are major advantages over central shunts. Although patency rates in infants were initially poor, improved microsurgical techniques have made patency acceptable, even in neonates. In the Birmingham experience, of 94 patients who received a Blalock-Taussig shunt in the first 2 years of life, many less than 3 months of age, only three shunts failed and required reoperation.[10] One of the 94 patients developed significant but nongangrenous arm ischemia.

Tyson and coworkers performed Blalock-Taussig shunts on 24 patients less than 2 years of age with 0% operative mortality and no late shunt failures.[9] Laks and associates had a 17.6% operative mortality in 17 babies less than 30 days of age.[8] Three shunts required early revision, and three patients had late shunt failure at a mean age of 15 months. No patients developed congestive failure.

Roh and associates reported a 26% mortality in children less than 3 months of age receiving a Blalock-Taussig shunt, with an 87% early patency rate, and 83% late patency.[11] In two other series of 28 total patients, 18 under one year of age, there were no operative deaths and no shunt failures.[7,12] Daily and coworkers found the Blalock-Taussig shunt to be the shunt of choice at any age for tetralogy patients, with a 0% operative mortality (versus 28.6% for central shunts) and much lower cumulative operative mortality (5.6% for Blalock-Taussig versus 41.9% for central shunts) when including the risk for subsequent total correction.[13] Severe hypoplasia of the pulmonary arteries was their main indication for an initial palliative shunt. With current anesthetic and surgical techniques, classic Blalock-Taussig shunts in infancy compare favorably with central shunts in terms of operative mortality and early and late patency, with substantially lower complication rates.

Several technical modifications of the classic Blalock-Taussig shunt have been reported. Laks and Castaneda described a subclavian arterioplasty at the aortic origin of the subclavian artery to avoid kinking on the side of the arch.[14] Khanna and Narayanan also used the subclavian artery on the side of the arch because of its greater length, using a single-clamp technique.[15] Pappas and Hawes described an intrapericardial approach (on the side opposite the arch) through an anterolateral thoracotomy, performing the anastomosis medial to the superior vena cava.[16] They cited minimal dissection and avoidance of the phrenic nerve as advantages, and reported 94% patency an average of 17 months later in 17 children less than 2 years of age.

The above modifications notwithstanding, the Blalock-Taussig shunt is usually performed through a posterior fourth interspace incision on the side opposite the arch. The subclavian artery is completely mobilized, as are the innominate and common carotid arteries. The subclavian is transected beyond the first branches and delivered through the sling of the vagus and recurrent laryngeal nerves. The azygos vein is divided and the pulmonary artery is mobilized well proximal and distal to the first upper lobe branch. After a low dose of heparin (1 mg/kg), the proximal pulmonary artery is clamped and the distal vessel controlled with silk loops on the first branch and main trunk. A longitudinal arteriotomy is made on the superior aspect of the main pulmonary artery, and an end-to-side anastomosis of subclavian to pulmonary artery performed with 6–0 polypropylene, using interrupted sutures on the anterior row. The distal subclavian may be spatulated through its first branches to enlarge the anastomosis. Once the clamps and slings are removed, a thrill should be easily palpable. Postoperative hypotension should be treated aggressively to avoid shunt thrombosis.

The most comprehensive evaluation of complications associated with Blalock-Taussig shunts was performed by Taussig and coworkers in 1971.[17] The three most common complications were subacute bacterial endocarditis (71 of 779 patients), brain abscess (38 patients), and pulmonary hypertension (29 of 685 patients, or 4.8%). Presumably some of these complications, particularly brain abscess, resulted more from the underlying cardiac pathology than the systemic–pulmonary artery shunt. Newfeld and associates also found a low incidence of pulmonary hypertension in 75 patients studied up to 23 years after Blalock-Taussig shunt, only three patients (4%) having histologic or hemodynamic evidence of pulmonary hypertension.[18] Hofschire and coworkers found no evidence of pulmonary hypertension for the first eight years after Blalock-Taussig

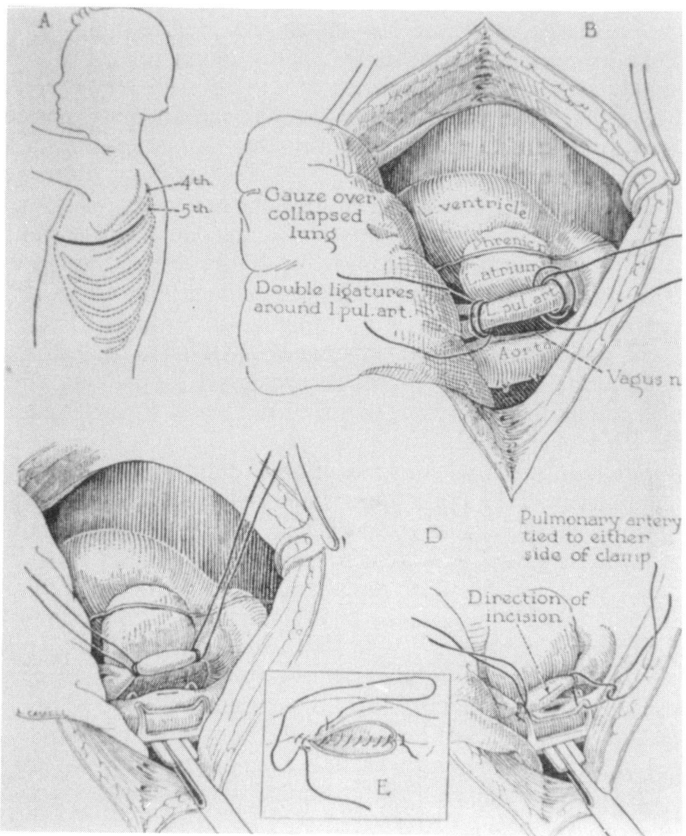

FIGURE 2. The Potts shunt. (Reprinted with permission from JAMA 132:627–631, 1946.)

shunts, after which some degree of pulmonary vascular obstructive disease (PVOD), mainly intimal fibrosis, occurred in 50% of those studied.[19] Rarely, aneurysms may develop late after Blalock-Taussig shunts. Scott and associates described two cases of aneurysmal degeneration of Blalock-Taussig shunts, and recommended a simple method of repair by an anterior approach.[20]

DESCENDING AORTA–LEFT PULMONARY ARTERY ANASTOMOSIS

The descending aorta to left pulmonary artery anastomosis was introduced by Potts and coworkers in 1946.[21] Use of the descending aorta had previously been discouraged by Blalock because of the risk of hindquarter paralysis,[3] but Potts and Smith used a specially-designed partially occluding clamp to allow distal flow (Fig. 2). They reported on three of these anastomoses in very ill and cyanotic children, two of whom survived. The third child died from congestive failure on the second postoperative day.

The Potts anastomosis became a popular alternative to the Blalock-Taussig shunt for nearly two decades, especially in children under 12 months of age with small subclavian arteries. Cole and associates presented results of the use of this shunt by Potts group in 340 patients by 1971.[22] Three major problems became apparent, however: (1) a high incidence of early congestive failure carrying a significant mortality; (2) a disturbing tendency to pulmonary hypertension 5–15 years postoperatively; and (3) difficulty closing the shunt at the time of subsequent definitive repair.

The tendency to excessive flow resulted partly because of initial efforts to create intentionally large shunts. Potts recommended in his initial report an aortic incision of 8–9.5 mm,[21] and congestive failure resulted in more than 20% of patients in reported series.[6,22,23] Pulmonary hypertension was found to be directly related to anastomotic size by Von Bernuth and associates,[24] and they found 39% of patients developed advanced PVOD. Newfeld and coworkers reported pulmonary hypertension rarely occurred in patients with a shunt duration of less than five years, but occurred in 18% of patients in an advanced form if followed longer.[18]

The difficulty of shunt takedown at time of definitive correction also led to decreasing popularity of the Potts shunt. Increased mortality rates were reported by many groups,[13,24–28] varying from 20[27] to 60%.[28] The Mayo Clinic group related the ratio of pulmonary to systemic vascular resistance (Rp/Rs) to mortality, and found four of nine patients with an Rp/Rs greater than 0.4 died at time of shunt takedown, whereas all 13 patients with Rp/Rs less than 0.4 survived.[24] Gross and coworkers found that three of eight (37.5%) patients died who had circumferential external ligation of a Potts shunt at time of repair, and of the five survivors four had a residual aortopulmonary shunt.[26]

Kirklin and Devloo described successful transpulmonary artery closure of the shunt, using hypothermic perfusion and circulatory arrest.[29] When Gross and associates used this technique, their mortality rate dropped from that noted above (37.5%) to 16.3%.[26]

Finally an additional problem with Potts shunts was the development of late aneurysms of the pulmonary artery.[30–32] Nwaneri and Fortune described a technique to repair the aneurysm at the time of total repair,[33] but this in addition to the other problems has led to virtual abandonment of the Potts shunt.

ASCENDING AORTA-RIGHT PULMONARY ARTERY SHUNT (WATERSTON SHUNT)

The ascending aorta-right pulmonary artery shunt was introduced by Waterston in 1962.[24] It gained popularity because it was easier to construct in infants than the Blalock-Taussig shunt, and easier to take down than the Potts shunt. The anastomosis was made by an approach behind the superior vena cava using a single clamp to control the proximal right main pulmonary artery and posterior portion of the ascending aorta (Fig. 3). In 1966, an intrapericardial approach anterior to the superior vena cava was recommended by Cooley and Hallman,[35] as well as a report by Edwards and coworkers supporting this shunt.[36]

Waterston subsequently reported in 1972 the first 100 patients to receive this shunt, 49% being less than 1 year of age.[37] Mortality was 43% in those under 12 months, primarily related to the severity and complexity of the heart lesion, and 12% in older children. He emphasized three important technical points, the first being an incision on the most posterior portion of the aorta. This minimized kinking and excessive flow to the ipsilateral lung (which received up to 75% of shunt flow in reported series for either the Blalock-Taussig or Waterston

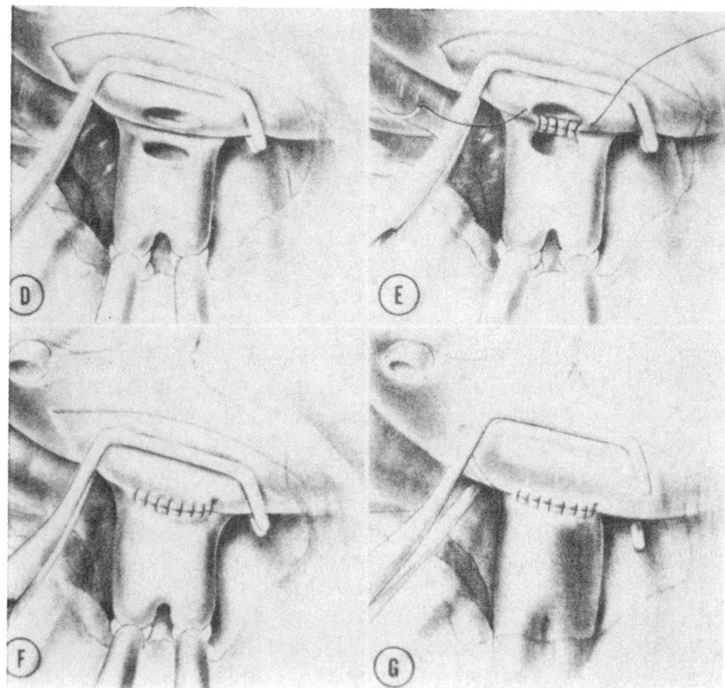

FIGURE 3. The Waterston shunt, illustrating anastomosis of the posterior ascending aorta side-to-side to the anterior right pulmonary artery. (Reprinted with permission from Surgery 72:897–904, 1972.)

shunts[38,39]). He consequently continued to use the retrocaval approach to facilitate the posterior aortotomy. The second point was a limitation of shunt size to prevent congestive failure, recommending an aortic incision of 4 mm in children under 12 months and 4.5 mm in older children. Third, precise suturing was critical, since postclamp suturing to control bleeding resulted in shunt failure and death in 6 patients.

The Waterston shunt is prone to a number of complications which have led to declining popularity over the last decade. Congestive heart failure has been reported in consistently more than 20% of patients,[2,23,40–44] and emphasizes the importance of limiting anastomotic size. Pulmonary hypertension and/or PVOD also may develop,[18,40,41,43,45] occurring in 8% of patients of Vetter et al.[40] Newfeld and associates found that PVOD was less likely in patients with Waterston as opposed to Potts shunts, rarely occurred in children under five years of age, and that the relatively small number of patients who developed PVOD was surprising, considering the large number of patients with excessive left-to-right shunts.[18]

Kinking of the right pulmonary artery is common following a Waterston shunt[41,44–52] and may lead to loss of right and left pulmonary artery continuity as well as severe right pulmonary artery stenosis. Tay and coworkers reported that 22 of 36 (61%) patients studied following Waterston shunts had kinking of the right pulmonary artery, 12 with severe stenosis and 8 with complete obstruction and discontinuity between right and left pulmonary artery.[41] Alfieri and coworkers found a 19% incidence of kinking and stenosis of the right pulmonary artery,[49] and Norberg and associates found a 64% incidence of postoperative structural abnormalities of the pulmonary arteries, primarily kinking or stenosis. Five of 33 (15%) had complete occlusion. They recommended recatheterization at 1 year post Waterston shunt to evaluate the pulmonary arteries. The cause of the kinking is partly due to not making the anastomosis directly posterior on the aorta,[37] as well as differences in growth and realignment of the great arteries.[51]

The technique of closure will depend upon pulmonary artery anatomy. In the absence of pulmonary artery distortion, a transaortic approach proximal to the aortic cross-clamp may be used, with either direct suture or patch insertion, depending on anastomotic size.[53] In cases of anastomotic kinking, reconstruction can be performed by formal takedown of the anastomosis and pulmonary artery repair by pericardial patch as described by Ebert and coworkers.[54] The same group subsequently reported recurrence of stenosis in some patients with pericardial patch reconstruction (4 of 5 patients), which did not occur in their experience when either prosthetic patch or conduit was utilized.[55] Finally, Ergin and Griepp described an extensive method of repair using complete transection of the ascending aorta to improve pulmonary artery exposure.[56]

Several groups have reported the presence of a Waterston anastomosis did not increase mortality at time of subsequent repair.[10,53,57] The University of Oregon group found a shunt patency of 92% at two years in 58 neonates using a 4-mm anastomosis, with an operative mortality of 35% (only three of 20 deaths were due to shunt failure).[57] The congestive failure rate was only 16%, which they ascribed to use of a calibrated clamp, and kinking occurred in only 7%. They still recommend Waterston shunts in infants using the calibrated clamp, with a policy of early definitive repair to limit pulmonary artery distortion. Nevertheless, for the reasons cited above, particularly problems with right pulmonary artery kinking and early congestive failure, the trend is away from Waterston anastomoses and toward classic Blalock-Taussig or modified shunts regardless of age.

SUPERIOR VENA CAVA-RIGHT PULMONARY ARTERY (GLENN) SHUNT

This shunt, in which the end of the right pulmonary artery is sutured to the side of the ligated superior vena cava, was introduced by Glenn in 1958 (Fig. 4).[58] Mathur and Glenn subsequently reported their long-term results in 63 patients in 1973, citing the advantages of this shunt over systemic artery-pulmonary artery shunts as (1) the delivery of only venous blood rather than mixed arterial and venous blood to the lungs, and (2) no added volume load on the heart.[59] The operative mortality for the entire series was 11% (7/63), with three late deaths all unrelated to the shunts. Over an average follow-up of 7.9 years, improved arterial oxygenation and lowered hematocrit were gratifying for 5–7 years, after which signs and symptoms of hypoxemia began to reappear.

The causes of late deterioration in their experience were (1) diminished shunt flow caused by increased pulmonary vascular resistance and increased blood viscosity, (2) expansion of venous collaterals rerouting blood to the inferior vena cava and right atrium around the shunt, and (3) diminished flow to the contralateral lung caused by closure of the pulmonary outflow tract. Additional operations used to improve oxygenation were SPAS to the contralateral lung, atrial septectomy, ligation of collateral venous connections, correction

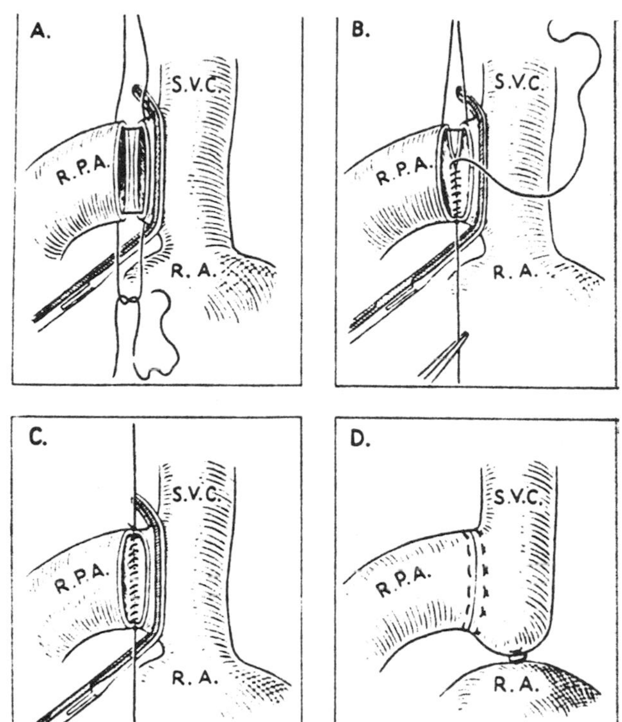

FIGURE 4. The Glenn shunt. (Reprinted with permission from N Engl J Med 259:117–120, 1958.)

of the cardiac defect, and, in situations where the contralateral lung could not be shunted and the lesion was uncorrectable, creation of an axillary arteriovenous fistula.[60] Their contraindications to Glenn shunts were (1) a correctable lesion, (2) pulmonary hypertension, and (3) age less than 6 months. Regarding the latter, a high operative mortality, peripheral edema, and superior vena cava syndrome had been observed in the very young, related to persistent elevation of pulmonary vascular resistance occurring normally in infancy. This led Edwards and Bargeron to recommend delayed ligation of the azygos vein.[61]

The principal complications of Glenn shunts may be grouped under those resulting from elevated venous pressure and those due to late shunt failure. Peripheral edema, superior vena cava syndrome,[62] chylothorax,[63] and protein-losing enteropathy[64] have all been described following Glenn shunts. They are more common, as one would expect, when pulmonary vascular resistance is elevated.[59]

The causes of late deterioration of Glenn shunts are multiple and include (1) development of venous collaterals, (2) decrease in left lung blood flow from spontaneous closure of ASD, VSD, or right ventricular outflow tract, (3) failure to securely close the vena caval-right atrial junction, (4) development of arteriovenous fistulae in the right lower lobe, (5) ventilation–perfusion mismatch of the right lung, (6) polycythemia, (7) thrombotic occlusion of small pulmonary arteries, and (8) unrecognized bilateral superior vena cava.[59,65–71]

McFaul and coworkers reported that significant arteriovenous fistulae developed in the right lower lobe in four patients more than 5 years following

Glenn shunts; they believed this to be a major cause of later shunt failure and difficult to correct.[67] The St. Louis University experience was different, however, in that systemic venous collaterals were found to be the major cause of shunt failure, with little evidence of intrapulmonary shunting at follow-up.[66,69] Results were best in patients with tricuspid atresia and univentricular heart, and poorest for Ebstein's anomaly, truncus arteriosus, transposition, and other complex defects. Di Carlo and associates also found no arteriovenous fistulae in 36 patients recatheterized late following Glenn shunt.[68]

The indications for Glenn shunts have declined considerably, due to their late failure rate, difficulty of take down, and lack of usefulness in those under 6 months of age (after which primary repair is often performed). Some groups avoid them altogether.[68,72] Di Carlo and coworkers found Glenn shunts most useful for patients over 5 years of age with complex heart disease not amenable to repair, and for patients over 18 months of age for whom future correction would involve Fontan correction, in which case the Glenn shunt is left intact.[68] Their operative mortality for the Glenn shunt was only 2% over the last decade.

Pennington and associates also recommended Glenn shunts as a staged procedure in selected patients prior to Fontan repair, when the latter would be direct right atrial to pulmonary artery anastomosis.[69] They contend that in the first few days following Fontan repair, the right atrium may perform more efficiently as a pump if volume load is less, especially in conditions such as univentricular heart when the right atrium may not be hypertrophied. In this situation, the presence of a Glenn shunt would lower right atrial volume by approximately one-third, since only inferior vena cava blood (approximately two-thirds of venous return) would then flow through the right atrium. The "selected" patients for staged Glenn procedures were patients with small-volume right atrium, or those with right pulmonary artery distortion from prior Waterston or Blalock-Taussig shunts. A potential disadvantage of this method of reconstruction is the diversion of two-thirds of venous return to the left lung, which represents only 40–45% of total lung volume. One other potential application of cavopulmonary shunt was described by Kawashima and coworkers for patients with cardiac anomalies such as tricuspid atresia associated with azygos or hemiazygous continuation when the inferior vena cava is absent.[73] In this situation, four patients were offered modifications of Glenn shunts, which they termed "total cavopulmonary shunt," with two long-term survivors.

Takedown of a Glenn shunt is difficult, requiring reconstruction of both the right pulmonary artery and superior vena cava-right atrial junction, either of which may require use of prosthetic material or pericardium.[72,74,75] Pacifico and Kirklin reported five Glenn shunts that were successfully taken down during repair of cardiac malfunctions in 1975.[72] They utilized a brief period of deep hypothermia with circulatory arrest to allow reconstruction of the superior vena cava and pulmonary artery, and recommended takedown of the shunt to avoid the long-term complications of Glenn shunts previously discussed. Currently the technique of takedown would be similar to that of Pacifico and Kirklin, although high cannulation of the superior vena cava with use of a right-angle cannula may allow complete reconstruction without requirement of circulatory arrest. The possibility of long-term complications when Glenn shunts are left intact was emphasized by Van den Bogaert and coworkers, who found multiple arteriovenous fistulae in the right lung five years after correction of tetralogy of Fallot (10 years after Glenn shunt, which was still intact).[76]

MODIFIED CENTRAL SHUNTS

Gazzaniga and coworkers introduced the "modified central shunt" in 1976.[77] They reported ten infants who received ascending aorta-pulmonary artery shunts with use of a 4 mm tube of microporous expanded polytetrafluoroethylene (PTFE), with graft length varying from 0.8–6 cm. One of two early deaths was due to shunt failure. They found the shunt applicable in infants in whom a Blalock-Taussig shunt was not possible, and found its advantages over Waterston or Potts shunts the ease of takedown and minimal tendency to produce pulmonary artery distortion. Disadvantages were the insertion of foreign material, the inability of the shunt to accommodate growth, and a tendency to kink if made too long. Jennings and coworkers used 4 mm-central shunts in seven infants and recommended it when a Blalock-Taussig shunt could not be performed.[78] There was no congestive failure in their series, but one patient died early of shunt thrombosis, and in addition there were two sudden, unexplained late deaths. Miyamoto and associates used 5–mm PTFE central shunts in 10 patients with a 90% patency, no shunt-related deaths, and a 50% incidence of congestive failure, 10% being uncontrollable.[79] They recommended the 5 mm graft to allow for growth, conceding the frequent need for digitalization to control congestive failure.

Despite the initial enthusiasm for the modified central shunt, this shunt has been criticized for being unpredictable regarding early and late patency, having a high rate of congestive failure and being outgrown in 12–24 months. Illustrative of this is the experience of Lamberti and associates, who had initial favorable experience similar to the above reports,[80] but subsequently found the shunt to have unacceptable rates of early and late thrombosis.[81] They found it had no advantage over the modified Blalock-Taussig shunt, and reserved it for situations in which a median sternotomy was required to perform concomitant surgical procedures. Donahoo and associates found the modified central shunt to be superior to either Waterston or Potts shunts, but did note in 30 patients two early shunt-related deaths and five failures that required revision.[82] Kusubara and coworkers used mostly 5 or 6 mm PTFE shunts, and had severe congestive failure develop in 9 of 33 (27%) infants, seven of whom died.[83] They devised a formula based upon body size to predict appropriate graft diameter and shunt flow. Danilowicz and associates reported favorable experience with PTFE central shunts, citing specifically the minimal dissection and bilateral pulmonary artery flow as advantages.[84] They did note occasional difficulty with graft kinking, however, which they remedied by using saphenous vein allograft in that situation because of its great pliability.

The above experience and the recent popularity of the modified Blalock-Taussig shunt in infants have resulted in declining use of modified central shunts except when median sternotomy is performed for other concomitant procedures or pulmonary arteries are hypoplastic. A very favorable recent report, however, by Barragry and coworkers recommended modified central shunts for pulmonary artery hypoplasia.[85] They used PTFE shunts, mostly 4 mm, in 23 neonates and avoided kinking by using side-to-side anastomosis of the ascending aorta–main pulmonary artery and a graft length of less than 1 cm. There was no shunt thrombosis in the 23 infants, no shunt-related deaths, and although congestive failure occurred in 40%, it was readily controlled by digoxin without requiring shunt takedown.

At time of shunt takedown the graft should be divided and the ends oversewn, as pulmonary artery distortion, graft dehiscence, and false aneurysm have been reported.[86]

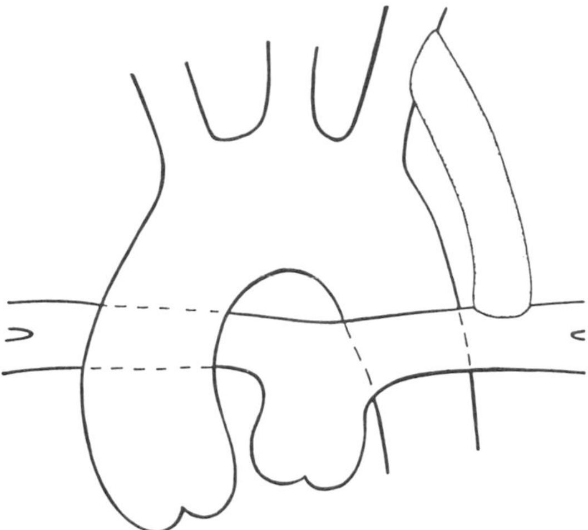

FIGURE 5. The modified Blalock-Taussig shunt by the Great Ormond Street method. (Reprinted with permission from J Thorac Cardiovasc Surg 81:112–119, 1981.)

MODIFIED BLALOCK-TAUSSIG SHUNT

The modified Blalock-Taussig shunt (MBTS), in which a prosthetic tube is interposed between the sides of the subclavian and pulmonary arteries, was popularized by de Leval and coworkers with their report in 1981 (Fig. 5).[87] It was originally described in 1962,[88] and in 1977 Allen and Cole reported 14 patients who were shunted with this technique using pericardial tube grafts.[89] The availability of PTFE, with its low thrombogenic characteristics, has stimulated wide application of this shunt recently.

De Leval and coworkers reported 86 MBTS using expanded PTFE, 44 (51%) in infancy, with an early overall failure rate of 8.1%, and a 2-year patency rate of 88.9%.[87] Their best results were with 5 mm grafts, and since the failure rate with 4 mm grafts was 66.6% at 2 years they cautioned against grafts smaller than 5 mm. They hypothesized that the subclavian artery orifice served as a "flow regulator," preventing congestive heart failure in the early postoperative period even with a 5-mm graft, whereas with growth the advantages of a larger graft and anastomosis were the potential to better serve the needs of a large child.

The operation can be performed on either side of the arch, and compared to the classic Blalock-Taussig shunt the advantages of the modified Blalock-Taussig shunt are minimal dissection time and risk of phrenic nerve injury, maintenance of normal blood flow to the arm and, in the case of infants with small subclavian arteries, a technically easier and larger anastomosis using a 5 mm graft. The exposure of the pulmonary artery is identical to a classic Blalock-Taussig shunt, and once the subclavian has been dissected, with careful avoidance of the vagus and recurrent laryngeal nerves, the mid portion of the vessel is isolated. An obliquely trimmed PTFE graft is then sewn end-to-side to a longitudinal incision in the inferior portion of the subclavian artery after which the anastomosis is checked for bleeding and the clamp reapplied. Heparin (1 mg/kg) is then administered, the graft cut to precise length to avoid kinking and distortion of the pulmonary artery, and an end-to-end anastomosis made to a longitudinal arteriotomy in the superior portion of the pulmonary artery. It is very important to maintain adequate systemic pressures throughout this period to prevent early shunt thrombosis, even if this requires infusion of vasopressors.

Since the introduction of the MBTS with PTFE in 1981, no fewer than 12 reports, all favorable, have appeared supporting the use of this shunt, particularly in neonates.[81, 90–100] Ilbawi and coworkers used the MBTS in 30 neonates (mean age 8.8 days, mean weight 3.24 kg) with an early shunt thrombosis and fatality rate of only 3.3%, and a 91% satisfactory shunt life at 3 years.[90] Nine patients recatheterized had no evidence of pulmonary artery distortion. Woulf and associates compared the MBTS with the classical Blalock-Taussig and Waterston shunts in 67 patients operated upon under 2 weeks of age at three institutions, and found the MBTS to be the safest and most effective shunt in neonates, although the late failure rate for the MBTS at 3.5 years was higher than with the other shunts.[91] Karpawich and coworkers had no shunt failures using 5-mm and 6-mm PTFE shunts, but two of four 4-mm shunts failed at 1 year.[92] Opie and coworkers found an 89% late patency rate with the MBTS, but recommend close follow-up for occasional complications including shunt thrombosis, graft infection related to pneumonia, and occasional pulmonary artery distortion.[93]

The effectiveness of the MBTS was analyzed according to patient weight and presence of pulmonary atresia by Bove and coworkers.[94] They cited an overall early and late mortality rate of 4% and 9% respectively. With weight greater than 3.6 kg and no pulmonary atresia, estimated shunt survival at 3 years was 92%; pulmonary atresia with weight greater than 3.6 kg, 76%; weight less than 3.6 kg without pulmonary atresia, 58%; and with both weight less than 3.6 kg and presence of pulmonary atresia, the 3-year estimated shunt survival was only 14%. Especially close follow-up would clearly be indicated in the last three subgroups.

Finally, the experience of Lamberti and associates is of interest in that the results of shunts in four groups were compared: classic Blalock Taussig, modified central, interposition (end of subclavian to side of pulmonary artery with interposition of PTFE), and MBTS by the Great Ormond Street method.[81] The latter shunt was superior to the others because of the lower operative risks, predictable patency (100% in 21 patients with MBTS), lack of distortion of pulmonary arterial anatomy, and technical ease of insertion and takedown. They concluded the MBTS most closely approaches the "ideal shunt" because it (1) predictably provides adequate pulmonary blood flow, (2) is easy to construct, (3) is reliable in short-term and long-term performance, (4) provides flow to both pulmomary arteries, (5) is easy to take down, (6) has a low incidence of pulmonary artery distortion, and (7) preserves normal arm blood flow.

Two complications have been reported for MBTS which should be noted. LeBlanc and associates reported an 18.8% incidence of seroma formation around the PTFE graft in 138 operations, four of which required reoperation.[101] This complication resulted from serous fluid leaking through the interstices of the graft, and was especially common when the graft was wrapped with silicone sheeting to facilitate subsequent takedown. The authors abandoned the latter practice. Caffarena and coworkers reported false aneurysm leading to massive hemoptysis 16 years following MBTS using Teflon conduit.[102] The aneurysm may have resulted from dissolution of silk suture, but since the graft had been ligated and not divided at time of total repair, development of anastomotic tension with growth may have been contributory. Certainly, as was discussed with modified central shunts, the grafts should be formally divided at time of takedown.

INTERNAL MAMMARY–PULMONARY ARTERY SHUNT

Use of the internal mammary artery in older children has been described, especially for hypoplastic pulmonary arteries.[103,104] The advantages of the internal mammary artery are its suitability for hypoplastic pulmonary arteries, the avoidance of prosthetic material, an anastomosis without tension which permits flow adaptation with growth, and a potential to last indefinitely. The smaller size of the internal mammary compared to the subclavian artery or prosthetic grafts is the main disadvantage.

PULMONARY ARTERY GROWTH

As hypoplastic pulmonary arteries are a common indication for shunts currently, it is reasonable to evaluate their effect on subsequent pulmonary artery growth. Gale and coworkers found the pulmonary annulus to descending aorta ratio increased substantially following Blalock-Taussig shunt, an average ratio increase of 0.19 when the original was less than one, and by 0.34 when the original ratio was less than 0.7 (mean follow-up was 28.9 months).[105] They concluded that Blalock-Taussig shunts were effective in facilitating growth of hypoplastic pulmonary arteries, allowing a lower right ventricular pressure after repair and, possibly, for tetralogy patients, a lower incidence of transannular patch compared to primary repair. Guyton and associates found that the ipsilateral and contralateral pulmonary artery to descending aorta ratios increased significantly following Blalock-Taussig shunt.[106] Rittenhouse and associates reported substantial pulmonary annulus growth in 130 tetralogy patients following shunts, most of which were Blalock-Taussig.[107] The mean pulmonary annulus to descending aorta ratio increased from 0.80 preshunt to 1.22 post shunt. The impression that preliminary shunts may lower the need for transannular patch subsequently was supported by this study, since only one transannular patch was necessary in the 30 patients with a preliminary shunt, compared to 5 of the 61 patients undergoing primary repair.

As four other reports also document substantial growth of the pulmonary valve annulus and pulmonary arteries after preliminary shunts,[90,108–110] the usefulness of shunts to enlarge hypoplastic pulmonary arteries is established. An interesting report by Rosenberg and coworkers examined the structural composition of central pulmonary arteries relative to growth potential after surgical shunts.[111] They found that in pulmonary arteries which failed to grow satisfactorily after a shunt, the most common structural abnormality was an inadequate proportion of elastin, suggesting that a deficiency of the volume of this important substance may prevent growth even in the presence of a satisfactory shunt.

NEW DEVELOPMENTS

Since the mid-1970s numerous reports have documented the usefulness of prostaglandin E_1 (PGE_1) in infants with cyanotic heart disease to maintain patency of the ductus arteriosus and to lower the risk of emergency neonatal shunts.[112–117] An extension of the effect of PGE_1 on the ductus was applied by Tokota and coworkers, who administered long-term (mean 47 days) intravenous PGE_1 at a low dose (0.02–0.03 μg/kg/min) in 16 cyanotic neonates with hypoplastic pulmonary arteries.[118] The average growth of pulmonary artery diameter by the time of shunt procedure was 4.5 mm, with 13 of 16 long-term survivors having patent shunts at a mean follow-up of 22 months. The major pathologic changes noted from the long-term PGE_1 were reversible hyperostosis of bones, and development of thin-walled pulmonary arteries. Their successful experience with long-term intravenous PGE_1 contrasts with that of MacMahon and associates, who noted failure of pulmonary artery growth in 4 of 11 patients receiving long-term oral PGE_1.[110]

The evaluation of shunt patency is at times difficult clinically, particularly when either no murmur is audible or murmurs may be due to primary cardiac lesions. Recently echocardiography has been successfully used to evaluate SPAS,[120] and especially pulsed Doppler echocardiography using suprasternal and high parasternal approaches.[121,122] Stevenson and associates found that pulsed Doppler accurately located and determined patency for 80% of Blalock-Taussig shunts and 91% of prosthetic shunts.[122] A recent report describing the ability of electrocardiogram-gated magnetic resonance imaging to successfully determine both patency and size of SPAS suggests that modality may be useful to evaluate questionable shunts.[123]

Several reports of percutaneous transcatheter balloon occlusion of incompletely ligated SPAS make that an option for the patient who otherwise requires no further surgery but has an unwanted persistent shunt.[124,125] Conversely, streptokinase has been successfully used to reopen occluded shunts, although bleeding was noted when applied in the early postoperative period.[126]

Finally the role of ductal ligation at time of SPAS is worth comment. With increasing numbers of shunts being performed on premature infants with ductal patency, several reports have described severe, and at times fatal, postoperative congestive failure occurring following SPAS when the ductus arteriosus did not close spontaneously.[81,118,127] Corno and coworkers found this to be a special problem for pulmonary atresia with intact ventricular septum, and postulated that excessive pulmonary artery runoff from two simultaneous shunts lowered the aortic diastolic pressure, which in their opinion contributed to a "steal" of blood into right ventricular sinusoids (and away from left ventricular myocardium), which commonly occur with this entity.[127] Lamberti and coworkers recommend ductal ligation at time of shunt procedure in premature infants, if the oxygen tension is over 80 mm Hg and the SPAS appears technically satisfactory.[81] The main argument against ductal ligation is that should the shunt subsequently close and need revision in the early postoperative period, the ductus can no longer be pharmacologically manipulated to stabilize the infant for reoperation, with potential for extreme pulmonary oligemia.

CONCLUSION

Due to increased emphasis on primary repair, the frequency of SPAS has declined appreciably during the last decade. The utility of shunting operations, however, to reverse life-threatening pulmonary oligemia and salvage a critically ill child has not changed since Blalock and Taussig's first report in 1945, and they remain especially important for the most tenuous of cyanotic patients, those under 1 year of age. The ability of shunts to enchance growth of hypoplastic pulmonary arteries and to allow later definitive repair is clearly documented. A relative advantage of initial shunts over primary repair in patients with tetralogy of Fallot may well be a lower incidence of transannular patch and lower post-repair right ventricular pressure when an initial SPAS is used.

As far as which shunt is "ideal," no shunt is applicable in all situations; each has potential inherent problems, and the need for versatility as demonstrated by Blalock remains important. Nevertheless, it is fair to conclude that, owing to improved microsurgical techniques and the major drawbacks of central shunts, the classic Blalock-Taussig shunt in now very applicable in infants under the age of 1 year compared to a decade or more ago. Moreover, the availability of PTFE and the numerous, excellent reports of the modified Blalock-Taussig shunt (5 mm or greater) in neonates would appear to make that the shunt of choice in the child under 30 days of age, weight less than 3.5 kg or dimunitive pulmonary or subclavian arteries, and on equal footing with the classic Blalock-Taussig shunt at any age. The role for central shunts would appear to be primarily when a median sternotomy is needed for other procedures, and then preferably as a modified shunt with a short (< 1–2 cm) 4-or 5-mm PTFE graft. The Glenn shunt remains contraindicated under 6 months of age. Owing to numerous drawbacks it is rarely indicated presently, but may still have a role as a supplement to Fontan repair (either concomitantly or staged) to lower postoperative right atrial volume loading, and in older patients who are otherwise inoperable.

REFERENCES

1. Blalock A, Taussig HB: The surgical treatment of malformations of the heart: In which there is pulmonary stenosis or pulmonary atresia. JAMA 128:189, 1945.
2. Lundsgaard C, Van Slyke DD: Cyanosis. Medical Monographs, Vol. 2. Baltimore, Williams & Wilkins, 1923.
3. Blalock A: Surgical procedures employed and anatomical variations encountered in the treatment of congenital pulmonic stenosis. Surg Gynecol Obstet 87:385, 1948.
4. Taussig HB, Crocetti A, Eshaghpour E, et al: Long-time observations on the Blalock-Taussig operation. II. Second operations, frequency and results. Johns Hopkins Med J 129:258, 1971.
5. Wood WC, McCue CM, Lower RR: Blalock-Taussig shunts in the infant. Ann Thorac Surg 16:454, 1973.
6. Neches WH, Naijeh JG, Park SC, et al: Systemic-pulmonary artery anastomoses in infancy. J Thorac Cardiovasc Surg 70:921, 1975.
7. Chopra PS, Levy JM, Dacumos GC, et al: The Blalock-Taussig operation: The procedure of choice in the hypoxic infant with tetralogy of Fallot. Ann Thorac Surg 22:235, 1976.
8. Laks H, Fagan L, Barner H, et al: The Blalock-Taussig shunt in the neonate. Ann Thorac Surg 25:220, 1978.
9. Tyson KR, Larrien AJ, Kirchmer JT: The Blalock-Taussig shunt in the first two years of life: A safe and effective procedure. Ann Thorac Surg 26:38, 1978.
10. Arciniegas E, Blackstone E, Pacifico A, Kirklin J: Classic shunting operations as part of two-stage repair for tetralogy of Fallot. Ann Thorac Surg 27:516, 1979.
11. Roh M, Hardesty RL, Siemers RD, et al: Blalock shunt: Procedure of choice in infants. J Cardiovasc Surg 25:1, 1984.
12. Marbarger JP, Sandza JG, Hartmann AP, Weldon CS: Blalock-Taussig anastomosis. The preferred shunt in newborns. Circulation 58(Suppl 1):73, 1978.
13. Daily PO, Stinson EB, Griepp RB, Shumway NE: Tetralogy of Fallot. Choice of surgical procedure. J Thorac Cardiovasc Surg 75:338, 1978.
14. Laks H, Castaneda AR: Subclavian arterioplasty for ipsilateral Blalock-Taussig shunt. Ann Thorac Surg 19:319, 1975.
15. Khanna SK, Narayanan PS: Single clamp technique of Blalock and Taussig's operation. J Cardiovasc Surg 21:239, 1980.
16. Pappas G, Hawes CR: Intrapericardial Blalock-Taussig shunt. J Thorac Cardiovasc Surg 83:422, 1982.
17. Taussig HB, Crocetti A, Eshaghpour E, et al: Long-time observations on the Blalock-Taussig operation. III. Common complications. Johns Hopkins Med J 129:274, 1971.
18. Newfeld EA, Waldman JD, Paul MH, et al: Pulmonary vascular disease after systemic-pulmonary arterial shunt operations. Am J Cardiol 39:715, 1977.
19. Hofschire PJ, Rosenquist GC, Ruckerman RN, et al: Pulmonary vascular disease complicating the Blalock-Taussig anastomosis. Circulation 56:124, 1977.
20. Scott WC, Zhao H, Allen M, et al: Aneurysmal degeneration of Blalock-Taussig shunts: Identification and surgical treatment options. J Am Coll Cardiol 3:1277, 1984.

21. Potts WJ, Smith S, Gibson S: Anastomosis of the aorta to a pulmonary artery. JAMA 132:627, 1946.
22. Cole RB, Mustar AJ, Fixler DE, et al: Long-term results of aorto-pulmonary anastomosis for tetralogy of Fallot. Circulation 43:263, 1971.
23. Truccone NJ, Bowman FO, Malm JR, Gersony WM: Systemic-pulmonary arterial shunts in the first year of life. Circulation 49:508, 1974.
24. von Bernuth G, Ritter DG, Frye RL, et al: Evaluation of patients with tetralogy of Fallot and Potts anastomosis. Am J Cardiol 27:259, 1971.
25. Azar H, Hardesty RL, Pontius RG, et al: A review of total correction in 200 cases of tetralogy of Fallot. Arch Surg 99:281, 1969.
26. Gross RE, Bernhard WF, Litwin SB: Closure of Potts anastomosis in total repair of tetralogy of Fallot. J Thorac Cardiovasc Surg 57:72, 1969.
27. Kirklin JW, Wallace RB, McGoon DC, et al: Early and late results after intracardiac repair of tetralogy of Fallot: 5 year review of 337 patients. Ann Surg 162:578, 1965.
28. Zerbine EJ, Macruz R, Bittencourt D, et al: Study of a series of 274 cases of pulmonic stenosis associated with interventricular septal defects corrected under extracorporeal circulation. J Cardiovasc Surg (Torino) 7:209, 1966.
29. Kirklin JE, Devloo RA: Hypothermic perfusion and circulatory arrest for surgical correction of tetralogy of Fallot with previously constructed Potts anastomosis. Dis Chest 39:87, 1961.
30. Stephens HB: Aneurysm of the pulmonary artery following a Potts' shunt operation. Report of death from rupture of an aneurysm of the pulmonary artery. J Thorac Cardiovasc Surg 53:642, 1967.
31. Ross RR, Taussig HB, Evans MH: Late hypothermic complication of anastomotic surgery for treatment of the tetralogy of Fallot. Circulation 18:553, 1958.
32. Cole RB, Muster AJ, Fixler DE, Paul MH: Long term results of aortopulmonary anastomosis for tetralogy of Fallot. Morbidity and mortality 1946–69. Circulation 11:263, 1971.
33. Nwaneri NJ, Fortune RL: Aneurysm of the pulmonary artery. Rare long term complication of central aorto-pulmonary shunts for congenital heart disease. J Cardiovasc Surg 27:94, 1986.
34. Waterston DJ, Stark J, Ashcraft KW: Treatment of Fallot's tetralogy in children under one year of age. Rozhl Chir 41:181, 1962.
35. Cooley DA, Hallman DL: Intrapericardial aortic-right pulmonary arterial anastomosis. Surg Gynecol Obstet 122:1084, 1966.
36. Edwards WS, Mohtashemi M, Holdefer WF Jr: Ascending aorta to right pulmonary artery shunt in infants with tetralogy of Fallot. Surgery 59:316, 1966.
37. Waterston DJ: Ascending aorta-to-right pulmonary artery shunts. Experience with 100 patients. Surgery 72:897, 1972.
38. Edmunds LH, Fishman NH, Heymann MA, Rudolph AM: Anastomoses between aorta and right pulmonary artery (Waterston) in neonates. N Engl J Med 284:464, 1971.
39. Fort L III, Morrow AG, Pierce GE, et al: The distribution of pulmonary blood flow after subclavian-pulmonary anastomosis. J Thorac Cardiovasc Surg 50:671, 1965.
40. Vetter VL, Rashkind WJ, Waldhausen JA: Ascending aorta-right pulmonary artery anastomosis. J Thorac Cardiovasc Surg 76:115, 1978.
41. Tay DJ, Engle MA, Ehleis KH, Levin AR: Early results and late developments of the Waterston anastomosis. Circulation 50:220, 1974.
42. Bernhard WF, Jones JE, Freidberg DZ, Litwin SB: Ascending aorta-right pulmonary artery shunt in infants with certain types of cyanotic congenital heart disease. Circulation 43:580, 1971.
43. Daicoff GR, Aslami A, Victorica BE, Shiebler GL: Ascending aorta-to-pulmonary artery anastomosis for cyanotic congenital heart disease. Ann Thorac Surg 18:260, 1974.
44. Reitman MJ, Galioto FM, El-Said G, et al: Ascending aorta to right pulmonary artery anastomosis. Circulation 49:952, 1974.
45. Somerville J, Yacoub M, Ross DW, Ross K: Aorta to right pulmonary artery anastomosis (Waterston's operation) for cyanotic heart disease. Circulation 49:952, 1974.
46. Gay WA, Ebert PA: Aorta-to-right pulmonary artery anastomosis causing obstruction of the right pulmonary artery. Ann Thorac Surg 16:402, 1973.
47. Ebert PA, Gary WA, Oldham HN: Management of aorta-right pulmonary artery anastomosis during total correction of tetralogy of Fallot. Surgery 71:231, 1972.
48. Idriss FS, Cavallo CA, Nikaidoh H, et al: Ascending aorta–right pulmonary artery shunt. J Thorac Cardiovasc Surg 71:49, 1976.
49. Alfieri O, Locatelli G, Bianchi T, et al: Repair of tetralogy of Fallot after Waterston anastomosis. J Thorac Cardiovasc Surg 77:826, 1979.

50. Norbert WJ, Tadavarthy M, Knight L, et al: Late hemodynamic and angiographic findings after ascending aorta-pulmonary artery anastomosis. J Thorac Cardiovasc Surg 76:345, 1978.
51. Rau PS, Ellison RG: The cause of kinking of the right pulmonary artery in the Waterston anastomosis—a growth phenomenon. J Thorac Cardiovasc Surg 76:126, 1978.
52. Berkoff HA, Chung KJ, Levy JM, et al: Intrapulmonary steal complicating repair of tetralogy of Fallot. Ann Thorac Surg 23:77, 1977.
53. Sade RM, Sloss L, Treves S, et al: Repair of tetralogy of Fallot after aortopulmonary anastomosis. Ann Thorac Surg 23:32, 1977.
54. Ebert PA, Gay WA Jr, Oldham HN: Management of aorta-right pulmonary artery anastomosis during total correction of tetralogy of Fallot. Surgery 71:231, 1972.
55. Wilson JM, Mack JW, Turley K, Ebert PA: Persistent stenosis and deformity of the right pulmonary artery after correction of the Waterston anastomosis. J Thorac Cardiovasc Surg 82:169, 1981.
56. Ergin MA, Griepp RB: Total correction of tetralogy of Fallot. How to deal with the complicated ascending aorta-right pulmonary artery anastomosis. J Thorac Cardiovasc Surg 77:469, 1979.
57. Garcia CE, Kay PH, Grunkemeier GL, et al: A current appraisal of the Waterston shunt. J Cardiovasc Surg (Torino) 27:604, 1986.
58. Glenn W: Circulatory bypass of the right side of the heart. IV. Shunt between superior vena cava and distal right pulmonary artery—report of clinical application. N Engl J Med 259:117, 1958.
59. Mathur M, Glenn WWL: Long-term evaluation of cava-pulmonary anastomosis. Surgery 74:899, 1973.
60. Glenn WWL, Fenn JE: Axillary arteriovenous fistula. A means of supplementing blood flow through a cava-pulmonary artery shunt. Circulation 46:1013, 1972.
61. Edwards WS, Bargeron LM Jr: The importance of the azygos vein in superior vana cava-pulmonary artery anastomosis. J Thorac Cardiovasc Surg 46:811, 1963.
62. Canent RV, Spach MS, Young WG: Cardiopulmonary dynamics in patients with anastomosis of the superior vena cava to the right pulmonary artery. Circulation 30:47, 1963.
63. Glenn WW, Ordway NK, Talner NS, et al: Circulatory bypass of the right side of the heart. Report of clinical application in thirty-eight cases. Circulation 31:172, 1965.
64. Gleason WA, Roodman ST, Laks H: Protein-losing enteropathy and intestinal lymphangiectasia after superior vena cava-right pulmonary artery (Glenn) shunt. J Thorac Cardiovasc Surg 77:843, 1979.
65. Bargeron LM Jr, Karp RB, Barcia A, et al: Late deterioration of patients after superior vena cava to right pulmonary artery anastomosis. Am J Cardiol 30:211, 1972.
66. Laks H, Mudd JG, Standeven JW, et al: Long-term effect of the superior vena cava-pulmonary artery anastomosis of pulmonary blood flow. J Thorac Cardiovasc Surg 74:253, 1977.
67. McFaul RC, Tajik AJ, Mair DD, et al: Development of pulmonary arteriovenous shunt after superior vena cava-right pulmonary artery (Glenn) anastomosis. Report of four cases. Circulation 55:212, 1977.
68. di Carlo D, Williams WG, Freedom RM, et al: The role of cava-pulmonary (Glenn) anastomosis in the palliative treatment of congenital heart disease. J Thorac Cardiovasc Surg 83:437, 1982.
69. Pennington DG, Nouri S, Ho J, et al: Glenn shunt: Long-term results and current role in congenital heart operations. Ann Thorac Surg 31:532, 1981.
70. Martin SP, Anabtawi IN, Selmonsky CA, et al: Long term follow-up after superior vena cava-pulmonary artery anastomosis. Ann Thorac Surg 9:339, 1970.
71. Boruchow IB, Swenson EW, Elliott LP, et al: Study of the mechanisms of shunt failure after superior vena cava-right pulmonary artery anastomosis. J Thorac Cardiovasc Surg 60:531, 1970.
72. Pacifico AD, Kirklin JW: Takedown of cava-pulmonary artery anastomosis (Glenn) during repair of congenital cardiac malformations. Report of five cases. J Thorac Cardiovasc Surg 70:272, 1975.
73. Kawashima Y, Kitamura S, Matsuda H, et al: Total cardiopulmonary shunt operation in complex cardiac anomalies. A new operation. J Thorac Cardiovasc Surg 87:74, 1984.
74. Saji I, Horiuchi T, Tanaka S, et al: Possibility of the second stage correction of tetralogy of Fallot following superior vena cava to right pulmonary artery shunt. J Cardiovasc Surg (Torino) 15:558, 1974.
75. Rohmer J, Quaegebeur JM, Brom AG: Takedown and reconstruction of cavopulmonary anastomosis. Ann Thorac Surg 23:129, 1977.

76. Van den Bogaert-Van Heesvelde AM, Derom F, Kunnen M, et al: Surgery for arteriovenous fistulas and dilated vessels in the right lung after the Glenn procedure. J Thorac Cardiovasc Surg 76:195, 1978.
77. Gazzaniga AB, Lamberti JJ, Siewers RD, et al: Arterial prosthesis of microporous expanded polytetrafluoroethylene for construction of aorta-pulmonary shunts. J Thorac Cardiovasc Surg 72:357, 1976.
78. Jennings RB, Innes BJ, Brickman RD: Use of microporous expanded polytetrafluoroethylene grafts for aorta-pulmonary shunts in infants with complex cyanotic heart disease. J Thorac Cardiovasc Surg 76:489, 1978.
79. Miyamoto K, Zavanells C, Lewin AN, et al: Aorto-pulmonary artery shunts with expanded polytetrafluoroethylene (PTFE) tube. Ann Thorac Surg 27:413, 1979.
80. Lamberti JJ, Campbell C, Replogle RL, et al: The prosthetic (Teflon) central aortopulmonary shunt for cyanotic infants less than three weeks old: results and long-term follow-up. Ann Thorac Surg 28:568, 1979.
81. Lamberti JJ, Carlisle J, Waldman JD, et al: Systemic-pulmonary shunts in infants and children. J Thorac Cardiovasc Surg 88:76, 1984.
82. Donahoo JS, Gardner TJ, Zahka K, Kidd BSL: Systemic-pulmonary shunts in neonates and infants using microporous expanded polytetrafluoroethylene: Immediate and late results. Ann Thorac Surg 30:146, 1980.
83. Kusuhara K, Miki S, Ueda Y, et al: Optimal flow of aorta-pulmonary artery shunt in patients with cyanotic heart disease. Ann Thorac Surg 44:128, 1987.
84. Danilowicz D, Ishmael RG, Doyle EF, et al: Use of saphenous vein allografts for aortopulmonary artery anastomosis in neonates with complex cyanotic congenital heart disease. Pediatr Cardiol 5:13, 1984.
85. Barragry TP, Ring WS, Blatchford JW, et al: Central aorta-pulmonary artery shunts in neonates with complex cyanotic congenital heart disease. J Thorac Cardiovasc Surg 93:767, 1987.
86. Evans VL, Hallman GL, Vargo TA, et al: False aneurysm of the ascending aorta from an expanded polytetrafluoroethylene (Gor-Tex) aortopulmonary shunt. Ann Thorac Surg 39:573, 1985.
87. de Leval MR, McKay R, Jones M, et al: Modified Blalocktaussig shunt. Use of subclavian artery orifice as a flow regulator in prosthetic systemic-pulmonary artery shunts. J Thorac Cardiovasc Surg 81:112, 1981.
88. Klinner W, Pasini M, Schaudig A: Anastomose zwichen system und lungenarterie mit hilfe von kunststoftprothesen bei cyanotischen Herzvitien. Thoraxchirurgie 10:68, 1962.
89. Allen RG, Cole FH Jr: Modified Blalock shunt utilizing pericardial tube grafts. J Pediatr Surg 12:287, 1977.
90. Ilbawi MN, Grieco J, De Leon SY, et al: Modified Blalock-Taussig shunt in newborn infants. J Thorac Cardiovasc Surg 88:770, 1984.
91. Woolf PK, Stephenson LW, Meijboom E, et al: A comparison of Blalock-Taussig, Waterston, and polytetrafluoroethylene shunts in children less than two weeks of age. Ann Thorac Surg 38:26, 1984.
92. Karpawich PP, Bush CP, Antillon JR, et al: Modified Blalock-Taussig shunt in infants and young children. J Thorac Cardiovasc Surg 89:275, 1985.
93. Opie JC, Traverse L, Hayden RI, et al: Experience with polytetrafluoroethylene grafts in children with cyanotic congenital heart disease. Ann Thorac Surg 41:164, 1986.
94. Bove EL, Kohman L, Sereika S, et al: The modified Blalock-Taussig shunt: analysis of adequacy and duration of palliation. Circulation 76(Suppl 3)III–19, 1987.
95. Benedetto GD, Tiraboschi R, Vanin V, et al: Systemic-pulmonary artery shunt using PTFE prosthesis (Gor-Tex). Early results and long-term follow-up in 105 consecutive cases. J Thorac Cardiovasc Surg 29:143, 1981.
96. Lawless CE, Smith EEJ, Hallidie-Smith K, et al: The modified Blalock-Taussig shunt using microporous polytetrafluoroethylene (PTFE). J Cardiovasc Surg (Torino) 23:287, 1982.
97. Wright J, Albrecht H, Beveridge J: Palliation in cyanotic congenital heart disease. Fifteen years' experience of various shunt procedures. Med J Aus 144:178, 1986.
98. Nanton MA, Roy DL, Murphy DM, et al: Polytetrafluoroethylene shunts in congenital heart disease. Can J Surg 25:134, 1982.
99. Bove EL, Sondheimer HM, Byrum CJ, et al: Pulmonary hemodynamics and maintenance of palliation following polytetrafluoroethylene shunts for cyanotic heart disease. Am Heart J 108:366, 1984.
100. Sanchez HE, Vosloo S: Blalock-Taussig shunts and modified Blalock-Taussig shunts. S Afr Med J 67:168, 1985.

101. LeBlanc J, Albus R, Williams WG, et al: Serous fluid leakage. A complication following the modified Blalock-Taussig shunt. J Thorac Cardiovasc Surg 88:259, 1984.
102. Caffarena JM, Llamas P, Otero-Coto E: False aneurysm of a palliative shunt producing massive hemoptysis. Chest 81:110, 1982.
103. Cobanoglu A, Abbruzzese P, Brunner D, et al: Therapeutic considerations in congenital absence of the right pulmonary artery. Use of the internal mammary artery as a preparatory shunt. J Cardiovasc Surg (Torino) 25:241, 1984.
104. Sievers H, Lange P, Heintzen P, et al: Internal mammary artery as a palliative systemic-pulmonary shunt in order to develop diminutive pulmonary arteries. Thorac Cardiovasc Surg 33:51, 1985.
105. Gale AW, Archiniegas E, Green EW, et al: Growth of the pulmonary annulus and pulmonary arteries after the Blalock-Taussig shunt. J Thorac Cardiovasc Surg 77:459, 1979.
106. Guyton RA, Owens JE, Waumett JD, et al: The Blalock-Taussig shunt. Low-risk, effective palliation, and pulmonary artery growth. J Thorac Cardiovasc Surg 85:917, 1983.
107. Rittenhouse EA, Mansfield PB, Hall DG, et al: Tetralogy of Fallot: Selective staged management. J Thorac Cardiovasc Surg 89:772, 1985.
108. Brandt III B, Camacho JA, Mahoney LT, et al: Growth of the pulmonary arteries following Blalock-Taussig shunt. Ann Thorac Surg 42:51, 1986.
109. Kirklin JW, Bargeron LM, Pacifico AD: The enlargement of small pulmonary arteries by preliminary palliative operations. Circulation 56:612, 1977.
110. Alfieri O, Blackstone EH, Parenzan L: Growth of the pulmonary annulus and pulmonary arteries after the Waterston anastomosis. J Thorac Cardiovasc Surg 78:440, 1979.
111. Rosenberg HG, Williams EG, Trusler GA, et al: Structural composition of central pulmonary arteries. Growth potential after surgical shunts. J Thorac Cardiovasc Surg 94:498, 1987.
112. Elliott RB, Starling MB, Neutze JM: Medical manipulation of the ductus arteriosus. Lancet 1:140, 1975.
113. Olley PM: E-type prostaglandins: A new emergency therapy for certain cyanotic congenital heart malformations. Circulation 53:728, 1976.
114. Neutze JM, Starling MB, Elliott RB, et al: Palliation of cyanotic congenital heart disease in infancy with E-type prostaglandins. Circulation 55:238, 1977.
115. Browdie DA, Norberg W, Agnew R, et al: The use of prostaglandin E_1 and Blalock-Taussig shunts in neonates with cyanotic congenital heart disease. Ann Thorac Surg 27:510, 1979.
116. Donahoo JS, Roland JM, Kan J, et al: Prostaglandin E_1 as a adjunct to emergency cardiac operation in neonates. J Thorac Cardiovasc Surg 81:227, 1981.
117. Freed MD, Heymann MA, Lewis AB, et al: Prostaglandin E_1 in infants with ductus arteriosus-dependent congenital heart disease. Circulation 64:899, 1981.
118. Yokota M, Muyaoka R, Aoshima M, et al: Modified Blalock-Taussig shunt following long-term administration of prostaglandin E_1 for ductus dependent neonates with cyanotic congenital heart disease. J Thorac Cardiovasc Surg 90:339, 1985.
119. MacMahon P, Gorham PF, Arnold R, et al: Pulmonary artery growth during treatment with oral prostaglandin E_1 in ductus dependent cyanotic congenital heart disease. Arch Dis Child 58:187, 1983.
120. Reitman M, Goldberg H, Boris G, et al: Echocardiographic assessment of a Blalock-Taussig shunt. J Clin Ultrasound 6:55, 1978.
121. Allen HD, Sahn DJ, Lange L, et al: Noninvasive assessment of surgical systemic to pulmonary artery shunts by range-gated pulsed Doppler echocardiography. J Pediatr 94:395, 1979.
122. Stephenson JG, Kawabori I, Bailey WW: Noninvasive evaluation of Blalock-Taussig shunts: Determination of patency and differentiation from patent ductus arteriosus by Doppler echocardiography. Am Heart J 106:1121, 1983.
123. Jacobstein MD, Fletcher BD, Nelson AD, et al: Magnetic resonance imaging: Evaluation of palliative systemic-pulmonary artery shunts. Circulation 70:650, 1984.
124. Florentine M, Wolfe RR, White RI Jr: Balloon embolization to occlude a Blalock-Taussig shunt. J Am Coll Cardiol 3:200, 1984.
125. Reidy JF, Baker E, Tyman M: Transcatheter occlusion of a Blalock-Taussig shunt with a detachable balloon in a child. Br Heart J 50:101, 1983.
126. Le Blanc JG, Culham AG, Chan K–W, et al: Treatment of grafts and major vessel thrombosis with low-dose streptokinase in children. Ann Thorac Surg 41:630, 1986.
127. Corno A, Mazzera E, Marino B, et al: Simultaneous patency of ductus arteriosus and surgical shunt in pulmonary atresia with intact ventricular septum. A cause of acute myocardial failure? Scand J Thorac Cardiovasc Surg 20:123, 1986.

A.D. PACIFICO, MD

SURGICAL CONSIDERATIONS IN REPAIR OF CLASSIC TETRALOGY OF FALLOT

Professor and Director
Division of Cardiothoracic Surgery
Department of Surgery
Alabama Congenital Heart Disease Diagnosis and Treatment Center
University of Alabama at Birmingham
Birmingham, Alabama

Reprint requests to:
A.D. Pacifico, MD
Department of Surgery
Division of Cardiothoracic Surgery
University of Alabama at Birmingham
University Station
Birmingham, AL 35294

The surgical management of the tetralogy of Fallot began with the palliative subclavian-pulmonary artery anastomosis introduced in 1945 by Blalock and Taussig.[1] Subsequent palliative procedures included a variety of systemic-pulmonary artery shunts,[2-5] and a closed palliative operation to reduce the magnitude of pulmonary stenosis.[6,7] Corrective repair was first accomplished using controlled cross-circulation in 1954 by Lillehei,[8] and using a pump oxygenator in 1955 by Kirklin.[9] For many years, the classical approach to repair of the tetralogy of Fallot has consisted of relieving pulmonary stenosis and closing the ventricular septal defect (VSD) through a right ventriculotomy incision.[10] Currently there is increased interest in accomplishing corrective repair via a transatrial (with or without a transpulmonary) approach,[11-13] which was first described in 1963 by Hudspeth, Cordell and Johnston.[14] This approach leaves the patient with an intact right ventricle when no ventriculotomy is used, or a more intact right ventricle when a limited ventriculotomy is required for transannular enlargement, both of which may increase the probability of preserved right ventricular function over the long term.

The basic approach used to repair tetralogy of Fallot is one important surgical consideration. Another is the guidelines employed to manage the pulmonary valve annulus. Transannular patching was employed in the early years of tetralogy surgery[15] and subsequently has been used conservatively by some,[10] liberally by others,[16] and according to a set of rules developed by us at the University of Alabama at Birmingham (UAB). These relate the measured size of the patient's pulmonary valve annulus to normal and permit an estimated prediction of the post-repair peak right/left ventricular pressure ratio ($P_{RV/LV}$) with and without transannular patching.[17-19]

This chapter focuses on the technical considerations involved in using the transatrial-transpulmonary approach to repair tetralogy of Fallot, including its indications and limitations, guidelines for transannular patching, and results.

GENERAL CONSIDERATIONS

The goal of corrective surgery for the tetralogy of Fallot is to accomplish complete and permanent closure of the VSD, providing as complete as possible relief of pulmonary stenosis and still leaving whenever possible an intact and functional pulmonary valve, with the avoidance of complete heart block and mortality. While accurate intraoperative methods are essential to achieve this goal, they rest upon complete and precise preoperative diagnostic studies. Currently Doppler echocardiography is widely used, enhanced by color flow mapping, to diagnose various forms of congenital heart defects. This excellent noninvasive method does permit diagnosis of the tetralogy of Fallot but does not provide accurate definition of the number, size, and location of the VSD (which are multiple in 3–15% of patients), or accurate delineation of the presence of bifurcation or branch pulmonary artery stenosis, or the anatomy of pulmonary artery arborization. Cineangiography with angled views[20] is still necessary to define the anatomy completely and accurately.

Signficiance of Post-repair Pulmonary Insufficiency

Pulmonary valve incompetence is present in all patients who have transannular patching as part of their repair, and in some patients without transannular patching because of incomplete coaptation of their diseased pulmonary valve leaflets or excision of a leaflet at the time of repair.

Wessel and colleagues have demonstrated that pulmonary valve incompetence results in reduced exercise capacity regardless of the post-repair right ventricular systolic pressure.[21] Fuster et al. evaluated the clinical status of 396 hospital survivors between 12 and 22 years postoperative.[22] Significant pulmonary valve incompetence contributed to some type of disability in only 1% of this group. It was associated with a 5% incidence of cardiomegaly. It must be recalled, however, that patients with isolated congenital absence of the pulmonary valve usually do not become symptomatic until the fourth decade of life.[23] This raises important questions concerning the effect of pulmonary valve incompetence 20-40 years or longer after repair. Bove et al. have demonstrated impaired right ventricular function in this group late postoperatively by radionuclide angiography.[24] Graham and colleagues have shown significantly greater right ventricular end-diastolic volumes in patients after transannular patching compared to those without this.[25] All of these considerations support the idea that a transannular patch should be used only when necessary and also raises serious concern regarding the *very* long-term effects of free pulmonary valve incompetence.

Preoperative Prediction of Post-repair $P_{RV/LV}$

Knowledge of the ratio of the diameter of the left and right pulmonary arteries before the upper lobe branch divided by the diameter of the aorta at the diaphragm (McGoon ratio) (Fig. 1) allows estimation of the post-repair $P_{RV/LV}$

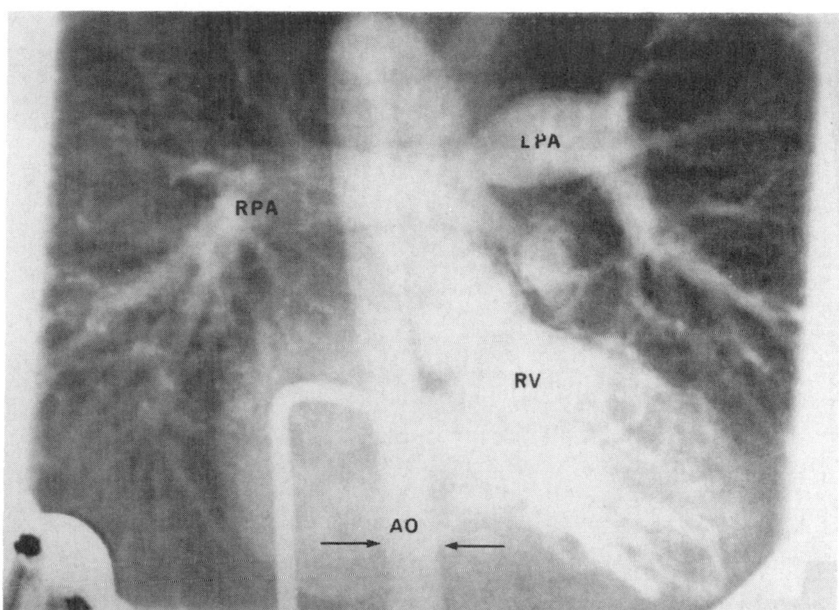

FIGURE 1. Right ventricular (RV) angiocardiogram displaying the branch pulmonary arteries and descending thoracic aorta. The diameter of the left (LPA) and right (RPA) pulmonary arteries prior to the upper lobe branch is added and divided by the diameter of the descending aorta (Ao) to determine the McGoon ratio. (From Blackstone EH, Kirklin JW, Bertranou EG, et al: Preoperative prediction from cineangiograms of postrepair right ventricular pressure in tetralogy of Fallot. J Thorac Cardiovasc Surg 78:542–552, 1979, with permission.)

(Fig. 2) when a transannular patch is employed.[26] An incremental increase in post-repair $P_{RV/LV}$ occurs when the pulmonary valve annulus is left intact, and its magnitude is related to the Z value of the annulus (Fig. 3). The Z values shown on the vertical axis in Figure 3 describe the number of standard deviations of the diameter of the patient's pulmonary valve annulus away from the mean normal value ($Z = 0$) of a similar sized patient (Table 1).[17,26]

In actual practice we estimate the post-repair $P_{RV/LV}$ (assuming that a transannular patch will be employed) from the preoperative cineangiogram (as in Fig. 1) and from the nomogram in Figure 2. The diameters of the left and right pulmonary arteries are separately measured just proximal to the takeoff of the upper lobe branch. The diameter of the descending aorta at the level of the diaphragm is also measured (arrows in Figure 1). The McGoon ratio is calculated as the sum of the right and left pulmonary artery diameters divided by the diameter of the descending thoracic aorta, and this is plotted on the horizontal axis of the nomogram shown in Figure 2. The predicted $P_{RV/LV}$ (with transannular patching) is thus determined. If the predicted $P_{RV/LV}$ is greater than about 0.75, then the pulmonary branches are considered too small for a satisfactory result from primary repair. In this circumstance we would recommend an initial systemic-pulmonary artery shunt, usually by Gor-Tex interposition, to simulate enlargement.[27] If the predicted post-repair $P_{RV/LV}$ is < 0.75, we proceed with definitive repair.

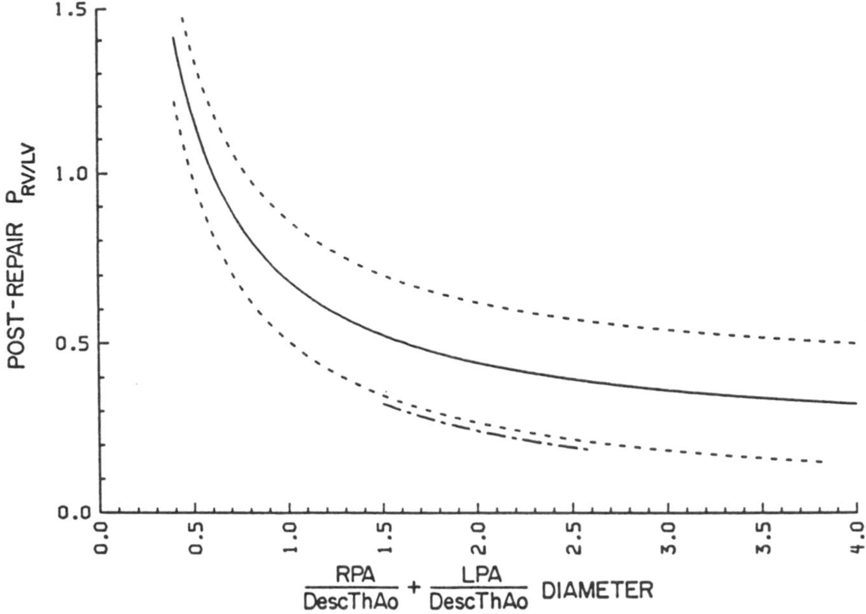

FIGURE 2. Nomogram relating the post-repair peak right/left ventricular pressure ratio ($P_{RV/LV}$) to the McGoon ratio. This nomogram assumes no residual pressure gradient from right ventricle to main pulmonary artery, as is present when transannular patching is employed. (From Blackstone EH, Kirklin JW, Bertranou EG, et al: Preoperative prediction from cineangiograms of postrepair right ventricular pressure in tetralogy of Fallot. J Thorac Cardiovasc Surg 78:542–552, 1979, with permission.)

Intraoperative Prediction of Post-repair $P_{RV/LV}$

Intraoperatively the pulmonary valve annulus is measured with Hegar dilators and the Z value established by using Table 1. The estimate of the competency of the pulmonary valve after valvotomy, as well as the resultant incremental increase in post-repair $P_{RV/LV}$ (Fig. 3) if the annulus is left intact, is considered when deciding upon the need for transannular patching and the resultant creation of pulmonary incompetence. When the pulmonary valve is normal, we prefer to leave the annulus intact as long as the resultant post-repair $P_{RV/LV}$ will be less than about 0.75. In general, a Z value larger than -1.5 is usually acceptable. Using these methods the surgeon can develop a reasonably accurate estimate of the post-repair $P_{RV/LV}$ and intelligently restrict the use of transannular patching to those situations in which it is truly necessary. This method also helps to avoid leaving residual right ventricular outflow tract obstruction from a small pulmonary valve annulus.

TRANSATRIAL-TRANSPULMONARY APPROACH

Right Ventricular Outflow Tract Anatomy

A long tubular and hypoplastic infundibulum (Fig. 4) is generally considered a contraindication to transatrial-transpulmonary repair. The right ventricular

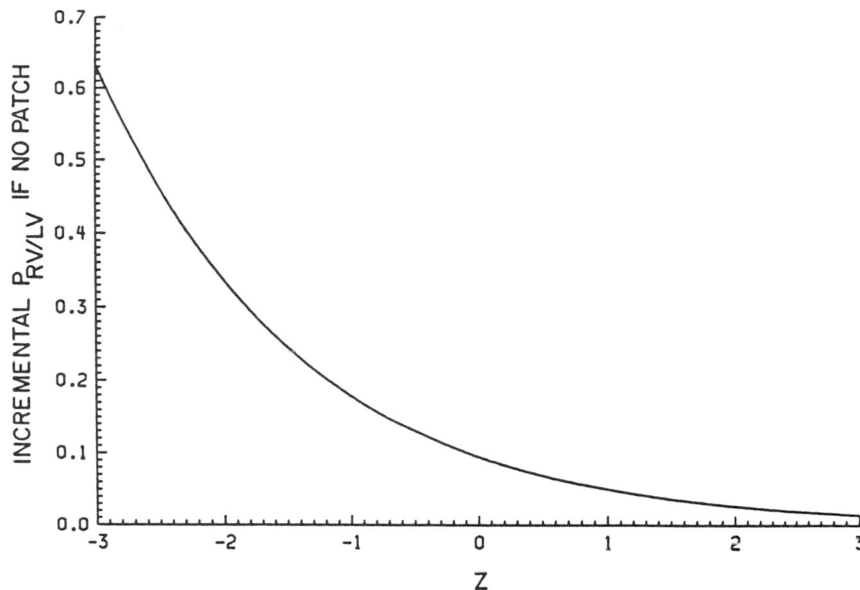

FIGURE 3. Nomogram relating the standard deviations from the mean normal pulmonary valve annulus (Z = 0) to the incremental increase in the post-repair $P_{RV/LV}$ if a transannular patch is not employed. (From Blackstone EH, Kirklin JW, Bertranou EG, et al: Preoperative prediction from cineangiograms of postrepair right ventricular pressure in tetralogy of Fallot. J Thorac Cardiovasc Surg 78:542–552, 1979, with permission.)

outflow tract obstruction produced by this type of infundibular anatomy cannot be adequately relieved solely by direct intraventricular muscle resection. It is best treated by placement of an enlarging patch within a vertical infundibular incision. Since this incision of necessity must be quite long, adequate exposure for patch closure of the VSD is provided, and therefore the cntire repair is

TABLE 1. Mean Normal Valve Diameters*

Body Surface Area (m^2)	Pulmonary Annulus Diameter (mm)†
0.25	8.4
0.30	9.3
0.35	10.1
0.40	10.7
0.45	11.3
0.50	11.9
0.60	12.8
0.70	13.5
0.80	14.2
0.90	14.8
1.0	15.3

* From Rowlatt et al: The quantitative anatomy of the normal child's heart. Pediatr Clin North Am 10:499–588, 1963, with permission.

† Approximate standard deviation for each annulus diameter = ±1.2.

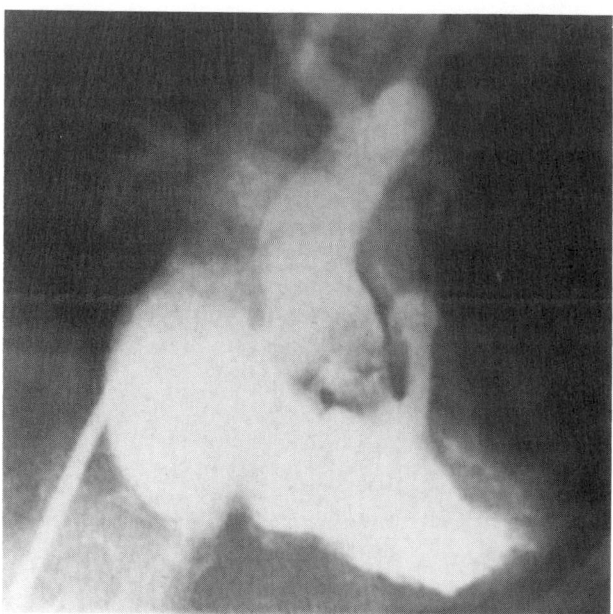

FIGURE 4. Right ventricular angiocardiogam demonstrating a long tubular and hypoplastic infundibulum, which is considered a contraindication to transatrial-transpulmonary repair. Description is provided in the text. (From Pacifico AD, Sand ME, Bargeron LM Jr, Colvin EC: Transatrial-transpulmonary repair of tetralogy of Fallot. J Thorac Cardiovasc Surg 93:919–924, 1987, with permission.)

accomplished by the classical transventricular approach. Although the pulmonary valve annulus appears very much smaller than the aortic valve annulus in Figure 4, intraoperative measurement yielded a Z value of 0.7 and repair was accomplished with infundibular patching, leaving the pulmonary valve annulus intact. The post-repair $P_{RV/LV}$ was 0.59.

Other types of infundibular anatomy can usually be managed by a transatrial-transpulmonary approach. Figure 5 shows the preoperative right ventricular angiocardiogram of a 10-month-old patient who underwent repair by a transatrial approach. Although the infundibulum is also rather long and tubular, it is not hypoplastic in the sense that the infundibular septum and its parietal and septal insertion are very thick. Mobilization and partial resection of them will produce an adequate infundibular area. In this patient, the parietal and septal insertions of the infundibular septum were mobilized and partially resected working through the tricuspid valve. The stenotic pulmonary valve commissures were incised and the annulus measured. It had a Z value of +1, and the post-repair $P_{RV/LV}$ measured in the operating room was 0.32.

In most patients with coexistent valvar pulmonary stenosis, pulmonary valvotomy is best accomplished working through an incision in the main pulmonary artery. Figure 6 shows the preoperative, right ventricular angiocardiogram of a 2-month-old patient. Pulmonary valvotomy was performed via a pulmonary arteriotomy, and the valve annulus had a Z value of 0. Working through the pulmonary valve orifice, the distal muscle bands of the parietal and septal insertion of the infundibular septum were mobilized and partially resected,

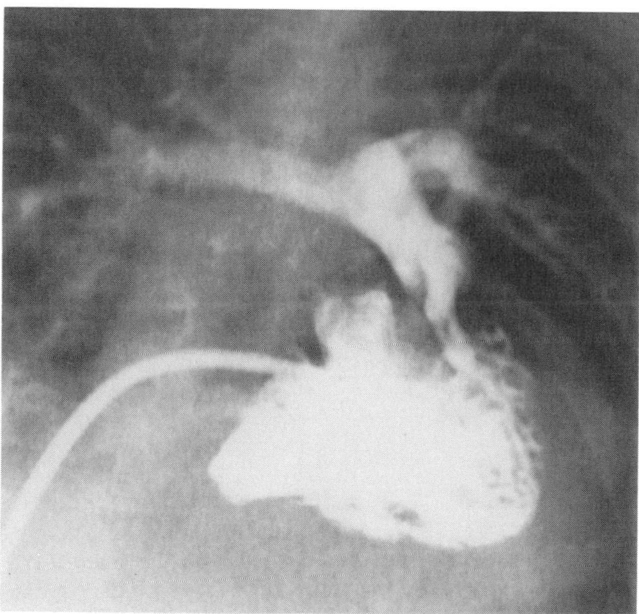

FIGURE 5. Right ventricular angiocardiogram of a 10-month-old patient who underwent repair by a transatrial approach. Although the infundibulum is rather long, the infundibular septum and its parietal and septal insertions are very thick. The pulmonary valve is stenotic. Additional description is provided in the text. (From Pacifico AD, Sand ME, Bargeron LM Jr, Colvin EC: Transatrial-transpulmonary repair of tetralogy of Fallot. J Thorac Cardiovasc Surg 93:919–924, 1987, with permission.)

after which the pulmonary arteriotomy was closed. Working through the right atrium and tricuspid valve, the infundibular dissection was completed and the VSD closed with a Dacron patch using continuous 4/0 polypropylene suture. The immediate postrepair $P_{RV/LV}$ was 0.31.

In some patients infundibular stenosis coexists with a small pulmonary valve annulus. Figure 7 shows the right ventricular angiocardiogram of a 16-month-old patient. Pulmonary valvotomy was performed through a longitudinal incision in the main pulmonary artery. The pulmonary valve annulus was measured and had a Z value of –3.5. The pulmonary artery incision was extended through the valve annulus for the maximal distance (8 mm in this example) required to allow passage of a Hegar dilator with a Z value of +2 into the right ventricle. Initial infundibular muscle mobilization and resection were carried out through this approach and the entire incision widened with a pericardial patch. Additional infundibular resection and VSD closure were performed via a right atrial approach, and the immediate post-repair $P_{RV/LV}$ was 0.55.

Surgical Technique

The surgical approach is through a median sternotomy incision. Pursestring sutures with tourniquets* are placed in the ascending aorta and separately in each

* DLP, Grand Rapids, Michigan

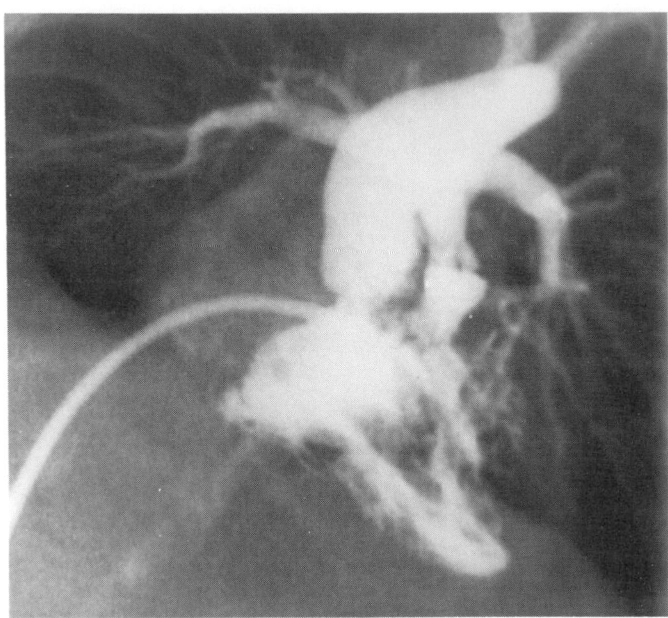

FIGURE 6. Right ventricular angiocardiogram of a 2-month-old patient who underwent repair by a transatrial-transpulmonary approach. Additional description is provided in the text. (From Pacifico AD, Sand ME, Bargeron LM Jr, Colvin EC: Transatrial-transpulmonary repair of tetralogy of Fallot. J Thorac Cardiovasc Surg 93:919–924, 1987, with permission.)

vena cava. The superior vena caval pursestring is placed anteriorly and distal to caval atrial junction to avoid injury to the sinus node artery. It is oval in shape, in the long axis of the cava, so that subsequent closure minimizes caval narrowing. When the vena cava is very small, the tourniquet is temporarily employed and the incision at the cannulation site later repaired with 6/0 polypropylene suture. The pursestring for the inferior vena caval cannula is placed laterally (not anteriorly) at the caval atrial junction so as not to interfere with the planned right atrial incision. The use of a short, thin-walled, arterial cannula* and thin-walled, angled, metal, venous cannulae* minimize clutter in the surgical field and enhance transatrial exposure. The aorta is mobilized away from the main pulmonary artery. After establishing cardiopulmonary bypass with direct cannulation of the ascending aorta and each vena cava, moderate hypothermia is induced, the aorta cross-clamped, and cold cardioplegic solution administered into the aortic root.[28]

The right atriotomy is made parallel to and about 2 cm to the right of the atrioventricular groove. Since the inferior vena caval cannula was placed to the right of the caval midline, the incision may be carried inferiorly to the left of or anterior to the caval cannulation site. Stay sutures of 4–0 silk are placed from the right atrial flap to the subcutaneous tissue on the left side of the incision and also from the atrial wall on the right side of the incision to the subcutaneous tissue on the right. This nicely exposes the right atrium. A disposable sump tip vent* is placed through a stab incision in the atrial septum to vent the left atrium. Silk

---

* DLP, Grand Rapids, Michigan

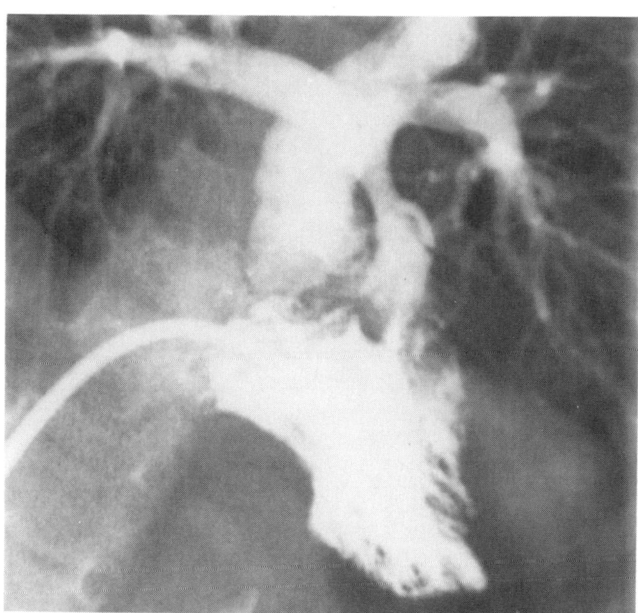

FIGURE 7. Right ventricular angiocardiogram of a 16-month-old patient showing a narrow ostium infundibulum, severely stenotic pulmonary valve, and narrow main pulmonary artery. Repair was accomplished using a transatrial-transpulmonary approach. The pulmonary valve annulus had a Z value of –3.5 and was enlarged by limited transannular patching. Additional description is provided in the text. (From Pacifico AD, Sand ME, Bargeron LM Jr, Colvin EC: Transatrial-transpulmonary repair of tetralogy of Fallot. J Thorac Cardiovasc Surg 93:919–924, 1987, with permission.)

(5/0) sutures are placed on the tricuspid valve leaflets and tagged with a shodded, curved clamp in order to provide gentle retraction. Usually two sutures are placed on the septal leaflet and two on the anterior leaflet. Exposure is facilitated by the use of cardioplegic solution, which provides a rather soft myocardium. In some patients additional retraction is required and is best obtained with small eyelid retractors or right-angle retractors.

The anatomy within the right ventricle is studied. The infundibular septum through this exposure is perpendicular to the operating table, quite different from its appearance through a right ventriculotomy incision when it is in a plane parallel to the operating table. This difference results from differing cardiac rotation induced by traction. The VSD and overriding aorta are easily visualized adjacent to the tricuspid valve annulus and to the right of the infundibular septum. The septal insertion is posterior and the parietal insertion anterior, both in a plane parallel to the operating table. Placement of a traction suture in the mid portion of the infundibular septum allows rightward retraction of it and improves visualization of the distal parietal and septal muscle bands, and the pulmonary valve and its annulus. Mobilization and partial resection of the parietal and septal insertions can usually be nicely accomplished from this exposure. The pulmonary valve annulus can be sized with Hegar dilators. The VSD is then closed using a patch of Dacron and a continuous 4/0 polypropylene suture beginning on the infundibular septum near its junction with the ventriculo-infundibular fold. The suture line is carried counterclockwise to the tricuspid valve where it penetrates the base of the anterior leaflet adjacent to the annulus, and is secured with a shodded clamp. The other arm of the suture is used in a clockwise direction, staying on the free edge of the VSD until reaching the area of the papillary muscle of the conus. Here the suture line leaves the free edge of the VSD and continues 7–10 mm inferiorly on the right ventricular side of the septum until it reaches the tricuspid septal leaflet, which it penetrates near its annular attachment. It then courses along the base of the septal leaflet and is ultimately tied to the initial arm of the suture. If any fragile areas are present in the suture line, they are secured with pledgetted mattress sutures.

When the pulmonary valve is stenotic, it is best exposed through a longitudinal incision in the main pulmonary artery. After valvotomy the pulmonary valve annulus is measured with a Hegar dilator, a Z value established from Table 1, and the post-repair $P_{RV/LV}$ estimated as described above. In general, when the Z value is smaller than −1.5, the annulus is usually enlarged,[13] unless the pulmonary valve is normal and the incremental increase in $P_{RV/LV}$ (Fig. 3) will leave the patient with a predicted $P_{RV/LV} \leq 0.75$. If the annulus is to be left intact, then, using small, right-angled retractors, the distal parietal and septal muscle bands are exposed and released by sharp dissection. If the annulus is to be enlarged, the pulmonary arteriotomy is extended through the annulus for a minimal distance, which permits insertion of a Hegar dilator with a Z value of +2 into the right ventricle. Through this limited right ventriculotomy incision (usually < 1.5 cm), the infundibular dissection is begun and the entire incision widened with a pericardial patch designed to leave the annulus and main pulmonary artery with a diameter 2 standard deviations larger than the mean normal pulmonary valve annulus ($Z = +2$). Transatrial exposure is then arranged, the infundibular dissection completed, and the VSD closed.

The vent is removed from the atrial septum and the incision closed. The right atriotomy is closed and the heart de-aired. When rewarming is complete, cardiopulmonary bypass is discontinued and the peak pressure in the right and left ventricles measured.

CONCLUSION

Transatrial-transpulmonary repair of tetralogy of Fallot can be applied to 90% of patients with the classic form of this malformation.[13] It is equally useful in infants as in older children and most adults. This method provides effective relief of right ventricular outflow tract obstruction and leaves a post-repair $P_{RV/LV}$ insignificantly different from that resulting after classical transventricular repair.

In a recent experience with this approach, the transatrial-transpulmonary approach was used in 61 of 70 consecutive patients; there were no hospital or late deaths and no reoperations during a follow-up period ranging between 2.3 and 53.8 months (mean 22.6) postoperatively.[13] Each patient was in New York Heart Association Functional Class I. Using the guidelines described above for deciding upon the need for transannular patching, only 16 (26%) of the 61 patients required this. Of the remaining 45 (74%), the pulmonary valve was normal in 22 (36%), and 23 (38%) required valvotomy or excision of one leaflet. The majority were left without severe pulmonary incompetence and with an intact right ventricle, which should result in a greater probability of preserved right ventricular function early postoperatively and over the very long term.[29]

REFERENCES

1. Blalock A, Taussig HB: The surgical treatment of malformations of the heart in which there is a pulmonary stenosis or pulmonary atresia. JAMA 128:189–2002, 1945.
2. Potts WJ, Smith S, Gibson S: Anastomosis of the aorta to a pulmonary artery. JAMA 132:627–631, 1946.
3. Davidson JS: Anastomosis between the ascending aorta and the main pulmonary artery in the tetralogy of Fallot. Thorax 10:348–350, 1955.
4. Waterston DJ: Treatment of Fallot's tetralogy in children under one year of age. Rozhl Chir 41:181–187, 1962.
5. De Leval MR, McKay R, Jones M, et al: Modified Blalock-Taussig shunt. Use of subclavian artery orifice as flow regulator in prosthetic systemic-pulmonary artery shunts. J Thorac Cardiovasc Surg 81:112–119, 1981.
6. Sellors TH: Surgery of pulmonary stenosis. A case in which the pulmonary valve was successfully divided. Lancet 1:988–989, 1948.
7. Brock RC: Pulmonary valvulotomy for relief of congenital pulmonary stenosis. Report of 3 cases. Br Med J 1:1121–1126, 1948.
8. Lillehei CW, Cohen M, Warden HE, et al: Direct vision intracardiac surgical correction of the tetralogy of Fallot, pentalogy of Fallot, and pulmonary atresia defects: Report of first ten cases. Ann Surg 142:418–455, 1955.
9. Kirklin JW, Dushane JW, Patrick RT, et al: Intracardiac surgery with the aid of a mechanical pump-oxygenator system (Gibbon type): Report of eight cases. Proc Staff Meet Mayo Clin 300:201–206, 1955.
10. Kirklin JW, Karp RB: The Tetralogy of Fallot. Philadelphia, W. B. Saunders Co., 1970.
11. Edmunds LH Jr, Saxena NC, Friedman S, et al: Transatrial repair of tetralogy of Fallot. Surgery 80:681–688, 1976.
12. Binet JP, Patane L, Nottin R: Correction of tetralogy of Fallot by combined transatrial and pulmonary approach. Mod Probl Pediatr 22:152–156, 1983.
13. Pacifico AD, Sand ME, Bargeron LM Jr, Colvin EC: Transatrial-transpulmonary repair of tetralogy of Fallot. J Thorac Cardiovasc Surg 93:919–924, 1987.
14. Hudspeth AS, Cordell AR, Johnston FR: Transatrial approach to total correction of tetralogy of Fallot. Circulation 27:796–800, 1963.
15. Kirklin JW, Ellis FH Jr, McGood DC, et al: Surgical treatment for the tetralogy of Fallot by open intracardiac repair. J Thorac Surg 37:22–46, 1959.
16. Castaneda AR, Norwood WI: Fallot's tetralogy. In Stark J, de Leval M (eds): Surgery for Congenital Heart Defects. London, Grune & Stratton, 1983.
17. Rowlatt UF, Rimoldi HJA, Lev M: The quantitative anatomy of the normal child's heart. Pediatr Clin North Am 10:499–588, 1963.
18. Pacifico AD, Kirklin JW, Blackstone EH: Surgical management of pulmonary stenosis in tetralogy of Fallot. J Thorac Cardiovasc Surg 74:382–395, 1977.
19. Blackstone EH, Kirklin JW, Pacifico AD: Decision-making in repair of tetralogy of Fallot based on intraoperative measurements of pulmonary arterial outflow tract. J Thorac Cardiovasc Surg 77:526–532, 1979.
20. Bargeron LM Jr, Elliott LP, Soto B, et al: Axial cineangiography in congenital heart disease. Circulation 56:1075–1083, 1977.
21. Wessel HU, Cunningham WJ, Paul MH, et al: Exercise performance in tetralogy of Fallot after intracardiac repair. J Thorac Cardiovasc Surg 80:582–593, 1980.
22. Fuster V, McGoon DC, Kennedy MA, et al: Long-term evaluation (12 to 22 years) of open heart surgery for tetralogy of Fallot. Am J Cardiol 46:635–642, 1980.
23. Shimazaki Y, Blackstone EH, Kirklin JW: The natural history of isolated congenital pulmonary valve incompetence: Surgical implications. Thorac Cardiovasc Surg 32:257–259, 1984.
24. Bove EL, Byrum CJ, Thomas FC, et al: The influence of pulmonary insufficiency on ventricular function following repair of tetralogy of Fallot. Evaluation using radionuclide ventriculography. J Thorac Cardiovasc Surg 85:691–696, 1983.
25. Graham TP Jr, Cordell D, Atwood GF, et al: Right ventricular volume characteristics before and after palliative and reparative operation in tetralogy of Fallot. Circulation 54:417–423, 1976.
26. Blackstone EH, Kirklin JW, Bertranou EG, et al: Preoperative prediction from cineangiograms of postrepair right ventricular pressure in tetralogy of Fallot. J Thorac Cardiovasc Surg 78:542–552, 1979.
27. Kirklin JW, Bargeron LM Jr, Pacifico AD: The enlargement of small pulmonary arteries by preliminary palliative operations. Circulation 56:612–617, 1977.

28. Pacifico AD: Cardiopulmonary bypass and hypothermic circulatory arrest in congenital heart surgery. In Grillo HC, Austen WG, Wilkins WE Jr, et al: Current Therapy in Cardiothoracic Surgery. Toronto, B.C. Decker, Inc., 1988.
29. Kawashima Y, Matsuda H, Hirose Hm, et al: Ninety consecutive corrective operations for tetralogy of Fallot with or without minimal right ventriculotomy. J Thorac Cardiovasc Surg 90:856–63, 1985.

CLARENCE S. WELDON, MD
JOHN C. LASCHINGER, MD

PULMONARY ATRESIA WITH INTACT VENTRICULAR SEPTUM

Clarence S. Weldon, MD
Formerly Professor of Surgery and Head
Division of Cardiothoracic Surgery
Department of Surgery
Washington University School of Medicine
St. Louis, Missouri

John C. Laschinger, MD
Chief Resident
Division of Cardiothoracic Surgery
Department of Surgery
Washington University School of Medicine
St.Louis, Missouri

Reprint requests to:
Clarence S. Weldon, MD
Division of Cardiothoracic Surgery
Department of Surgery
Washington University School of Medicine
Suite 3108 Queeny Tower
4989 Barnes Hospital Plaza
St. Louis, MO 63110

Hearts designated as pulmonary atresia with intact ventricular septum (PA:IVS) share in common a completed interventricular septum and an imperforate membrane replacing a normal pulmonary valve. Such designated hearts differ each from the other through a wide spectrum of variant right ventricular morphology. The spectrum extends from greatly dilated and thin-walled ventricles through near normal ones to severely hypoplastic ventricles, which seem to have no trabeculated body and no infundibulum. A significant number of these abnormal ventricles contain persistent sinusoidal communications between the right ventricular cavity and the coronary arteries which may or may not be attached to the aorta. It is this enormous variation of right ventricular morphology and consequent function which makes the design of therapy for PA:IVS complex and which renders the evaluation of reported results of therapy so difficult.

CARDIAC ANATOMY

PA:IVS occurs in hearts that are left sided, that have an atrial situs which is solitus, and that have atrioventricular and ventriculoarterial connections which are concordant. Exceptions are extremely rare.[45,46] The atrial septum is always incomplete. True secundum type atrial septal defects occur in about 20% of cases.[15] Primum type defects have not been recognized,[21] and atrial septal defects are restrictive in about 5–10% of cases. When this restriction is severe, primum tissue can protrude aneurysmally into the left atrium.[43]

The tricuspid valve is abnormal and exceptions to this, if they exist at all, are also extremely rare. The abnormal tricuspid valve may, in fact, be the principal determinant of PA:IVS *(vide infra).* Functionally, the tricuspid valve may be stenotic, competent, or regurgitant. Many patients display a combination of both valve stenosis and regurgitation.[41] Anatomically, the tricuspid valve may be unguarded;[9] that is, there may be no evidence of valve tissue and support mechanism. An Ebstein's type abnormality, when seen with PA:IVS, is usually severe.[54] Other forms of regurgitant valves occur with severe dysplasia or displacement or are verrucous without evidence of commissural development.[3] Stenotic valves reveal a varying amount of dysplasia.[3] The valve margins may attach directly to primitive papillary muscles without cordal development.[19] Severe stenosis has been described with an Ebstein's deformity in which the orifice of displaced tricuspid membrane was only a tiny perforation.[54] Parachute deformities of the tricuspid valve exist with PA:IVS.[19]

The right ventricle in PA:IVS may, on occasion, have a normal size with a near normal tricuspid valve, but this is uncommon. Most PA:IVS hearts display gross distortions of global anatomy, including the inlet, the trabecular, and the infundibular zones. Davignon's always-cited report from 1961 divided hearts with PA:IVS into those with small right ventricles and those with large right ventricles.[11] This classification is too simple to be useful. More recently, Bull and associates[6] have revived the 1975 tripartite concept of ventricular organization provided by Goor and Lillehei[24] in 1975. This system recognizes three parts of the right ventricle: an inlet section, a trabecular portion, and an infundibulum or subarterial outlet zone. This concept has a sound basis in right ventricular morphogenesis *(vide infra).* From angiographic analyses, Bull and associates[6] then recognized among PA:IVS hearts those which have all three zones present (Fig. 1A), those which have an absence of the trabecular portion (Fig. 1B), and those which have an absence of both the infundibular and the trabecular portion with only an inlet zone remaining (Fig. 1C). This system of classification is worthy in that it permits a more definitive design of therapy and allows a more critical evaluation of results. It is deficient in that it ignores those hearts with PA:IVS which have global dilatation of the right ventricle with extreme compressive cardiomegaly. This scheme furthermore suggests that certain portions of the right ventricle are congenitally absent or inappropriately developed, whereas obliteration of both the infundibulum and the trabecular portions are probably a secondary phenomenon consequent to muscular hypertrophy. Careful necropsy examination of specimens has demonstrated that an infundibulum and an apical trabecular zone are always present no matter how severely attenuated.[21]

The pulmonary valve is represented by a membrane that contains commissural markings, sometimes confined to the periphery of the valve, and sometimes meeting in the center of the valve. Intermediate forms have been described.[53] The pulmonary arteries are confluent and connect to a main pulmonary artery, which extends all the way back to the imperforate membrane. Van Praagh and associates[48] have described hypoplasia of branch pulmonary arteries. Pulmonary venous connections and the mitral valve are usually normal. The left ventricle is normally formed but usually demonstrates hypertrophy of the wall and dilatation of the cavity.[53] Valvar aortic stenosis has been noted in a few patients with PA:IVS.[40] Discontinuity of one or both coronary arteries from the aorta have been described as associated with PA:IVS.[34]

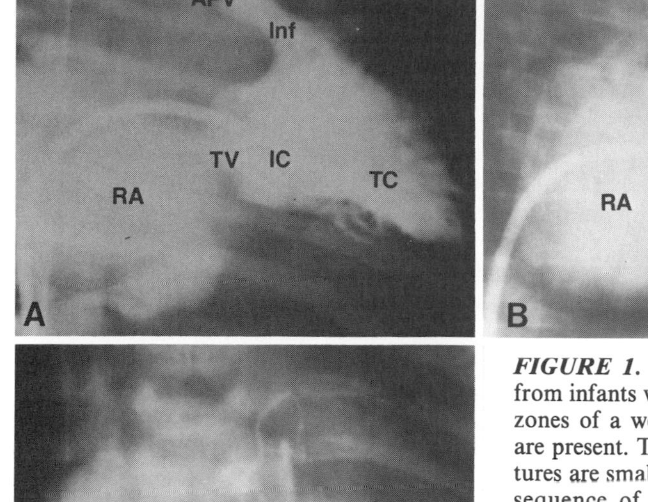

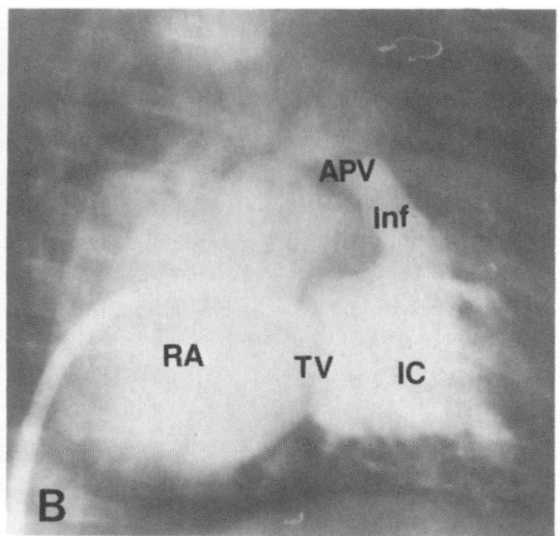

FIGURE 1. Right ventriculograms from infants with PA:IVS. *A,* All three zones of a well-formed right ventricle are present. The cavities of these structures are smaller than normal as a consequence of obliterative myocardial hypertrophy or incomplete fetal development. RA = right atrium, TV = tricuspid valve, IC = inlet cavity, TC = trabecular cavity, Inf = infundibulum, APV = atretic pulmonary valve. *B,* The degree of right ventricular hypoplasis is more severe than that seen in A. The infundibulum cavity is smaller, although still patent. The trabecular zone is obliterated by myocardial hypertrophy. *C,* The degree of right ventricular hypoplasia is profound. There is severe stenosis of the tricuspid valve. The trabecular zone which is obliterated is not apparent. The infundibulum is atretic and not apparent. Fistulas that connect the diminutive right ventricular cavity by way of myocardial sinusoids to the coronary arteries are filled with contrast and are readily apparent. S = sinusoids, PDA = posterior descending branch of right coronary artery.

PA:IVS associated with severe right ventricular hypoplasia is frequently complicated by fistulous communications between the hypertensive right ventricular cavity and the coronary arteries by way of myocardial sinusoids.[51] These communications can be recognized grossly or seen histologically[26] and have been studied extensively by angiography.[33] Incidence of their existence and association with PA:IVS is estimated at between 10–40% of patients.[40] Channels that constitute these fistulas may communicate singly or multiply[18] with coronary arteries and with one or both of the coronary arteries. In patients who have discontinuity between a coronary artery and the aorta, coronary artery flow is retrograde and dependent upon the persistence of the fistula. The presence of these fistulous communications is associated with a sclerosis of the coronary artery, always with the one being supplied by the fistulous communications, but in certain instances also the coronary artery not so supplied.[16] Endocardial fibrosis developing in these diminutive right ventricles is common and has been cited as having a potential for obliterating the origin of the fistulas.[39] Therefore, it has been proposed that there is a reciprocal relationship between the severity of coronary artery sclerosis and endocardial fibroelastosis.[5] Both Bull and associates[6] and Freedom and Harrington[18] have extensively studied these fistulous communications between the right ventricular cavity myocardial sinusoids and the coronary arteries as well as the resulting changes that occur in the coronary arteries and in the right ventricular endocardium. The results of their work indicate that these are remnants of the sinusoidal spaces which nourish the myocardium before the development of coronary arteries and that they persist in response to the hypertension that develops in the right ventricular cavity following abnormal pulmonary valve development with resulting atresia. There is no question that the sinusoids are more prominent in severely hypoplastic and hypertensive ventricles and are rarely seen in dilated ventricles that are associated with tricuspid insufficiency.[22] The rapidly developing sclerosis seen in the coronary arteries is thought to be a pure stress phenomenon resulting from the high-pressure systolic flow. Freedom's studies[21] suggest a fibromuscular intimal hyperplasia, which is the sort of injury reaction seen when veins are used as arteries or in ordinary developing coronary atherosclerosis.

ETIOLOGY

Santos and colleagues[44] studied ductal angles in patients with pulmonary atresia with intact ventricular septum and in patients with pulmonary atresia associated with ventricular septal defects. Kutsche and Van Mierop[32] similarly studied these two groups of patients, examining the anatomy of the proximal pulmonary circulation. Both groups concluded from their studies that in PA:IVS total obstruction at the valve level was a late developing phenomenon and that, through much of fetal life, flow was antegrade through the proximal pulmonary circulation and ductus arteriosus. They therefore felt that PA:IVS was a late and progressive obstructive development. Kutsche and Van Mierop evoked the possibility of an intrauterine inflammatory process.

Arom and Edwards[2] described the relationship between the right ventricular muscle bundles and the pulmonary valve and have discovered that in PA:IVS there is an exaggeration of the prominence of the infundibular muscle bundles related to the right and left posterior cusps and an exaggerated significance of the anterior muscle bundle.

The right ventricular infundibulum forms with conal septation. The trabeculated portion of the right ventricle is a result of outpouching from the bulbar heart. The inlet portion of the right ventricle forms with migration of the atrioventricular canal. It is not possible to say how much of the abnormal right ventricular morphology seen in PA:IVS is a result of attenuation of these various processes and how much is a consequence of hypertrophic myocardial obliteration of formed parts. Furthermore, morphology may be a consequence of hemodynamic molding. Thus, abnormal flow patterns and abnormal volumes in the developing right ventricle may produce abnormal structure. Both flow patterns and volumes are dictated primarily by the function of structures at the atrioventricular junction and secondarily by the structures at the ventricular outlet. It is likely that all three factors are operative.

It is possible to conceive of the development of pulmonary atresia as a result of null flow or reduced flow at the pulmonary valve level (retrograde flow through the ductus and antegrade flow through the proximally obstructed right ventricle meeting at the ventricular outlet). One fact remains clear: an analysis of right ventricular morphology and tricuspid function in PA:IVS[21,53] indicates that there is linear relationship between the severity of stenosis of the tricuspid valve and hypoplasia of the right ventricle and a similar linear relationship between dilatation of the right ventricle and regurgitation at the tricuspid valve. In patients with PA:IVS, therefore, it seems probable that the principal determinant of both the anatomical and functional expression of PA:IVS is the distortion at the right atrioventricular junction.

FETAL CIRCULATION IN PA:IVS

As stated earlier, it is not possible to determine precisely whether pulmonary atresia results from faulty valve formation or whether initially the pulmonary valve is functional and permits a right ventricular outflow and antegrade ductal flow, with the atresia being a progressive and late phenomenon. In any case, once the pulmonary valve is critically stenotic or atretic, a stage is set for abnormal dynamics. In the case of tricuspid insufficiency, venous blood will slosh back and forth between the right atrium and the obstructed right ventricle, dilating and thinning these structures, producing an enlargement that in severe cases produces a cardiomegaly of such a degree that the heart occupies almost the entire thorax. When the tricuspid valve is competent, whether stenotic or not, the right ventricular cavity becomes hypertensive, encouraging the persistence and enlargement of fistulas between the cavity and myocardial sinusoids and the coronary arteries if these are still in existence, and initiates the process of myocardial hypertrophy resulting from isometric contractions with its potential for obliterating both the trabecular and infundibular portions of the formed right ventricle.

Independent of the function of the tricuspid valve, blood returning to the fetal heart must cross the foramen ovale to reach the systemic circulation. The entire output of the heart is through the aortic root; the left ventricle, therefore, undergoes a degree of dilatation and hypertrophy which is greater than normal, and the aortic root enlarges beyond a normal diameter. The admixture of blood in the left atrium produces a lower than normal saturation of blood perfusing the brain and coronary arteries and a higher than normal oxygen saturation of blood perfusing the pulmonary circulation. Whether or not these changes in PO_2 produce developmental abnormalities of the brain, the coronary circulation, or the lungs has not been established. Efforts to produce pulmonary stenosis experimentally by pulmonary banding in fetal lambs[42] demonstrate that when bands are placed during late gestation, interference with placental blood flow produces fetal death. However, bands placed early in gestation result in increase in the right ventricular wall thickness and a decrease in right ventricular cavity size. These experiments support the hypothesis that the morphology of the right ventricle is related to the time during gestation when fusion of the pulmonary valve occurs. Thus early fusion could produce developmental abnormalities, and later fusion hypertrophic obliteration of a well-formed right ventricle. In summary, therefore, although it is recognized that pulmonary atresia in the developing fetal heart are associated with: (1) suprasystemic abnormal pressures in the right ventricle; (2) increased flow through the left ventricle and the preductal aorta; (3) decreased and retrograde flow through the ductus; and (4) oxygen desaturation within the coronary circulation, it is impossible to relate precisely these physical and chemical abnormalities to such events as myocardial cell multiplication, maturation, and regression of cardiac chamber components or to the development of the coronary circulation and the connective tissue components of the heart.

POSTNATAL CIRCULATION

With expansion of the lungs at birth, pulmonary blood flow in the presence of PA:IVS is entirely retrograde through the ductus arteriosus. Thus, the magnitude of the pulmonary circulation at birth is related directly to the length and cross-sectional diameter of the ductus arteriosus. Blood entering the obstructed right ventricle either regurgitates through the tricuspid valve or, in the presence of persistent right ventricular coronary sinusoids, enters the coronary circulation during systole. Elevations of right atrial pressure may produce signs of systemic venous congestion and may represent some obstruction to flow at the foramen ovale. Although this pathway was obviously adequate during fetal life, it is possible that with the elevation of left atrial pressures and partial closure of foramen ovale, it becomes inadequate. Balloon septostomy in infants with pulmonary atresia and high right atrial pressure has therefore been employed. Because of the absolute dependence of all pulmonary blood flow on patency of ductus arteriosus, the primary form of therapy in infants with pulmonary atresia is pharmacologic maintenance of ductal patency with E-type prostaglandins. This therapy is always instituted at the time of diagnosis. However, because it is a temporary form of therapy, continued survival depends upon replacement of the ductus arteriosus with a surgical shunt constructed between the pulmonary circulation and the systemic circulation or relief of the obstruction at the pulmonary valve level.

CLINICAL SYNDROME

The principal clinical feature is rapidly developing cyanosis in the newborn with progression to metabolic acidemia. Heart failure is not uncommon. Heart murmurs are variable and depend upon ductal flow and tricuspid regurgitation. The electrocardiogram is varied and depends upon the size of the right ventricle. The chest roentgenogram demonstrates a decrease in pulmonary vascular markings and usually enlargement of the heart. A diagnosis can be established by Doppler echocardiography, which adequately demonstrates the size of the three parts of the right ventricle, the total obstruction at the pulmonary valve, and the size of the tricuspid valve as well as the degree of its competence. Cardiac catheterization is necessary to determine the presence of right ventricular coronary sinusoids and whether or not there is continuity between the aorta and the coronary circulation. A two-catheter technique has been advised for demonstrating the length of an atretic infundibulum.[20] The double catheter technique is no longer necessary because of the availability of high fidelity echocardiography.

PALLIATIVE OPERATIONS

Infants with PA:IVS and associated tricuspid insufficiency that produces gross enlargement and thinning of the right ventricle, those with discontinuity between the aorta and the coronary arteries, and those with associated aortic atresia have not been successfully managed by any form of palliative therapy. We are unaware of any attempts to treat such patients with neonatal allogeneic cardiac transplantation, but on the basis of their inoperability by reconstructive techniques, such a trial certainly would be justified. Neither of the methods for establishing a nonductal pulmonary blood flow (pulmonary valvotomy and/or shunting) will have any beneficial effect on structural tricuspid regurgitation, right ventricular failure that complicates right ventricular dilatation in the presence of regurgitation, coronary ischemia resulting from a sinusoidal-based circulation or aortic-coronary discontinuity, or the noncompliant nature of persistent spongy myocardium or massively hypertrophied myocardium.

Many institutional reports of experience with the palliative management of infants with PA:IVS, including one from our own,[50] are available.[4,8,12–14,17,28,29,36,37,47] For the most part, these reports extend back over a period of 20–25 years and reflect an ongoing evolutionary search for improved methods of palliation. They precede the advent of prostaglandin therapy, and frequently include the period during which the only available neonatal shunting procedures were laterally constructed Potts-type or Waterston-type anastomoses. These reported series differ one from the other in that there is no uniform system of classifying PA:IVS according to tricuspid valve size, tricuspid function, or the degree of right ventricular hypoplasia. Bull and associates[6] made their recommendation for a classification according to the Gore and Lillehei tripartite scheme in 1982. Generally, survival figures hover around 50%, but it is likely that differences in survival figures reflect more accurately the right ventricular morphologic types that constitute an individual institutional series than they reflect differences in surgical skill or excellence in the perioperative management of patients.

Early reports of valvotomy for PA:IVS demonstrated very few survivors. Several authors, however, were able to accumulate series in which the survivors approached 50%.[7,14] The reason for these dismal results is that incision or excision of the pulmonary valve with relief of obstruction at the valve level does not always restore a normal or near-normal pulmonary blood flow. The right ventricle, which is a thick-walled, noncompliant structure often with a small cavity lined with thick fibrous endocardium, cannot fill and thus constitutes a site of residual obstruction. The obstructive role of the hypoplastic tricuspid valve has been debated.[19] In the reported series of patients with pulmonary atresia combined from Columbia University and the University of Maryland,[38] 11 infants with PA:IVS were treated by valvotomy alone. There was a single survivor. In our own series of 30 patients, eight infants with recognizable tripartite right ventricles were treated by transventricular valvotomy. All patients survived the operation, but only two maintained a satisfactory pulmonary blood flow and arterial saturation. The remainder (75%) required a secondary shunt procedure to relieve pulmonary oligemia. All eight infants initially treated by valvotomy, including five treated secondarily with shunts, survived to childhood. Of these eight, four have now undergone successful secondary repairs.

Because valvotomy and valvectomy fail to produce a satisfactory pulmonary blood flow, other investigators recommended an aortic-pulmonary shunt as the primary palliative procedure for all infants with PA:IVS. Early reports from centers adopting this policy documented improved survival.[14] Valvotomy, of course, is impossible when there is infundibular obliteration, and so successes with shunting were observed in these previously untreatable patients. Our own experience with shunting as an initial procedure indicates that shunting alone as a palliative operation produces initial success but eventually unacceptable results. Eleven patients in our series of 30 were so treated. There were no operative deaths and only two deaths within 30 days of the procedure. However, there were six late deaths between 3 and 6 months following the procedure. Three patients only survived. Similarly, among eight patients so managed with neonatal shunts at Columbia University and the University of Maryland,[38] there has been only one long-term survivor. In 1971, Bolman and colleagues[4] recommended a combined transventricular valvotomy and shunting procedure performed concomitantly as an ideal palliative operation. They suggested that the reestablishment of transventricular flow is essential for the salvage of right ventricular function and that shunting is essential to reestablish an adequate pulmonary blood flow in the neonatal period. Their report demonstrated improved results with this approach. Nine patients in our series of 30 had concomitant shunts and valvotomy procedures. There were four operative deaths, all of which occurred before the introduction of prostaglandin therapy. One patient died within 30 days of the operation, and one died 3 months following the procedure. Four of the nine patients survived long term. The most recent report from the Columbia group indicates that of 19 infants who underwent simultaneous concomitant valvotomy and shunt, there were four early deaths and five late deaths, with 10 long-term survivors. The effort to develop a satisfactory palliative operation for all infants with PA:IVS, therefore, has not been successful. It has been suggested[10] that in patients who have tripartite anatomy or at least a patent infundibulum and are candidates for valvotomy, and who also have proven right ventricular–sinusoidal–coronary artery communications, relief of the right ventricular hypertension at the time of valvotomy will produce a coronary artery hypoperfusion and resulting myocardial ischemia or infarction. This suggestion, however, has not been properly documented.

From the accumulated data and from a more complete appreciation of the right ventricular morphologic variants that occur in PA:IVS, it is possible to make the following recommendations.

1. Infants with a tricuspid valve area 75% of normal or greater will have tripartite anatomy, rare persistence of sinusoids, and only mild right ventricular hypoplasia. Such patients can be managed by valvotomy or valvectomy alone, provided the procedure is accompanied by judicious use of prostaglandin therapy in the early postoperative period. Furthermore, satisfactory growth of the right ventricle will ensue following the valvotomy or valvectomy and permit secondary reparative operations by repeat valvotomy or more often by a right ventricular outflow tract reconstruction.

2. Infants whose tricuspid valve orifice has an area of between 50 and 75% of normal will usually have tripartite anatomy, although the degree of right ventricular hypoplasia will be more severe and the infundibulum may be severely narrowed. Valvotomy or valvectomy alone is not dependable. However, valvotomy can be performed and always should be performed in this group of patients. The reason why this is so is that no subsequent ventricular growth can be expected unless transventricular flow has been established. Shunts are not always essential in this group, and certain patients can be maintained following valvotomy alone along with judicious withdrawal of prostaglandins. Therefore, the recommendation for concomitantly performed shunts and valvotomy does not seem reasonable. Unfortunately, improvement in the arterial saturation that is recognized immediately following valvotomy is often not sustained. Reasons for this phenomenon are not clear, but cyanosis and hypoxemia reappear with cessation of prostaglandin therapy. A policy of sequential shunting in patients who have had a valvotomy but who do not sustain a satisfactory oxygenation

has been adopted by us as stated above and has been successful in all five patients in whom it was employed.

3. Patients who have a tricuspid valve orifice that is smaller than 50% of normal but who have demonstrated some patency of the infundibulum will have a degree of right ventricular hypoplasia with a reduction in right ventricular compliance that is incompatible with a large transventricular flow. Valvotomy should always be performed to encourage transventricular flow, as certain of these patients have demonstrated a phenomenal growth of the right ventricle which allows later reconstruction. More often, however, such growth does not obtain and patients who survive this form of therapy become candidates for a Fontan-type operation. In addition, valvotomy should be performed in an effort to relieve right ventricular hypertension in the presence of persistent fistulas. However, it is in this group of patients that a shunt is required to establish a near-normal pulmonary blood flow, and therefore the recommendation is for concomitantly performed shunt and valvotomy.

4. Infants with an atretic infundibulum always have gross hypoplasia of the right ventricle, often with absence of the trabecular portion. Transventricular valvotomy is not possible and transpulmonary artery valvotomy is useless. These patients are managed by an initial shunt procedure, and although this procedure produces pulmonary blood flow with elevation of the arterial PO_2, the incidence of early and late death is so high that alternative forms of therapy are needed. The cause of the early and late death is still obscure but is probably not related to shunt failure. It is this group of patients in which persistent right ventricular, sinusoidal, coronary artery fistulas are most common. The cause of early and late mortality has been related to myocardial ischemia and infarction, which are consequences of a developing endocardial fibroelastosis which narrows the origin of these fistulas and of the ensuing coronary sclerosis which complicates high pressure flow in the coronary arteries. Fyfe and colleagues[23] have documented such infarctions and evidence of myocardial ischemia in 17 autopsy specimens of infants who died following palliative surgery. They demonstrated this ischemia and infarction with and without the presence of fistulas. Similar studies have been reported by Hansdorf and colleagues[27] at the University of Hamburg, by Becker[3] in 1981, and by Freedom's group[21] using an autofluorescence technique.

Waldman and associates[49] have provided a remarkable case report of an infant with PA:IVS with right ventricular coronary artery communications through sinusoids. Only a shunt procedure was performed at 2 days of age, even though the infundibulum was apparently not atretic. There were communications from the right ventricle through sinusoids to the coronary artery, and these were demonstrated to be persistent at a later catheterization. At 5 months of age, the right ventricle was plicated and a patch was sewn over the tricuspid valve. One year following surgery, neither the right ventricle nor the sinusoids could be demonstrated by angiography.

TYPES OF PALLIATIVE OPERATIONS

Pulmonary valvotomy may be performed through a left thoracotomy, approaching the pulmonary valve through a pulmonary arteriotomy. A similar operation can be performed through a median sternotomy. Zollinger and coworkers[52] have recently advised a transpulmonary artery valvectomy using a punch designed to create aortic defects for coronary-aortic anastomoses. Transventricular valvotomies can be performed through an incision in the

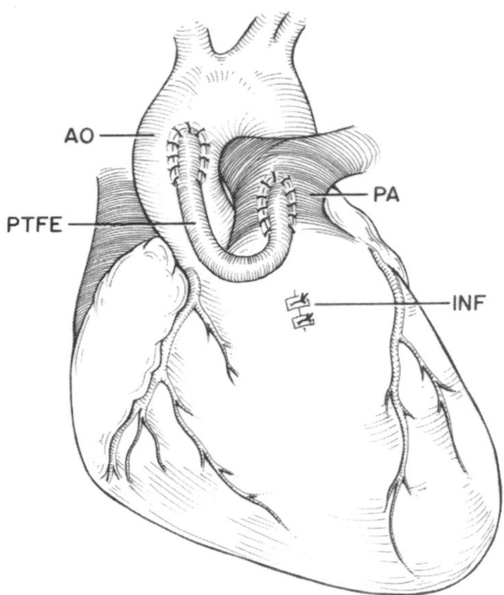

FIGURE 2. Artist's rendering of a satisfactory method for combining a valvotomy and shunt for the palliative management of pulmonary atresia with intact ventricular septum. The approach is through a median sternotomy. The valve is incised by introducing knives and dilators through a right ventricular infundibulotomy. A shunt is constructed by interposing a loop of 4-mm PTFE graft between the main pulmonary artery and the aorta. Side-biting clamps may be used on both great vessels. The main pulmonary artery may be totally occluded with impunity. Inf. = sutured infundibulotomy, PA = pulmonary artery, Ao = aorta, PTFE = loop of prosthetic graft.

infundibulum with the introduction of knives and dilators placed through the valve. Transventricular valvotomies are most easily performed through a median sternotomy. This approach permits better control of potential hemorrhage and provides and opportunity for resuscitative massage. There is no evidence to recommend either of the approaches to the right ventricular outflow tract or either of the approaches to the imperforate membrane, or for that matter to recommend valvectomy over valvotomy.

Concerning shunting operations, we have a strongly held opinion that there is no role for lateral shunts whether these be Waterston-type shunts, Potts-type shunts, classic Blalock-Taussig shunts, or modified Blalock-Taussig shunts performed with the use of polytetrafluoroethylene (PTFE) grafts constructed between the subclavian artery and the left pulmonary artery. The reason is that such laterally constructed shunts have a potential for tenting and narrowing the involved pulmonary artery or encasing it in a scar, thus rendering the patient an unsuitable candidate for Fontan's procedure. There are two acceptable types of shunting procedures. We have employed a central shunt constructed of a loop of 4-mm PTFE graft between the aorta and the main pulmonary artery. While there is ductal patency, the main pulmonary artery can be clamped completely to construct the pulmonary end of the shunt, and with the enlargement of the neonatal aortic root, an aortic anastomosis can easily be accomplished with a side-biting clamp (Fig. 2). Joshi[29] recommended the use of a PTFE tube shunt with the tube interposed between the left subclavian artery and the main pulmonary artery, the operative field provided by left thoracotomy (Fig. 3). Kantor and associates[30] have championed this approach.

SECONDARY PROCEDURES FOLLOWING SUCCESSFUL PALLIATION

Several reports of serial angiography obtained in children surviving valvotomy and reestablishment of transpulmonary flow have demonstrated a remarkable

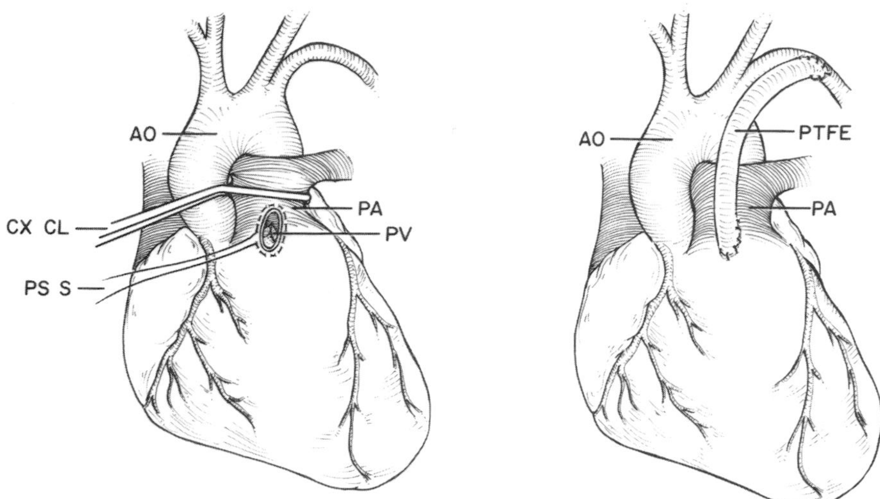

FIGURE 3. Artist's rendering of another satisfactory method for combining a pulmonary valvotomy and shunt for the palliative management of pulmonary atesia with intact ventricular septum. The approach is through an anterolateral or posterolateral left thoracotomy. The main pulmonary artery is clamped distally. The valve is incised directly through a pulmonary arteriotomy guarded by a pursestring suture. The shunt of PTFE graft is interposed between the pulmonary arteriotomy and the left subclavian artery. PA = pulmonary artery, PV = pulmonary valve, PSS = pursestring suture, Cx. Cl. = cross clamp, Ao = aorta, PTFE = 4 mm-PTFE graft.

increase in the size of the right ventricular cavity with regression of myocardial hypertrophy.[25,35] These reports provide the most substantial evidence that a principal cause of right ventricular hypoplasia in PA:IVS is hypertrophic myocardial overgrowth with obliteration of a reasonably well-formed right ventricular cavity. Patients with restoration of right ventricular function are suitable candidates for corrective procedures that further enlarge the capacity of the right ventricle and eliminate all residual obstruction. It is possible to restore pulmonary valve function by the insertion of a prosthetic pulmonary valve. The development of Fontan's operation for bypass of the right ventricle now provides a secondary procedure for infants who survive palliation but have little or no restoration of right ventricular function. In our series of 30 patients, eight children have now undergone such secondary corrective procedures. There were no operative deaths. Five operations were done to enlarge a small but functioning right ventricle by myomectomy and prosthetic or homograft enlargement of the right ventricular wall (Fig. 4). An effort was made to remove fibrous tissue from the endocardium. Normal right ventricular pressure and normal arterial saturations were recorded at the conclusion of the five operations. There was one late death 10 months following repair done at the age of 4½ years. This child developed sepsis, pulmonary embolic occlusion of the right pulmonary artery, and pulmonary insufficiency with severe congestive failure. A third operation was done to insert a pulmonary valve, and death followed within 24 hours from a bleeding diathesis which produced pulmonary hemorrhage. Three patients who had inadequate growth of the right ventricle and who had palliative procedures

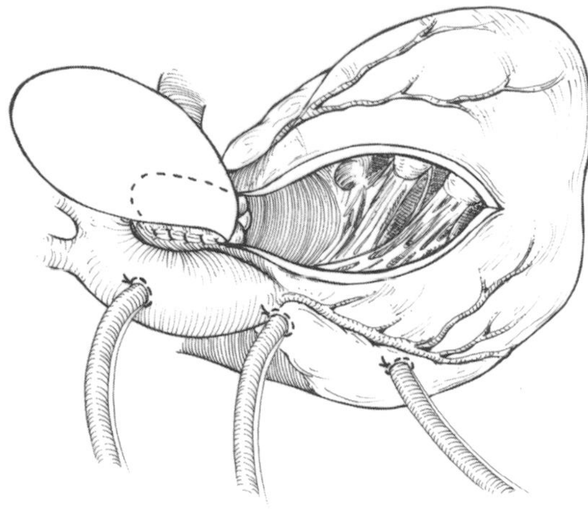

FIGURE 4. Artist's rendering of the technique used for both primary and secondary definitive repair of cavitary hypoplasia of the right ventricle. The pulmonary artery, pulmonary valve infundibulum, and anterosuperior trabecular portion of the right ventricle are opened. In neonates, fibrous tissue and hypertrophied muscle are removed. In older children with cavitary growth, lesser myomectomies suffice. A patch of prosthetic cloth is fashioned to enlarge the pulmonary annulus, the infundibulum, and the anterosuperior portion of the trabecular right ventricular sinus. The reconstruction can be done with cryopreserved aortic root homograft tissue.

using central PTFE shunts between the aorta and the main pulmonary artery underwent secondary Fontan procedures, with an interruption of a previously placed shunt and a patch closure of the tricuspid valve, suture of the foramen ovale, and interposition of a valved conduit between the right atrial appendage and the pulmonary artery. These operations were performed at age 15 months, 21 months, and 3½ years. The tricuspid valve was closed to prevent tricuspid regurgitation, which is asynchronous with atrial systole and which would have caused an atrial overload. Normal systemic arterial saturations have persisted in all three patients. At the present time, we would recommend Kreutzer's[3] modification of Fontan's procedure, as this has the enormous advantage of placing the right atrial pulmonary artery anastomosis in the lateral, rather than the anterior, mediastinum and therefore may be applicable at an even earlier age (Fig. 5). De Leval and associates'[12] early report in 1981 followed the course of 60 patients with PA:IVS presenting during the decade 1970–80. Definitive repairs were done for nine patients. Five patients had right ventricular outflow tract reconstructions and four had modified Fontan procedures. There were two early deaths. The largest series of definitive operations has been provided by Alboliras and associates[1] and documents 20 patients. Right ventricular outflow reconstruction with atrial septal defect closure and shunt removal was done in 10 patients with two deaths, and a modified Fontan operation was performed in 10 patients with one early and one late death.

THE ROLE OF PRIMARY CORRECTIVE OPERATIONS

Although a variety of open operations to relieve obstruction at the imperforate valve have been performed, primary corrective repairs have not been sufficiently explored. The development of the technique of circulatory arrest at profound hypothermia makes this exploration feasible. We have operated successfully upon two infants at age 3 days and 6 days. An operation similar to the one done for secondary repairs was carried out with a prosthetic enlargement involving the pulmonary artery, the pulmonary annulus, the infundibulum, and the anterosuperior trabecular portion of the right ventricle. Myomectomy to enlarge the cavity was combined with a resection of endocardial fibroelastosis. In one infant, satisfactory blood flow

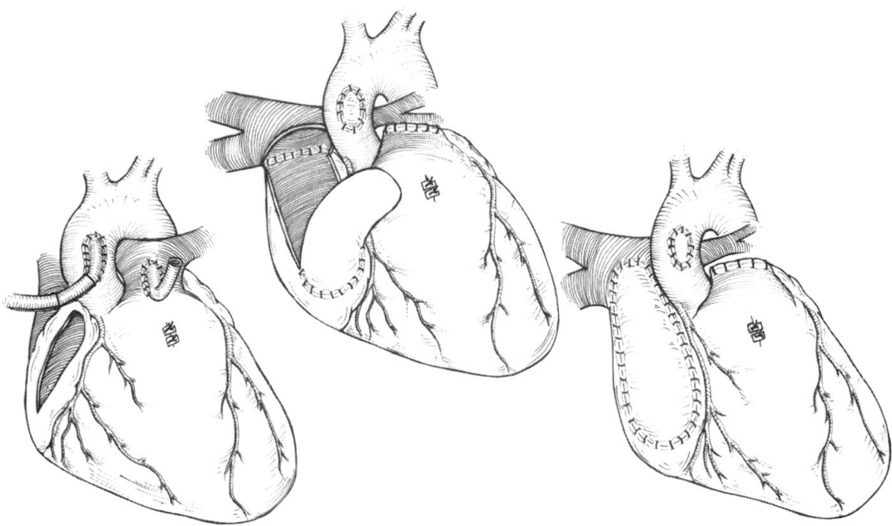

FIGURE 5. Artist's rendering of the steps taken to definitively repair a heart with pulmonary atresia with intact ventricular septum which has failed to undergo satisfactory right ventricular growth. The conversion is from a palliative arrangement (central shunt with or without valvotomy) to a modified Fontan circulation. The central shunt is divided: the aortic end may be used as a cannulation site. A large incision is made in the enlarged right atrium. The pulmonary artery is divided from the heart. The proximal pulmonary artery is oversewn. The anterior wall of the main pulmonary artery containing the pulmonary end of the central shunt is excised. The divided main pulmonary artery is drawn rightward beneath the ascending aorta into approximation with the right atrial appendage. The opened appendage is sutured to the posterior wall of the divided distal pulmonary artery to create the posterior circumference of a large stoma. A patch of pericardium is sutured into the large right atrial incision. The pericardial patch is used to close the remaining opening into the right atrium and the excised portion of the anterior wall of the pulmonary artery. The atriopulmonary anastomosis lies in the lateral mediastinum and is not subject to compression by the sternum.

was established by the operation. In the other, a central PTFE shunt had to be added at the end of the procedure in order to provide sufficient pulmonary blood flow. This patient developed pulmonary over-circulation within two weeks. The repair was then tested by a balloon obliteration of the shunt and completed by ligation of the shunt through a small anterior thoracotomy. This same patient has subsequently undergone a third operation to close an atrial septal defect. Both patients were excellent candidates for the primary repair, in that there was tripartite anatomy. Ishizawa and coworkers[28] have recently reported primary repairs done in four infants with PA:IVS. Two of the four patients died. Most congenital heart surgeons have been reluctant to explore primary corrective operations, believing that the mortality will be higher than that obtained with valvotomies or combined valvotomies and shunts. However, this belief has not been adequately tested.

SOME THOUGHTS FOR THE FUTURE

The end results of neonatal shunting for patients with the most severe degree of right ventricular hypoplasia, that is, those in whom there is only an inlet

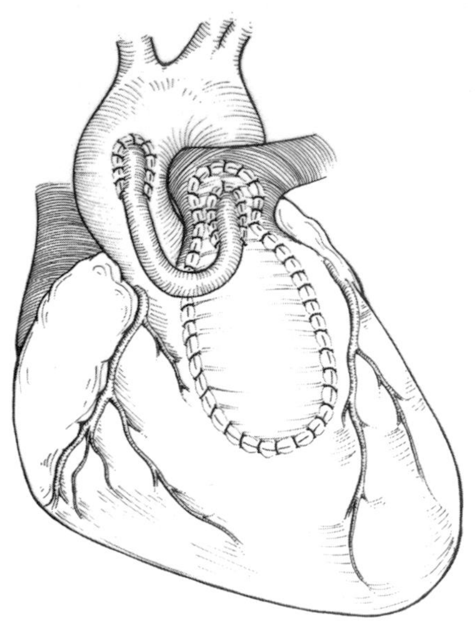

FIGURE 6. Artist's rendering of a proposed operation worthy of trial for the management of neonates with pulmonary atresia with intact ventricular septum having the most severe degree of hypoplasia, including atresia of the infundibulum, absence of the trabecular cavity, and fistulous communications between the right ventricular cavity, myocardial sinusoids, and the coronary circulation. Working under circulatory arrest at profound hypothermia, an incision is made from the pulmomary artery through the pulmonary valve annulus through the atretic infundibulum into the diminutive right ventricular cavity. Hypertrophic muscle and fibrous tissue are excised to create a larger cavity. A composite patch with a built-in central shunt is used to close the incisions. The built-in shunt is attached to the aorta. The shunt provides pulmonary flow. The patch and fibromyomectomy permit some transventricular flow and provide relief of right ventricular hypertension.

portion (atresia of the infundibulum and hypertrophic overgrowth of the trabecular portion), have been so dismal that alternative forms of therapy must be sought. These patients, of course, have the highest incidence and the most severe degree of persistent right ventricular, sinusoidal, coronary fistulas. Three approaches deserve some trial. The first approach involves neonatal open operation performed under circulatory arrest at deep hypothermia in which the entire outflow tract of the right ventricle is incised through the proximal main pulmonary artery through the atretic valve annulus through the atretic infundibulum all the way into the hypoplastic and diminutive right ventricular cavity. A large prosthetic patch is placed over this incision. The patch has a built-in central prosthetic shunt to be attached to the aorta to provide additional pulmonary flow (Fig. 6). The purpose of such operation would be to reduce the hypertension in the right ventricular cavity and encourage closure of fistulous connections to the coronary arteries as well as theoretically to encourage some growth of the ventricle. A second proposal involves the performance of a Kreutzer-modified Fontan procedure as soon as careful follow-up indicates a satisfactory lowering of pulmonary vascular resistance. The third approach involves the idea of secondarily closing the tricuspid valve orifice to eliminate fistulas between the right ventricle and the coronary circulation. All three approaches deserve a larger exploration than they have been given.

REFERENCES

1. Alboliras ET, Julsrud PR, Danielson GK, et al: Definitive operation for pulmonary atresia with intact ventricular septum. J Thorac Cardiovasc Surg 93:454, 1987.
2. Arom KV, Edwards JE: Relationship between right ventricular muscle bundles and pulmonary valve. Significance in pulmonary atresia with intact ventricular septum. Circulation 54:III-79, 1976.
3. Becker AE, Becker MJ, Edwards JE: Pathologic spectrum of dysplasia of the tricuspid valve. Arch Pathol 91:167, 1971.

4. Bowman FO, Malree JR, Hayes CJ, et al: Pulmonary atresia with an intact ventricular septum. J Thorac Cardiovasc Surg 61:85, 1969.
5. Bryan CS, Oppenheimer EH: Ventricular endocardial fibroelastosis. Basis for its presence or absence in cases of pulmonic and aortic atresia. Arch Pathol 87:82, 1969.
6. Bull C, de Leval M, Mercanti C, et al: Pulmonary atresia and intact ventricular septum: A revised classification. Circulation 66:266, 1982.
7. Celemajor JM, Bowder JD, Gengos DC, et al: Pulmonary valve function with intact ventricular septum. Am Heart J 76:452, 1968.
8. Cobanoglu A, Metzdorff MT, Pinson CW, et al: Valvotomy for pulmonary atresia with intact ventricular septum. A disciplined approach to achieve a functioning right ventricle. J Thorac Cardiovasc Surg 89:482, 1985.
9. Cole RB, Muster AJ, Leu M, Paul MH: Pulmonary atresia with intact ventricular septum. Am J Cardiol 21:23, 1968.
10. Cooper N, Brazier J, Buckberg G: Effects of systemic-pulmonary shunts on regional myocardial blood flow in experimental pulmonary stenosis. J Thorac Cardiovasc Surg 70:166, 1965.
11. Davignon AL, Greenwald WE, Dushane JW, Edwards JE: Congenital pulmonary atresia with intact ventricular septum: Clinicopathological correlation of two anatomic types. Am Heart J 62:591, 1961.
12. de Leval M, Bull C, Stark J, et al: Pulmonary atresia and intact ventricular septum: Surgical management based on a revised classification. Circulation 66:272, 1982.
13. Dhanavaravibul S, Nora JJ, McNamara DG: Pulmonary valvular atresia with intact ventricular septum: Problems in diagnosis and results of treatment. J Pediatr 77:1010, 1970.
14. Dobell ARC, Grignon A: Early and late results in pulmonary atresia. Ann Thorac Surg 24:264, 1977.
15. Elliott LP, Adams P, Edwards JE: Pulmonary atresia with intact ventricular septum. Br Heart J 25:489, 1963.
16. Essed CE, Klein HW, Krediet P, Vorst EJ: Coronary and endocardial fibroelastosis of the ventricles in the hypoplastic left and right heart syndromes. Virchows Arch Path Anat Histol 368:87, 1975.
17. Foker JE, Braunlin EA, St Cyr JA, et al: Management of pulmonary atresia with intact ventricular septum. J Thorac Cardiovasc Surg 92:706, 1986.
18. Freedom RM, Harrington DP: Contributions of intramyocardial sinusoids in pulmonary atresia and intact ventricular septum to a right-sided circular shunt. Br Heart J 36:1061, 1974.
19. Freedom RM, Dische MR, Rowe RD: The tricuspid valve in pulmonary atresia and intact ventricular septum. Arch Pathol Lab Med 102:28, 1978.
20. Freedom RM, White RJ Jr, Ho CS, et al: Evaluation of patients with pulmonary atresia and intact ventricular septum by double catheter technique. Am J Cardiol 33:892, 1974.
21. Freedom RM, Wilson G, Trusler GA, et al: Pulmonary atresia and intact ventricular septum. Scand J Thorac Cardiovasc Surg 17:1, 1983.
22. Freedom RM: The morphologic variations of pulmonary atresia with intact ventricular septum: Guidelines for surgical interventions. Pediatr Cardiol 4:183, 1983.
23. Fyfe DA, Edwards WD, Driscoll DJ: Myocardial ischemia in patients with pulmonary atresia and intact ventricular septum. J Am Coll Cardiol 8:402, 1986.
24. Goor DA, Lillehei CW: Congenital Malformations of the Heart. New York, Grune & Stratton, 1975, p 11.
25. Graham TJ Jr, Bender HW, Atwood GF, et al: Increase in right ventricular volume following valvulotomy for pulmonary atresia or stenosis with intact ventricular septum. Circulation 49 & 50:II–69, 1974.
26. Guidici C, Becu L: Cardio-aortic fistula through anomalous coronary arteries. Br Heart J 22:729, 1960.
27. Hausdorf G, Gravinghoff L, Keck EW: Effects of persisting myocardial sinusoids on left ventricular performance in pulmonary atresia with intact ventricular septum. Eur Heart J 8:291, 1987.
28. Ishizawa E, Horiuchi T, Tadokoro M, et al: Surgical management of pulmonary atresia and critical pulmonary stenosis with intact ventricular septum. Tohoku J Exp Med 150:135, 1986.
29. Joshi SV, Brawn WJ, Mee RBB: Pulmonary atresia with intact ventricular septum. J Thorac Cardiovasc Surg 91:192, 1986.
30. Kanter KR, Pennington DG, Nouri S, et al: Concomitant valvotomy and subclavian-main pulmonary artery shunt in neonates with pulmonary atresia and intact ventricular septum. Ann Thorac Surg 43:490, 1987.
31. Kreutzer GD, Vargas FJ, Schlichter AJ, et al: Atriopulmonary anastomosis. J Thorac Cardiovasc Surg 83:427, 1982.

32. Kutsche LM, Van Mierop LHS: Pulmonary atresia with and without ventricular septal defect: A different etiology and pathogenesis for the atresia in the 2 types? Am J Cardiol 51:932, 1987.
33. Lauer RM, Fink HP, Petry EL, et al: Angiographic demonstration of intramyocardial sinusoids in pulmonary valve atresia with intact ventricular septum and hypoplastic right ventricle. N Engl J Med 271:68, 1964.
34. Lenox CC, Briner J: Absent proximal coronary arteries associated with pulmonary atresia. Am J Cardiol 30:666, 1972.
35. Lewis AB, Wells W, Lindesmith GG: Right ventricular growth potential in neonates with pulmonary atresia and intact ventricular septum. J Thorac Cardiovasc Surg 91:835, 1986.
36. Malm JR, Bowman FO, Hayes CJ, et al: Results of surgical treatment of pulmonary atresia with intact ventricular septum. Adv Cardiol 11:18, 1974.
37. Milliken JC, Laks H, Hellenbrand W, et al: Early and late results in the treatment of patients with pulmonary atresia and intact ventricular septum. Circulation 72:II–61, 1985.
38. Moulton AL, Bowman FO Jr, Edie RN, et al: Pulmonary atresia with intact ventricular septum. Sixteen-year experience. J Thorac Cardiovasc Surg 78:527, 1979.
39. O'Connor WN, Cottrill CM, Johnson CL, et al: Pulmonary atresia with intact ventricular septum and ventriculocoronary communications: Surgical significance. Circulation 65:805, 1982.
40. Patel RG, Freedom RM, Moes CAF, et al: Right ventricular volume determination in 18 patients with pulmonary atresia and intact ventricular septum. Analysis of factors influencing right ventricular growth. Circulation 61:428, 1980.
41. Rowe RD, Freedom RM, Mehrizi A, Bloom KR: The Neonate with Congenital Heart Disease. Philadelphia, W.B. Saunders, 1981, pp 328–349.
42. Rudolph AM: Congenital Diseases of the Heart. Chicago, Yearbook Medical Publishers, 1974, p 363.
43. Sahn DJ, Alleu HD, Anderson R, Goldberg SJ: Echocardiographic diagnosis of atrial septal aneurysm in an infant with hypoplastic right heart syndrome. Chest 73:727, 1978.
44. Santos MA, Moll JN, Drumond C, et al: Development of the ductus arteriosus in right ventricular outflow tract obstruction. Circulation 62:818, 1980.
45. Shimazu T, Ando M, Takao A: Pulmonary atresia with intact ventricular septum and corrected transposition of the great arteries. Br Heart J 45:471, 1981.
46. Steeg CN, Ellis K, Bransilver B, Gersony WM: Pulmonary atresia and intact ventricular septum complicating corrected transposition of the great arteries. Am Heart J 82:382, 1971.
47. Trusler GA, Yamamoto N, Williams WG, et al: Surgical treatment of pulmonary atresia with intact ventricular septum. Br Heart J 38:957, 1976.
48. Van Praagh R, Ando M, Van Praagh S, et al: Pulmonary atresia: Anatomic considerations. In Kidd BSL, Rowe RE (eds): The Child with Congenital Heart Disease after Surgery. Mt. Kisco, NY, Futura Publishing Co., 1976, p 103.
49. Waldman JD, Lamberti JJ, Mathewson JW, George L: Surgical closure of the tricuspid valve for pulmonary atresia, intact ventricular septum and right ventricle coronary artery communications. Pediatr Cardiol 5:221, 1984.
50. Weldon CS, Hartmann AF, McKnight RC: Surgical management of hypoplastic right ventricle with pulmonary atresia or critical pulmonary stenosis and intact ventricular septum. Ann Thorac Surg 37:12, 1984.
51. Williams RR, Kent GB Jr, Edwards JE: Anomalous cardiac blood vessels communicating with the right ventricle: Observations in a case of pulmonary atresia with an intact ventricular septum. Arch Pathol 52:480, 1951.
52. Zollinger RW II, Culpepper WS III, Ochsner J: Simplified technique for the surgical palliation of pulmonary atresia with right ventricular hypoplasia and intact septum. Ann Thorac Surg 41:222, 1986.
53. Zuberbuhler JR, Anderson RH: Morphological variations in pulmonary atresia and intact ventricular septum. Br Heart J 41:281, 1979.
54. Zuberbuhler JR, Allwork SP, Anderson RH: The spectrum of Ebstein's anomaly of the tricuspid valve. J Thorac Cardiovasc Surg 77:202, 1979.

ROSS M. UNGERLEIDER, MD
DAVID C. SABISTON, JR, MD

DOUBLE OUTLET RIGHT VENTRICLE

Department of Surgery
Duke University Medical Center
Durham, North Carolina

Reprint requests to:
Ross M. Ungerleider, MD
Department of Surgery
Duke University Medical Center
Box 3178
Durham, NC 27710

The term double outlet right ventricle (DORV) was first used at the Mayo Clinic in 1957 during a procedure on a patient thought to have a large VSD with excessive pulmonary blood flow.[16,17] At that time, the salient anatomic hallmark of this entity—origin of both great arteries from the right ventricle—was correctly identified and a successful repair performed using an intraventricular tunnel procedure similar to current techniques.[34] Several reports followed, corroborating the morphologic characteristics of DORV with description of a variety of anatomic subtypes.[2,5,9,22,29,31,32,45,49,58,59]

Rather than being a specific entity with a predictable clinical presentation, DORV is a type of ventriculoarterial connection associated with a broad spectrum of clinical manifestations. To meet the requirements for DORV, the whole of one and more than 50% of the other great vessel must originate from the morphologic right ventricle.[17,22,35] By this definition, the placement of a congenital heart lesion into the DORV classification is in part dependent upon subjective judgment of the surgeon and the cardiologist, and several criteria for making distinctions between DORV and related conditions have been presented.[12,14,17,22] Although it has been suggested that the diagnosis requires discontinuity between the aortic and mitral leaflets, elongation of the anterior mitral leaflet may be present[31] and there may be normal fibrous connection between the aortic and mitral valves in patients with DORV.[22,55] Furthermore, careful examination at autopsy of normal hearts demonstrates that aortomitral discontinuity can be present in otherwise normal hearts.[41]

Therefore, the presence of aortomitral discontinuity does not appear to be an essential feature for the accurate diagnosis of DORV.[22,40] The relationship of the great arteries to each other may be variable and range from normal to d or l malposition with side by side or anterior-posterior configuration.[14] This feature may greatly impact upon surgical decision making but does not influence the diagnosis as long as both arteries arise for the most part from the right ventricle.

The vast majority of patients with DORV have a large VSD which allows the left ventricle to return oxygenated blood into the right ventricle where it flows into the great arteries. It is the location of this VSD with respect to the great vessels that influences the physiologic features of the lesion, its clinical course, and the recommended repair. An additional factor that influences prognosis is the association of other cardiac anomalies. Although the incidence of chromosomal and other noncardiac abnormalities is only 12.5%, the association of DORV with other cardiovascular defects can be as high as 85%.[44,61] Cardiovascular defects usually include subpulmonic or subaortic stenosis, coarctation or interruption of the aorta, total anomalous pulmonary venous connection, mitral valve abnormalities, coronary artery anomalies, and endocardial cushion defects.[17,22,44,46,47,61]

TYPES OF DORV AND CLINICAL PRESENTATIONS

The four most common locations of the VSD in DORV in relation to the great arteries are shown in Figure 1. Although the VSD is usually large, it can be smaller than the aortic root (and restrictive to LV outflow) in 10% of patients.[21,25,27,42] Patients with multiple VSDs and rarely, absence of a VSD altogether, have been encountered.[30,45]

The most common location of the VSD is subaortic[17,44] (Fig.1A). These patients frequently have associated pulmonary stenosis, and the presence of pulmonary outflow obstruction greatly impacts upon the physiologic behavior of this lesion. When pulmonary stenosis is present, the lesion is very similar to tetralogy of Fallot, which because of aortic overriding can give the appearance of DORV.[12] The distinction is often difficult to categorize, and several authors suggest that in this circumstance the malformation should not be characterized as DORV unless 90% of the aorta arises from the right ventricle.[17,35] Others do not regard TOF and DORV as mutually exclusive, and define TOF as a form of DORV with a specific anatomic placement of the infundibular septum.[12] In this respect, nomenclature of congenital heart lesions may overlap and lead to confusion. This emphasizes the importance of understanding the patterns (rather than the names) of congenital lesions as they relate to physiologic features and to options for correction.[46,50,51,58] Patients with DORV (TOF variety) who have a large subaortic VSD and pulmonary stenosis present with cyanosis of varying degrees depending upon the amount of pulmonary outflow obstruction. Likewise, patients with DORV and pulmonary stenosis whose VSDs are in other locations (Fig. 1) can present with cyanosis, since the net physiologic defect is reduced pulmonary blood flow.

When the VSD is subpulmonic in location (Fig. 1B), left ventricular outflow is directed toward the pulmonary artery, and the clinical behavior is very similar to transposition of the great arteries (TGA). This type of DORV was first described by Taussig and Bing in 1949[49] and has since borne this eponym, although its place in the spectrum of DORV as distinct from hearts with TGA was not fully appreciated at that time.[17,54] In these patients an important

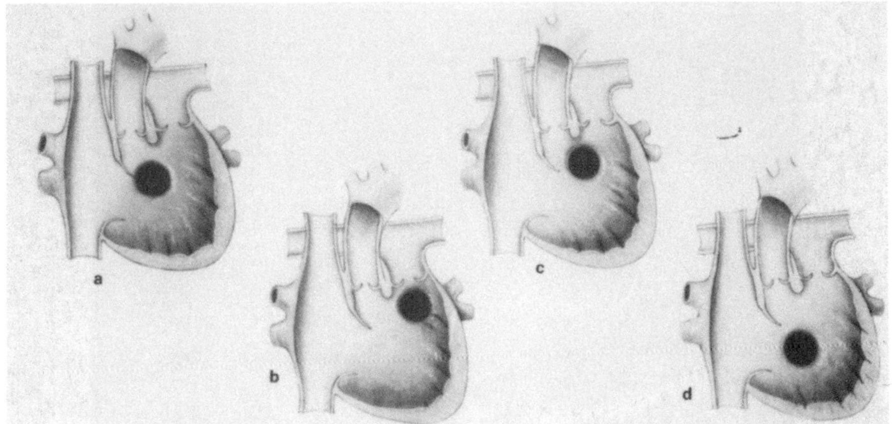

FIGURE 1. Anatomic types of DORV as determined by location of ventricular septal defect. *A,* Subaortic. *B,* Subpulmonary (Taussig-Bing). *C,* Doubly committed. *D,* Noncommitted. (From Stark J: Double outlet ventricles. In Stark J, De Leval M (eds): Surgery for Congenital Heart Defects. New York, Grune & Stratton, 1983, with permission.)

anatomic feature is the possible presence of a discrete band of muscular tissue separating the aortic and mitral valves (infundibular septum). This band not only tends to separate the right and left ventricular flow patterns but can create a degree of subaortic stenosis, further augmenting pulmonary blood flow. In this presentation of DORV, there is streaming of systemic venous blood (unsaturated) into the aorta and of pulmonary venous blood (oxygenated) into the pulmonary artery. Right ventricular pressure equals systemic pressure, and this increases flow and pressure in the pulmonary arterial bed. The physiology of this presentation is identical to that of TGA with a large VSD. Because of the characteristics of blood flow in this type of DORV (TGA variety), patients are often cyanotic with increased pulmonary blood flow and are at risk for the early development of pulmonary vascular disease.[46,47,61]

Whenever DORV occurs in the absence of pulmonary stenosis, pulmonary blood flow is increased. If the VSD is in the subaortic, doubly committed, or uncommitted position (Fig. 1A, C, and D respectively), the clinical presentation is usually that of a large, isolated VSD with predominant left to right shunting. This is potentiated by low pulmonary arterial resistance, compared with systemic resistance, and in these children there is an unfortunate tendency for the changes of pulmonary vascular obstruction to develop at an early age,[28,47,51] probably secondary to the high flow at high pressure generated across the pulmonary vascular bed. Although these patients initially present in congestive heart failure, these symptoms resolve as pulmonary hypertension develops and pulmonary blood flow diminishes. Eventually, cyanosis occurs as pulmonary blood flow is restricted by irreversible pulmonary hypertension and can be termed an *Eisenmenger type* of DORV.[46]

DIAGNOSIS

With the variety of anatomic subtypes of DORV and spectrum of physiologic change that may occur, the clinical presentation is highly inconsistent. Patients without pulmonary stenosis usually present with some degree of heart failure and with recurrent pulmonary infections. Pulmonary stenosis limits pulmonary blood

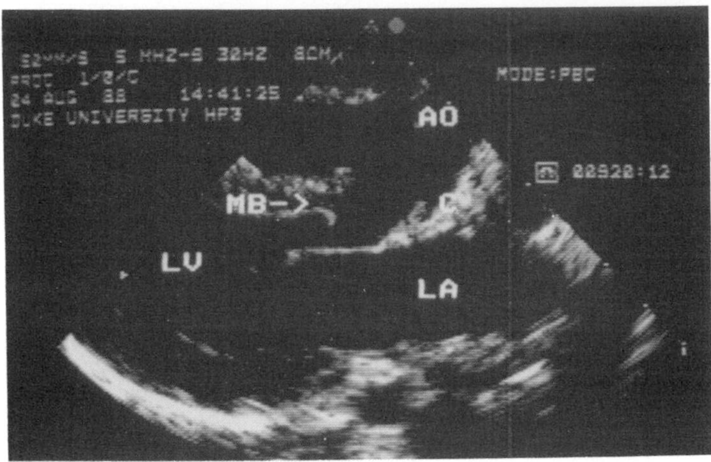

FIGURE 2. Long axis echocardiogram demonstrating discrete muscle bundle (MB) in left ventricular outflow tract. This image was obtained from the epicardial surface at the time of repair and directed resection of this anomalous tissue during the time of intracardiac correction. (AO = aorta; LV = left ventricle; LA = left atrium; MB = subaortic muscle bundle.)

flow and, depending upon its severity, can produce various degrees of cyanosis. These children may have a history of dyspnea on exertion, and parents may describe a squatting behavior by these children after exercise. Patients with subpulmonic VSDs are usually cyanotic and are difficult to distinguish from those with TGA. Infants who become cyanotic shortly after birth may improve with the utilization of prostaglandins to maintain patency of the ductus arteriosus, particularly if they have the TOF type of DORV. Infants with DORV and a subpulmonary VSD usually have increased pulmonary blood flow with mild cyanosis and congestive heart failure. Since left ventricular output is directed via the VSD into the pulmonary artery and right ventricular output streams toward the aorta, pulmonary artery oxygen saturations are usually higher than aortic saturations.[57] In the absence of significant pulmonary stenosis, DORV with VSDs located anywhere but the subpulmonic region are indistinguishable from large isolated VSDs in presentation. It is interesting, and probably fortunate, that these VSDs seldom close spontaneously,[26] and the true diagnosis usually becomes evident at the time of more specific evaluation.

Although there are no characteristic signs on physical examination suggesting DORV, chest films may occasionally reveal malposition of the great arteries and provide an initial impression suggesting DORV.[23,55] The increasing technical advances in two-dimensional echocardiography, especially when coupled with color flow imaging, can generate a substantial amount of information, which not only reveals the correct diagnosis but also localizes the position of the VSD and demonstrates the physiology of blood flow.[20] In addition, echo can provide critical information about other intra- or extracardiac anomalies, some of which are not as well delineated by angiographic techniques (i.e., mitral valve or endocardial cushion abnormalities) (Fig. 2).[13,20,24,53]

Cardiac catheterization with cineangiography is necessary to enhance the preoperative information and to provide crucial information regarding the

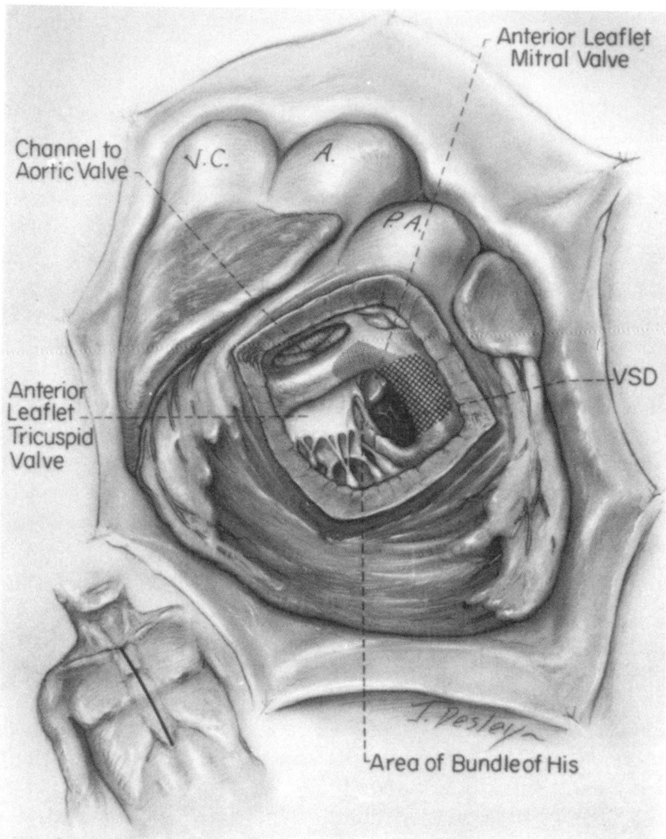

FIGURE 3. View of subaortic ventricular septal defect in a patient with DORV as viewed through the right ventriculotomy. Cross-hatched area demonstrates the region for safe enlargement of the ventricular septal defect. Stippled area indicates the region in the infundibular septum that might need to be enlarged to prevent subaortic obstruction in the intracardiac tunnel. (From Judson JP, Danielson GK, Puga FJ, et al: Double outlet right ventricle. J Thorac Cardiovasc Surg 85:32, 1983, with permission.)

presence and reversibility of pulmonary hypertension. Angiograms help to define the relationships of the great vessels and to display the anatomy of the coronary arteries so that appropriate decisions can be made regarding options for surgical repair.

Most patients with DORV require a surgical procedure since, if left untreated, those with unobstructed pulmonary blood flow will rapidly develop irreversible pulmonary hypertension and succumb to the complications of pulmonary vascular disease. Those whose pulmonary vascular bed is protected by pulmonary stenosis follow a clinical course similar to those with untreated tetralogy of Fallot and become increasingly cyanotic and restricted in their activity.

SURGICAL MANAGEMENT

The fact that these lesions can be complex is demonstrated by the study of Wilcox et al.[58] Among 63 hearts with DORV, it was determined that 23 (36.5%)

were inoperable as a result of the extent of their anatomic aberrancy. This group of hearts had associated lesions such as straddling valves, multiple septal defects, left ventricular hypoplasia, or other combinations of complex lesions that made the possibility of successful operation unlikely. In an autopsy series of 50 hearts with DORV,[46] 26 were found to be so severely abnormal that surgical correction could not have been performed. Despite these discouraging figures, DORV is often a correctable lesion with an increasingly improving surgical outlook.

To plan suitable surgical repair, the surgeon must know the orientation of the great vessels, the location (and size) of the VSD and its relationship to the great arteries, the distribution and location of the coronary arteries, whether there is pulmonic or aortic stenosis, and the nature of any associated intra- or extracardiac anomalies.[58] These data must be combined with information regarding hemodynamics obtained from echocardiographic examination and cardiac catheterization.[40] The goal of operation is to separate the systemic and pulmonary circulations. This can be accomplished by the use of intraventricular tunnels or extracardiac conduits. These types of repair require the use of cardiopulmonary bypass (CPB). In infants, deep hypothermia with total circulatory arrest may be desirable, but the procedure can also be performed with moderate hypothermia and cardioplegia. Palliation in infancy (i.e., placement of systemic-pulmonary artery shunt) may be appropriate in those patients requiring an extracardiac conduit as part of the eventual repair. This permits achievement of a size that will allow placement of a larger conduit.

The most common form of DORV is that associated with a subaortic VSD with or without pulmonary stenosis. Repair of this lesion proceeds in a manner similar to that for repair of tetralogy of Fallot. Repair can be performed in infancy if the caliber of the pulmonary arteries is acceptable. After the patient is placed on CPB, the right ventricle is opened in a region that avoids the coronary arteries. The orifices of both great arteries are identified and areas of subpulmonic, infundibular stenosis are relieved. Because the infundibular septum, which separates the aortic and pulmonary valves, can be oriented in a more sagittal plane than normal (depending on the orientation of the great vessels), care must be taken to avoid incising this area and damaging the aortic valve. The VSD is identified and its borders clearly visualized. If the VSD is smaller than the orifice of the aortic valve, it can usually be safely enlarged in an anterior and superior direction (Fig. 3).[14,25] Once again, caution is necessary when enlarging the VSD so that enough border is maintained to allow secure placement of sutures for the intracardiac baffle. In most cases of subaortic and doubly committed VSDs, a patch can usually be fashioned that directs left ventricular outflow into the aorta while avoiding the orifice to the pulmonary artery (Figs. 4 and 5). Reconstruction of the right ventricular outflow tract is then accomplished to complete the repair. This can usually be performed during rewarming so that CPB time is reduced. RV outflow can be augmented in several ways, including simple closure of the ventriculotomy, RV outflow patching (with pericardium or prosthetic material), which can extend across the pulmonary valve annulus if necessary to relieve pulmonary valvar stenosis, or even with the use of a valved external conduit (as might be necessary in the case of severe pulmonary stenosis that is not amenable to transannular patching because of an anomalous coronary artery). In addition, patients with pulmonary hypertension requiring transannular patching may do better with a valved conduit—preferably homograft—to protect the right ventricle.[10] It is crucial that the surgeon be alerted to any additional cardiac defects

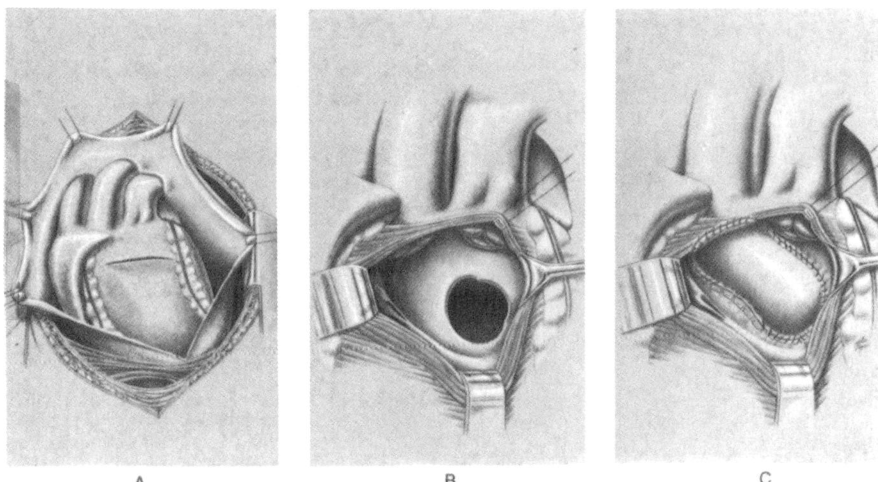

FIGURE 4. Typical intracardiac tunnel repair for DORV with a subaortic or doubly committed ventricular septal defect. The aorta is d-malposition in relation to the pulmonary artery. *A,* Ventricular incision is made. *B,* Ventricular septal defect is enlarged if necessary. *C,* An intracardiac tunnel (patch) is placed in a manner that directs left ventricular outflow through the VSD into the aorta. The right ventricle is then closed primarily or with a patch. (From Replogle RL, Campbell DJ, Campbell CD, Arcilla RA: Double-outlet ventricles. In Arciniegas E (ed): Pediatric Cardiac Surgery. Chicago, Year Book Medical Publishers, 1985, with permission.)

that might need simultaneous correction. The incidence of associated cardiac anomalies is high,[44,61] especially if ASDs and PDAs are included in this definition. The use of routine intraoperative epicardial echo with color flow imaging is becoming an invaluable adjunct to the repair of these types of complex lesions because of its ability to depict accurately and clearly intracardiac structures and disclose previously unappreciated details of anatomy at the time of surgical correction (Fig. 2).[53] Complications of this type of repair include obstruction to LV outflow from a poorly configured patch,[8,17] hemolysis across the patch (which usually disappears within 6 weeks after the surface of the baffle endothelializes),[43] heart block and other arrhythmias, bleeding, and heart failure (usually right ventricular if there is substantial pulmonary hypertension). In patients with significant pulmonary hypertension, repair can be accomplished through the right atrium.[3,10,17] Because of the potential for dysrhythmias, it is recommended that temporary atrial and ventricular pacing wires be left prior to closure of the chest. When DORV is associated with a noncommitted VSD, repair follows the same principles but is usually more difficult because the length and configuration of the patch may increase the risk of subaortic, baffle obstruction to LV outflow. This problem can be diminished, in part, by generous enlargement of the VSD away from the conduction tissue. When the patient has an associated complete AV canal defect, repair of the entire lesion can usually be performed, but once again, careful attention must be given to the intraventricular baffle with anterior-superior enlargement of the inlet type VSD if necessary (Fig. 6). DORV can also commonly occur in association with abnormalities of the aortic arch (i.e., coarctation). It is usually preferable to repair the

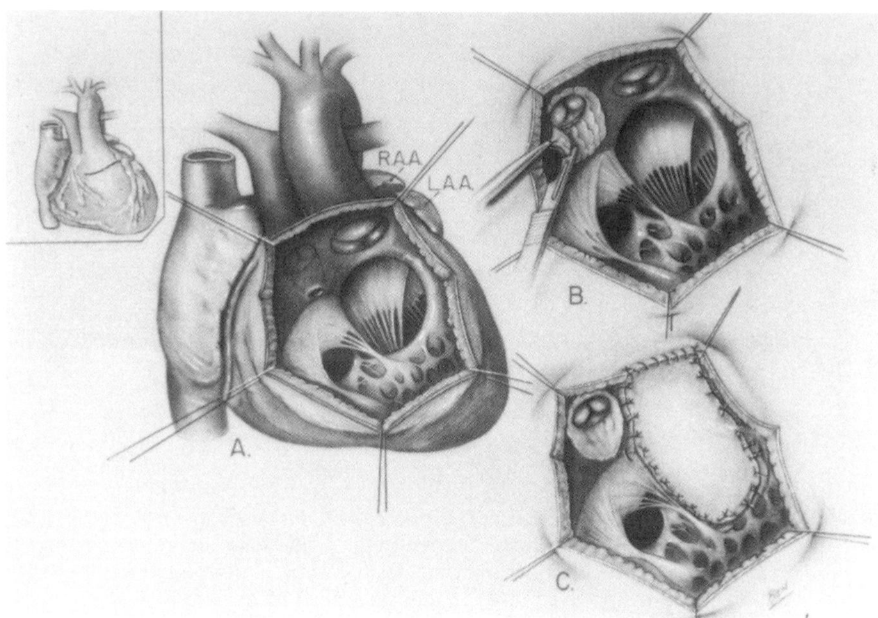

FIGURE 5. Double outlet right ventricle with a large subaortic ventricular septal defect (VSD), subpulmonic stenosis, and l-malposition of the aorta in relation to the pulmonary artery. *A,* Exposure via the right ventriculotomy (inset). Mitral valve can be seen through the VSD. *B,* Resection of subvalvar pulmonary stenosis. *C,* Patch over the VSD directing left ventricular blood into the aorta. The right ventriculotomy can be closed primarily if the pulmonary stenosis is relieved. Other options for repairing the outflow tract include a transannular patch or a valved conduit from the ventricle to the distal pulmonary artery depending on specific defects encountered (see text). (From Pacifico AD, Kirklin JW, Bargeron LM: Complex congenital malformations: Surgical treatment of double outlet right ventricle and double outlet left ventricle. In Kirklin JW (ed): Advances in Cardiovascular Surgery. New York, Grune & Stratton, 1973, with permission.)

arch anomaly at the time of DORV repair and this can be achieved easily through a median sternotomy (Fig. 7).[37,52]

The surgical repair of DORV with subpulmonary VSD has evolved through several modifications because, until recently, a consistently reliable method of repair had not been available. Although placement of an intracardiac baffle to direct LV outflow toward the aorta remained a favorable option, the location of the VSD in proximity to the pulmonary orifice and the presence of the frequently present muscle bands from the infundibular septum could make construction of this baffle technically demanding or even impractical. Nevertheless, careful resection of muscle and placement of the suture line may allow this type of repair in selected patients (Fig. 8).[60] It is usually advisable to inspect the anatomical features through a right atriotomy to ascertain the potential for this type of repair prior to performing a right ventriculotomy. If the patient proves to have findings incompatible with an intracardiac baffle, it may be possible to close the VSD through the right atrium in a manner that directs LV outflow into the pulmonary artery. The patient can then be treated as one with TGA, and an atrial or an arterial switch can be performed.[38] Because of the increasing success with the

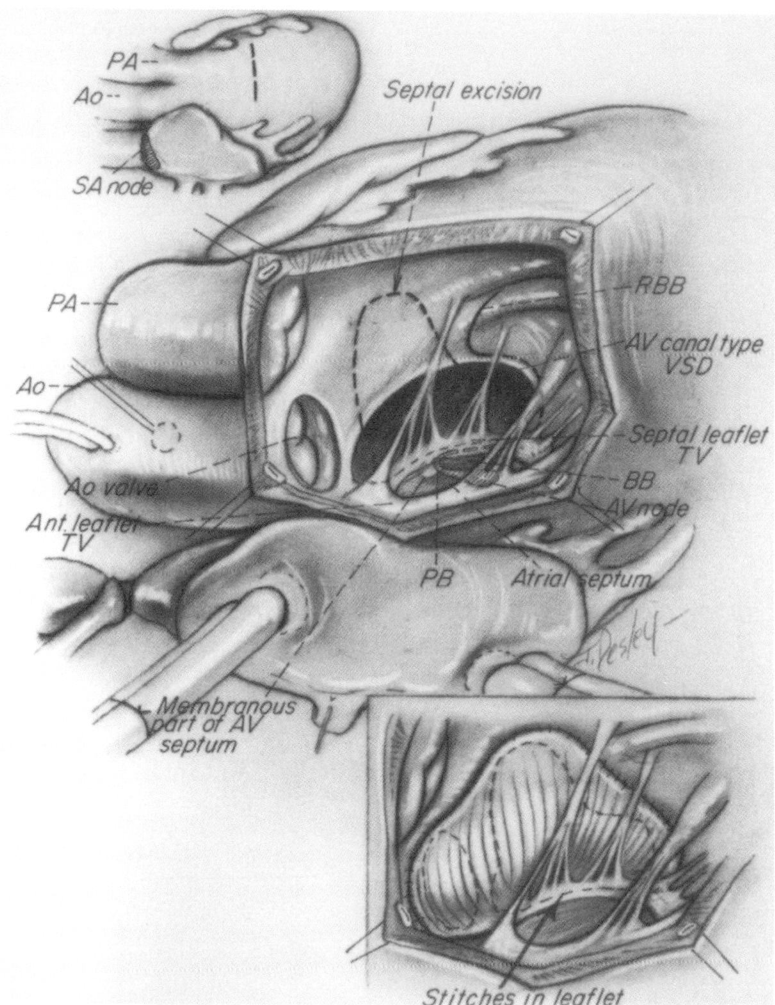

FIGURE 6. Repair of DORV with a subaortic VSD of the inlet or AV canal type. Dashed line indicates the area of septal excision for safe VSD enlargement. Inset demonstrates the location of the patch to direct left ventricular outflow towards the aorta. (From Bharati S, Lev M, Kirklin JW: Cardiac Surgery and the Conduction System. New York, John Wiley & Sons, Inc., 1983, with permission.)

arterial switch procedure,[39] it is becoming the operation of choice for these patients and is preferred at this institution as well as several others.[6,15] If this operation is chosen, it can be performed in infancy, although not with the same urgency as with simple TGA, since the VSD can be depended on to maintain left ventricular pressures until the actual time of operation (as in TGA with large VSD). If an atrial switch procedure is chosen, then it is probably important to try to avoid a right ventriculotomy. However, when an arterial switch is chosen, then the VSD can be repaired through the atrium, the proximal pulmonary artery (neo-aorta; although it is important to keep the sutures on the RV side of

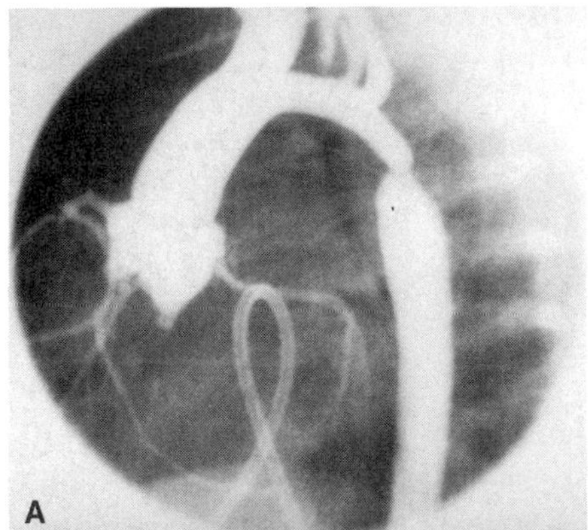

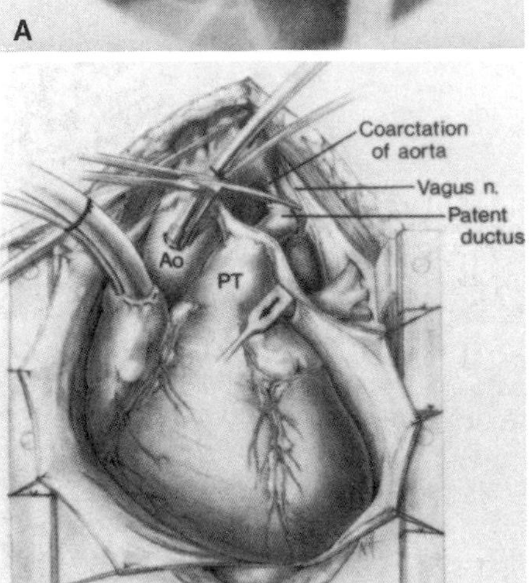

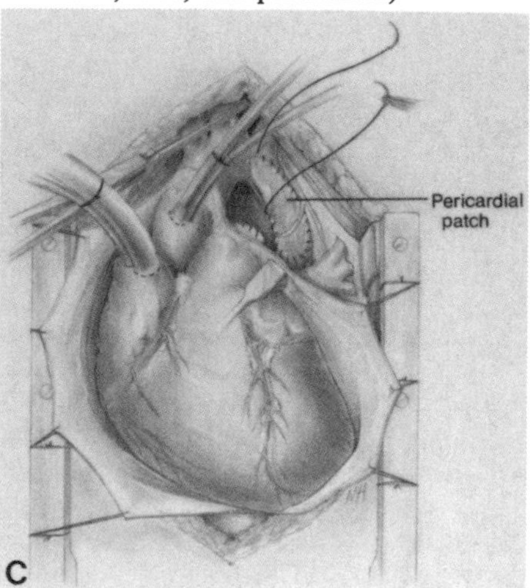

FIGURE 7. *A,* Aortogram from patient with DORV and doubly committed VSD with a hypoplastic aortic arch and discrete aortic coarctation. *B,* Technique for simultaneous repair of aortic arch defect during complete correction of the DORV. Under total circulatory arrest, the patent ductus arteriosus is ligated and the aorta is opened through the area of narrowing. *C,* The aorta is repaired with a patch of pericardium. Attention can then be directed toward repair of the intracardiac defect with reinstitution of cardiopulmonary bypass flow when appropriate. (B and C from Ungerleider RM, Ebert PA: Ann Thorac Surg 44:517, 1987, with permission.)

the inferior part of the septum to avoid creation of heart block), or through a right ventriculotomy.[39] If the VSD is closed through a right ventriculotomy, this can be done during rewarming after the coronary transfer has been completed (Fig. 9).

There are instances in which the arterial switch may not be appropriate. The presence of significant subaortic stenosis might contraindicate the performance of arterial switch, depending upon the feasibility of opening the right ventricular outflow into the aorta (neo-pulmonary artery). In these patients, arterial switch without coronary translocation (Damus-Kaye-Stansel procedure) can be performed.[10] This requires patching of the VSD into the pulmonary artery, and diversion of the proximal pulmonary artery end-to-side into the aorta. RV to PA continuity is restored with the use of an external conduit (Fig. 10). If severe subpulmonic stenosis is present, then arterial switch is contraindicated and the lesion should be repaired using the Rastelli procedure. In this operation, the VSD is baffled to the aorta (through a right ventriculotomy) and the pulmonary artery is divided. The proximal pulmonary artery is oversewn, and RV to PA continuity

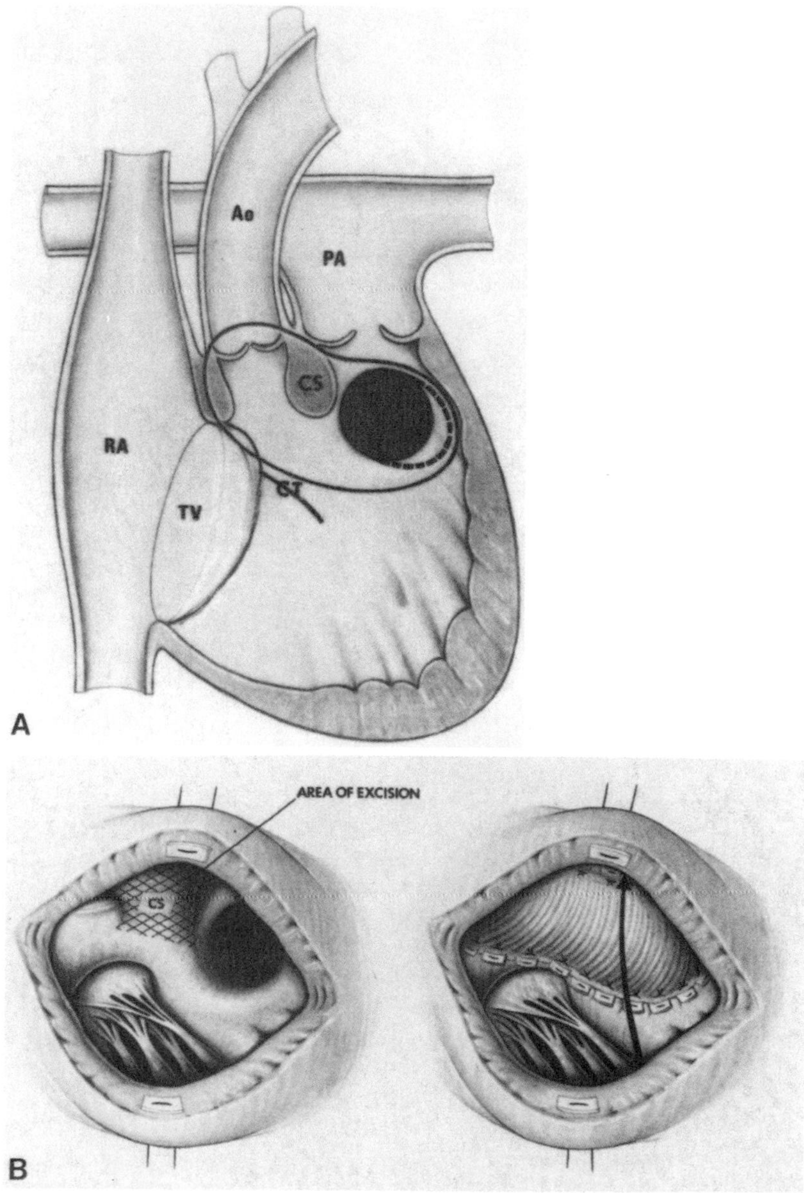

FIGURE 8. *A,* Schematic demonstrating obstruction imposed by conal septum (CS) to intracardiac tunnel repair for patients with DORV and subpulmonary VSD. *B,* Excision of muscle from the infundibular septum may allow redirection of left ventricular flow through a properly placed intraventricular baffle towards the aorta while still preserving the integrity of the pulmonary valve. (From Yacoub MH, Radley-Smith R: Anatomic correction of the Taussig-Bing anomaly. J Thorac Cardiovasc Surg 88:380, 1984, with permission.)

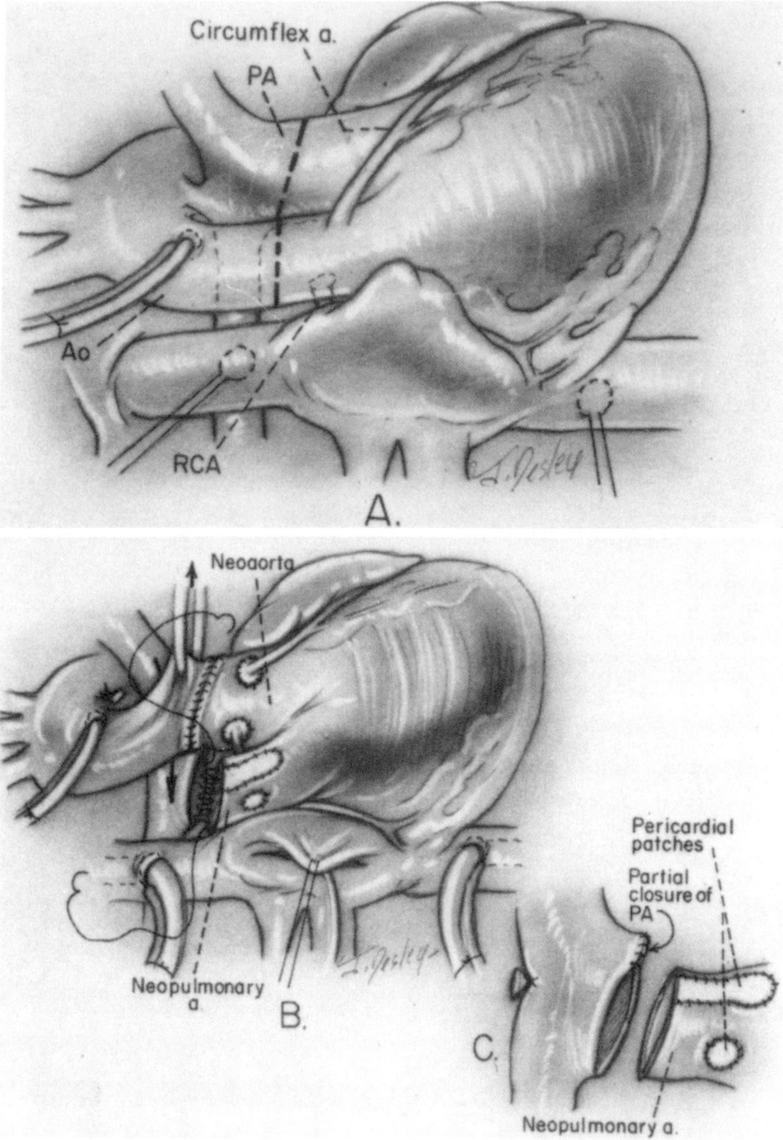

FIGURE 9. Technique for arterial switch with coronary translocation in patients with DORV and side-to-side malposition of the great arteries. The LeCompte maneuver may not be necessary after transection of the great vessels (A). The VSD may be repairable through the semilunar valves. If not, the VSD can be closed after reconstruction of the aorta with coronary transfer (B) through either a right atriotomy or a ventriculotomy. In patients with DORV and subpulmonary VSD, there is often great size discrepancy between the aorta and pulmonary artery (with the aorta being much smaller). This size discrepancy can be resolved during anastomoses of the great vessels (C). (From Quaegebeur JM: The arterial switch: An eight-year experience. J Thorac Cardiovasc Surg 92:361, 1986, with permission.)

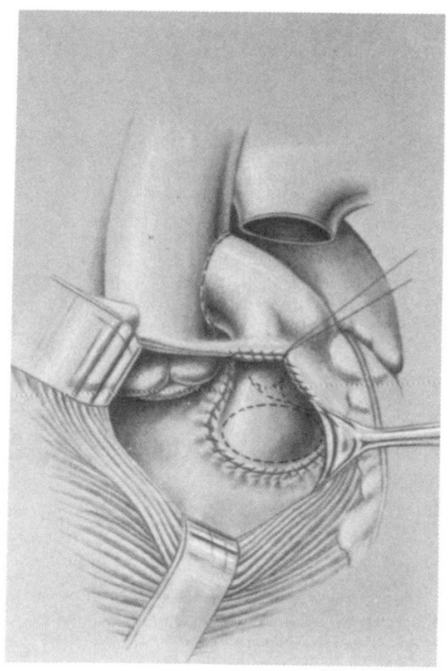

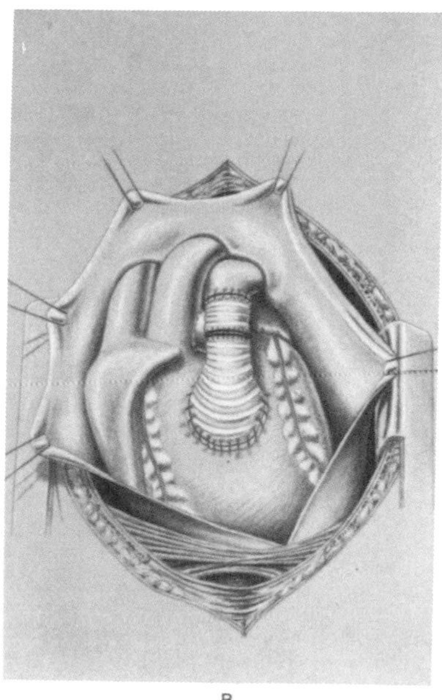

FIGURE 10. Technique for the Damus-Kaye-Stansel procedure for DORV with subpulmonary VSD. This technique is useful when there is severe subaortic or aortic valvar obstruction. *A,* The VSD is directed toward the pulmonary valve with an intracardiac patch. The pulmonary artery is then transected and the proximal pulmonary artery anastomosed to the aorta end to side. *B,* RV-PA continuity is established utilizing a valved conduit, preferably a homograft. The aortic valve should not need to be closed unless RV pressure approaches LV pressure. (From Replogle RL, Campbell DJ, Campbell CD, Arcilla RA: Double outlet ventricles. In Arciniegas E (ed): Pediatric Cardiac Surgery. Chicago, Year Book Medical Publishers, 1985, with permission.)

is established with the use of an external conduit (Fig. 11). Because symptomatic infants with DORV and subpulmonary VSDs usually require a combination of banding and shunting[35] (if palliation is chosen), our preference is to attempt early total repair, preferably with arterial switch, but with the recognition that external conduits can be safely applied to the infant population.[11] The ready availability and excellent performance of allografts further favor this approach.[1,33] In patients with severe atrioventricular valve abnormalities (i.e., straddling chordae) or other complicated pictures, it may be necessary to stage the patient toward a modified Fontan procedure.[17]

RESULTS

The trend in surgery for patients with all forms of DORV is total correction earlier in life with better survival and long-term quality of life.[19] This reflects the impact of technology on the field of pediatric cardiac surgery as a whole and is dramatically exemplified by the change in outlook for patients with complex congenital heart disease such as DORV.

Prior to the "current era," the overall risk of hospital mortality for repair of DORV (all forms) ranged from 11–40%, and was largely influenced by the type of DORV (patients with subaortic and doubly committed VSDs having a

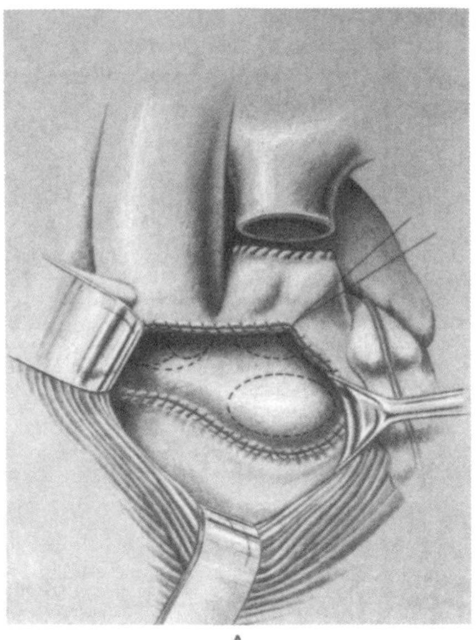

A

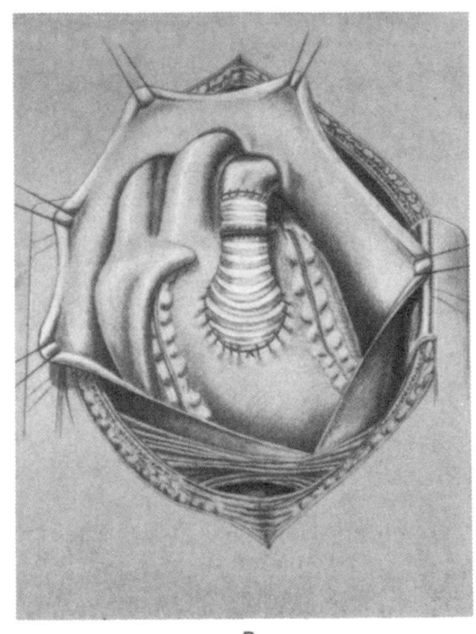

B

FIGURE 11. Technique for Rastelli repair for DORV. This is useful in cases of DORV with subpulmonary VSD associated with severe subpulmonary obstruction. *A,* The VSD is patched so that LV outflow is directed to the aortic valve. *B,* RV-PA continuity is reestablished using a valved conduit, preferably a homograft. (From Replogle RL, Campbell DJ, Campbell CD, Arcilla RA: Double outlet ventricles. In Arciniegas E (ed): Pediatric Cardiac Surgery. Chicago, Year Book Medical Publishers, 1985, with permission.)

better prognosis than those with subpulmonary VSDs), as well as by age at operation (young age being a risk factor), type of operation performed (intraventricular tunnel repairs leading to better results than atrial switch and external conduit procedures), and the presence of severe associated cardiac anomalies or of significant pulmonary hypertension.[18,36,44,47] Because of the high risk of early repair, it was considered reasonable to palliate patients: with systemic to pulmonary artery shunts (if pulmonary stenosis was present), with pulmonary artery bands (if there was no pulmonary stenosis), and with a combination of the two (for patients with subpulmonary VSDs who presented with cyanosis in the face of high pulmonary blood flow).[35] Despite these protocols, the long-term survival for patients with DORV remained a dismal 38% at 12 years (and is as low as 22% over 10 years for patients with noncommitted VSDs).[18] Late mortality was influenced by conduit stenoses, late dysrhythmias, and heart-failure—often due to progressive pulmonary hypertension.[14,17,28,47]

More recently inspected data, however, reveal an exceptionally improved prognosis for patients with all forms of DORV,[40] with the possible exception of the relatively unusual cases of remote, noncommitted VSDs.[6,18,28,39] Using intraventricular repair, as described in this chapter, for infants with subaortic or doubly committed VSDs (with VSD enlargement if indicated), an operative mortality of 5–10% should be anticipated, and can approach less than 5% if the patient is between 6 and 12 months of age.[18,28,40] Furthermore, long-term outlook for these patients after successful intraventricular patch repair is exceptionally good, with a 10-year survival of approximately 97% and an excellent quality of life.[17]

The most remarkable turnabout has been for patients with DORV and subpulmonary VSD (Taussig-Bing malformation). As recently as the mid-1980s, procedures employing VSD closure with atrial level switch (Mustard or Senning), intraventricular tunnel repair, or Damus-Kaye-Stansel reconstruction were still producing high mortality (as high as 70%).[40] This dismal outlook was further influenced by the association of this lesion with coarctation of the aorta and the tendency for these patients to develop severe pulmonary hypertension early in the course.[17,51] With adoption of protocols that offer atrial switch with coronary translocation in early infancy, 90% of infants with DORV and subpulmonary VSDs can be expected to survive the surgical repair, and the long-term outlook appears to be remarkably good.[6,15,39,60] Improved techniques for reconstruction of hypoplastic aortas in neonates has further improved the outlook for these patients.[37] Although infants with this lesion usually do not require arterial switch in the first week of life, the rapid progression to pulmonary vascular obstructive changes compels that repair be performed by 3 months of age, and this is especially true in infants with anomalies of the aortic arch. Patients with subpulmonic or subaortic stenosis may still require reconstruction using valved conduits (Rastelli or Damus-Kaye-Stansel procedure), and in these instances, early palliation may be indicated to allow placement of a larger conduit.[17] With the growing experience in allografts used as external cardiac conduits, it appears that they may last for at least 20 years before the need for replacement.[1,17] It is becoming clear that use of an atrial level switch should be avoided in these patients,[36,40] but techniques for intraventricular repair have improved.[60]

Variations of DORV exist, such as double outlet left ventricle (DOLV)[4] and DORV with atrioventricular discordance (ventricular inversion).[48] The physiologic aspects of these anomalies parallel those of DORV, and methods of repair employ many of the same concepts.[17,40]

Overall, the results for most forms of DORV include an operative mortality of 10% (or less) with excellent long-term survival and quality of life. Surgical repair early in life helps to avoid the risk of irreversible pulmonary hypertension and reduces the complications of multiple operative procedures associated with initial palliation.

REFERENCES

1. Angell WW, Angell JD, Oury JH, et al: Long-term follow-up of viable frozen aortic homografts. A viable homograft valve bank. J Thorac Cardiovasc Surg 93:815–22, 1987.
2. Barratt-Boyes BG, Lowe JB, Watt WJ, et al: Initial experiences with extracorporeal circulation in intracardiac surgery. Br Med J 2:1826, 1960.
3. Binet JP; Discussion of Judson JP, Danielson GK, Puga FJ, et al: Double-outlet right ventricle: Surgical results 1970–1980. J Thorac Cardiovasc Surg 85:32, 1983.
4. Brandt PWT, Calder AL, Barratt-Boyes BG, Neutze JM: Double-outlet left ventricle: Morphology, cineangiocardiographic diagnosis and surgical treatment. Am J Cardiol 38:897, 1976.
5. Brawn K, De Vries A, Feingold DS, et al: Complete dextroposition of the aorta, pulmonary stenosis, interventricular septal defect, and patent foramen ovale. Am Heart J 43:773, 1952.
6. Brawn WJ, Mee RBB: Early results for anatomic correction of transposition of the great arteries and for double-outlet right ventricle with subpulmonary ventricular septal defect. Ann Thorac Surg 38:433, 1984.
7. Ceithaml EL, Puga FJ, Danielson GK, et al: Results of the Damus-Stansel-Kaye procedure for transposition of the great arteries and for double-outlet right ventricle with subpulmonary ventricular septal defect. Ann Thorac Surg 38:433, 1984.

8. Chaitman BR, Grondin CM, Theroux P, Bourassa MG: Late development of left ventricular outflow tract obstruction after repair of double-outlet right ventricle. J Thorac Cardiovasc Surg 72:265, 1976.
9. Cheng TO: Double-outlet right ventricle: Diagnosis during life. Am J Med 32:637, 1962.
10. Cherian KM, John TA, Abraham KA: Transatrial correction of origin of both great vessels from the right ventricle with pulmonary hypertension. J Thorac Cardiovasc Surg 84:783, 1982.
11. Ebert PA, Robinson SJ, Stanger P, Engle MA: Pulmonary artery conduits in infants younger than six months of age. J Thorac Cardiovasc Surg 72:351, 1976.
12. Edwards WD: Double-outlet right ventricle and tetralogy of Fallot. Two distinct but not mutually exclusive entities. J Thorac Cardiovasc Surg 82:418, 1981.
13. Huhta JC (ed): Pediatric Imaging/Doppler Ultrasound of the Chest. Philadelphia, Lea & Febiger, 1986.
14. Judson JP, Danielson GK, Puga FJ, et al: Double-outlet right ventricle: Surgical results 1970–80. J Thorac Cardiovasc Surg 85:32, 1983.
15. Kanter KR, Anderson RH, Lincoln C, et al: Anatomic correction for complete transposition and double-outlet right ventricle. J Thorac Cardiovasc Surg 90:690, 1985.
16. Kirklin JW, Harp RA, McGoon DC: Surgical treatment of origin of both vessels from right ventricle, including cases of pulmonary stenosis. J Thorac Cardiovasc Surg 48:1026, 1964.
17. Kirklin JW, Barratt-Boyes BG (eds): Cardiac Surgery. New York, Wiley Medical Publications, 1986.
18. Kirklin JW, Pacifico AD, Blackstone EH, et al: Current risks and protocols for operations for double-outlet right ventricle. J Thorac Cardiovasc Surg 92:913, 1986.
19. Kirklin JW: The movement of cardiac surgery toward the very young. Presidential Address, First World Congress of Pediatric Cardiac Surgery. Diagnosis and treatment of C.H.D., Bergamo, Italy, June 19, 1988.
20. Kisslo J, Adams DB, Belkin RB (eds): Doppler Color Flow Imaging. New York, Churchill Livingstone, 1988.
21. Lavoie R, Sestier F, Gilbert G, et al: Double-outlet right ventricle with left ventricular outflow tract obstruction due to small ventricular septal defect. Am Heart J 82:290, 1971.
22. Lev M, Bharati S, Meng CCL, et al: A concept of double-outlet right ventricle. J Thorac Cardiovasc Surg 64:271, 1972.
23. Lincoln C, Anderson RH, Shinebourne EA, et al: Double-outlet right ventricle with L-malposition of the aorta. Br Heart J 37:453, 1975.
24. Ludomirsky A, Huhta JC: Color Doppler of Congenital Heart Disease in the Child and Adult. Mt. Kisco, New York, Futura Publishers, 1987.
25. Marin-Garcia J, Neches WH, Park SC, et al: Double-outlet right ventricle with restrictive ventricular septal defect. J Thorac Cardiovasc Surg 76:853, 1978.
26. Marino B, Loperfido F, Sardi CS: Spontaneous closure of ventricular septal defect in a case of double-outlet right ventricle. Br Heart J 49:608, 1983.
27. Mason DT, Morrow AG, Elkins RC, Friedman WF: Origin of both great vessels from the right ventricle associated with severe obstruction to left ventricular outflow. Am J Cardiol 24:118, 1969.
28. Mazzucco A, Faggian G, Stellin G, et al: Surgical management of double-outlet right ventricle. J Thorac Cardiovasc Surg 90:29, 1985.
29. McGoon DC: Origin of both great vessels from the right ventricle. Surg Clin North Am 41:1113, 1961.
30. McMahon JE, Lips M: Double-outlet right ventricle with intact ventricular septum. Circulation 30:745. 1964.
31. Neufeld HN, DuShane JW, Wood EH, et al: Origin of both great vessels from the right ventricle. I. Without pulmonary stenosis. Circulation 23:399, 1961.
32. Neufeld HN, DuShane JW, Edwards JE: Origin of both great vessels from the right ventricle. II. With pulmonary stenosis. Circulation 23:603, 1961.
33. O'Brien MF, Stafford EG, Gardner MAH, et al: A comparison of aortic valve replacement with viable cryopreserved and fresh allograft valves, with a note on chromosomal studies. J Thorac Cardiovasc Surg 94:812, 1987.
34. Pacifico AD, Kirklin JW, Bargeron LM: Complex congenital malformations: Surgical treatment of double outlet right ventricle and double outlet left ventricle. In Kirklin JW (ed): Advances in Cardiovascular Surgery. New York, Grune & Stratton, 1973.
35. Pacifico AD: Double outlet right ventricle: In Sabiston DC Jr (ed): Davis-Christopher Textbook of Surgery, 12th ed. Philadelphia, W.B. Saunders Co., 1981.

36. Piccoli G, Pacifico AD, Kirklin JW, et al: Changing results and concepts in the surgical treatment of double-outlet right ventricle: Analysis of 137 operations in 126 patients. Am J Cardiol 52:549, 1983.
37. Pigott JD, Chin AJ, Weinberg PM, et al: Transposition of the great arteries with aortic obstruction: Anatomical review and report of surgical management. J Thorac Cardiovasc Surg 94:82, 1987.
38. Quaegebeur JM: The optimal repair for the Taussig-Bing heart. J Thorac Cardiovasc Surg 85:276, 1983.
39. Quaegebeur JM, Rohmer J, Ottenkamp J, et al: The arterial switch operation. An eight-year experience. J Thorac Cardiovasc Surg 92:361, 1986.
40. Replogle RL, Campbell DJ, Campbell CD, Arcilla RA: Double-outlet ventricles. In Arciniegas E (ed): Pediatric Cardiac Surgery. Chicago, Year Book Medical Publishers, 1985.
41. Rosenquist GC, Clark EB, Sweeney LJ, et al: The normal spectrum of mitral and aortic valve discontinuity. Circulation 54:298, 1976.
42. Serratto M, Arevalo F, Goldman EJ, et al: Obstructive ventricular septal defect in double-outlet right ventricle. Am J Cardiol 19:457, 1967.
43. Singh A, Letsky EA, Stark J: Hemolysis following correction of double-outlet right ventricle. J Thorac Cardiovasc Surg 71:226, 1976.
44. Sondheimer HM, Freedom RM, Olley PM: Double-outlet right ventricle: Clinical spectrum and prognosis. Am J Cardiol 39:709, 1977.
45. Sridaromont S, Ritter DG, Feldt RH, et al: Double-outlet right ventricle. Anatomic and angiocardiographic correlations. Mayo Clinic Proc 53:555, 1978.
46. Stark J, de Leval M (eds): Surgery for Congenital Heart Defects. London, Grune & Stratton, 1983.
47. Stewart RW, Kirklin JW, Pacifico AD, et al: Repair of double-outlet right ventricle: An analysis of 62 cases. J Thorac Cardiovasc Surg 78:502, 1979.
48. Tabry IF, McGoon DC, Danielson GK, et al: Surgical management of double-outlet right ventricle associated with atrioventricular discordance. J Thorac Cardiovasc Surg 76:336, 1978.
49. Taussig HB, Bing JF: Complete transposition of the aorta and a levoposition of the pulmonary artery: Clinical, physiological, and pathological findings. Am Heart J 37:551, 1949.
50. Tynan MJ, Becker AE, Macartney FJ, et al: Nomenclature and classification of congenital heart disease. Br Heart J 41:544, 1979.
51. Ungerleider RM, Sabiston DC Jr: Double-outlet right ventricle. In Sabiston, DC Jr (ed): Essentials of Surgery. Philadelphia, W.B. Saunders Co., 1987.
52. Ungerleider RM, Ebert PA: Midline approach to aortic coarctation in infants and children. Ann Thorac Surg 44:517, 1987.
53. Ungerleider RM, Greeley WJ, Philips J, Kisslo A: Routine intraoperative color flow imaging prevents surgically unacceptable results in the repair of congenital heart lesions. In press.
54. Van Praagh R: What is the Taussig-Bing malformation? (editorial). Circulation 38:445, 1968.
55. Van Praagh R, Perez-Trevino C, Reynolds JL, et al: Double-outlet right ventricle (S.D.L.) with subaortic ventricular septal defect and pulmonary stenosis. Pediatr Cardiol 35:42, 1975.
56. Venables AW, Campbell PE: Double-outlet right ventricle: A review of 16 cases with 10 necropsy specimens. Br Heart J 28:461, 1966.
57. Wedemeyer AL, Lucas RV, Castaneda AR: Taussig-Bing malformation, coarctation of the aorta, and reversed patent ductus arteriosus. Circulation 42:1021, 1970.
58. Wilcox BR, Ho SY, Macartney FJ, et al: Surgical anatomy of double-outlet right ventricle and situs solitus and atrioventricular concordance. J Thorac Cardiovasc Surg 82:405, 1981.
59. Withan AC: Double-outlet right ventricle: A partial transposition complex. Am Heart J 53:928, 1957.
60. Yacoub MH, Radley-Smith R: Anatomic correction of the Taussig-Bing anomaly. J Thorac Cardiovasc Surg 88:380, 1984.
61. Zamora R, Moller JH, Edwards JE: Double-outlet right ventricle. Anatomic types and associated anomalies. Chest 68:672, 1975.

L. DOUGLAS COWGILL, MD

TRICUSPID ATRESIA

A. Presentation and Palliative Procedures

From the Department of Surgery
Dean Clinic
Madison, Wisconsin

Reprint requests to:
L. Douglas Cowgill, MD
Department of Surgery
Dean Clinic
1313 Fish Hatchery Rd.
Madison, WI 53715

Tricuspid atresia is an uncommon cause of cyanotic heart disease, occurring when there is absence or imperforation of the tricuspid valve. There may be many anatomical variations, with three additional abnormalities always present: (1) patency of the interatrial septum, (2) hyperplasia of the mitral valve and left ventricle, and (3) hypoplasia or absence of the right ventricle.

Tricuspid atresia was reported in 1817 by Kreysig,[1] and constitutes approximately 3% of congenital heart anomalies seen post mortem (Table 1).[2] It is the most common cause of hypoplasia of the right ventricle.

EMBRYOLOGY

The embryologic cause of tricuspid atresia is uncertain, but according to Van Praagh and coworkers it results from developmental arrest during formation of the right ventricle, leading to rightward shift of the ventricular septum, thereby obliterating the right atrioventricular orifice.[3] The observation by Rosenquist and associates that the dimple on the floor of the right atrium (the presumed center of the atretic valve) transilluminates into the left ventricle supports this concept of right ventricular hypoplasia causing rightward shift of the ventricular septum.[4] With further rightward shift of the septum, the tricuspid valve is spared and double-inlet left ventricle or common ventricle with right-sided outflow chamber results.

The embryologic morphology of the ventricular chambers in tricuspid atresia is controversial. Bharati and associates believe that tricuspid atresia is a variant of the hypoplastic

TABLE 1. Incidence of Tricuspid Atresia in Postmortem Cases

Author	No. of Autopsies	Tricuspid Atresia	Percent
Abbott (1936)	1000	21	2.1
Gibson and Clifton (1938)	105	1	1.0
Edwards and Burchell (1949)	212	4	1.9
Sommers and Johnson (1951)	141	6	4.3
Donzelot and D'Allaines (1954)	95	5	5.3
Hospital for Sick Children, Toronto (1954)	574	29	5.1
Nadas and Fyler (1972)	1017	29	3
Total	3144	95	3.02

From Keith JD, Rowe RD, Vlad R: Heart Disease in Infancy and Childhood. New York, MacMillan, 1967, p. 644, with permission.

right heart complex, comparable to hearts with tricuspid stenosis or pulmonary atresia with intact ventricular septum.[5] Their subsequent report on the conduction system in tricuspid atresia supported this view, in that it differs from that found in univentricular heart with outlet chamber.[6]

On the other hand, Anderson and colleagues contend that the majority of cases of tricuspid atresia are univentricular heart, the anterior chamber being a rudimentary chamber of right ventricular type comparable to that seen in single ventricle with outlet chamber, but distinguishable from a true right ventricle by the absence of valvular tension apparatus, normal conduction pathways, and potential communication between the rudimentary chamber and right atrium.[7] Only in the minority of cases of tricuspid atresia, where a fibrous membrane separates the right atrium from a truly hypoplastic right ventricle, do the latter features exist.[7,8] A subsequent report supported this view by finding similar coronary artery and ventricular morphology patterns between tricuspid atresia and univentricular heart, both being different from those seen in pulmonary atresia with intact ventricular septum.[9]

Currently, it seems unlikely that any classification grouping tricuspid atresia with other entities will ever be totally successful. More recently Anderson and associates have recommended a change in terminology for univentricular hearts, since this term is imprecise.[10] They argue that in most hearts having received this label it is not the ventricle that is univentricular (as there is also a rudimentary chamber) but the atrioventricular connection, and recommend the term univentricular atrioventricular connection for hearts in which the atria connect to only one ventricle (which would include most cases of tricuspid atresia as well as double-inlet ventricle).

ANATOMY

Common Features

There is complete agenesis of the tricuspid orifice, but this may be variable in type. Van Praagh and associates[3] first described three types: (1) muscular, (2) fibrous (membranous) and (3) Ebstein's, and subsequently added two additional types: (4) valvular, and (5) atrioventricular canal type.[11] This classification was subsequently used by Weinberg.[12]

The most common type is muscular atresia in which there is no evidence of valve tissue and a solid muscular atrial floor is present, often with a central dimple opposite the morphologic left ventricle. This type represented 84%[3] and 76%[12] of the cases of tricuspid atresia in the series cited. A similar type is membranous or fibrous atresia, in which the atrioventricular portion of the membranous septum (between the right atrium and left ventricle) appears in the usual location of the tricuspid valve, representing 8%[8] and 12%[12] of cases in these series. This type is commonly associated with juxtaposition of the atrial appendages. The valvular type was present in 6% of Weinberg's cases,[12] and is characterized by a thin membrane of valve tissue, sometimes with rudimentary chordae but with no atrioventricular orifice. The valvular type is distinguished from the membranous type in that the former is located above the right ventricle, not the left ventricle. Ebstein's type (in which there is downward displacement of an atretic valve, opposite the right ventricle) was present in 8% of Van Praagh's cases[3] and in 6% of Weinberg's.[12] Others have found this type as infrequently as 2.5% of cases of tricuspid atresia.[7,13] The atrioventricular canal type was mentioned briefly by Van Praagh,[11] and occurs when a leaflet of the common atrioventricular valve completely seals the only entrance into the right ventricle. This type is exceedingly rare, and was not found in Van Praagh's original series[3] or in the others cited.[7,12]

It has been noted that this classification has limited clinical value in that the muscular, membranous, and valvular types are indistinguishable hemodynamically and angiographically, and are treated identically surgically.[14] The Ebstein variety can usually be distinguished angiographically, and may be amenable to valvular excision and replacement with a prosthetic valve.

The interatrial septal defect is usually of the fossa ovalis type and is not usually restrictive. Bharati and colleagues found the atrial septal defect was a secundum (fossa ovalis) type in 87% of patients with tricuspid atresia without transposition, a patent foramen ovale in 7%, an ostium primum defect in 2%, sinus venosus in 1%, and common atrium in 3%.[5] Rarely aneurysmal dilatation of the interatrial septum may develop and has been associated with mitral valve[15,16] and pulmonary venous[17] obstruction.

The mitral valve and left ventricle are always large, reflecting the chronic volume overload of the left heart. The mitral valve is normally situated, typically bicuspid and competent, rarely with more than two cusps. The left ventricle is thick, finely trabeculated, and deviates the left anterior descending coronary artery and ventricular septum well to the right.

The right ventricle is always hypoplastic, but can vary according to size of ventricular septal defect, presence of transposition, amount of pulmonary blood flow, and type of atretic valve. Since the left anterior descending coronary artery is shifted rightward, the small right ventricle lies between the right atrium and left anterior descending coronary artery. The anterior free wall is thin, and there is a two-compartment ventricle, infundibular and trabecular. The infundibular chamber is superior and tubular, has a smooth, thin endocardium, and its diameter is closely related to that of the pulmonary valve and artery to which it leads. The more proximal trabecular portion of the right ventricle is rough and coarse, contains the ventricular septal defect (usually single but occasionally multiple), and may be separated from the infundibular portion by a narrow opening resembling an os infundibulum. Usually the larger the ventricular septal defect, the larger the right ventricle. The ventricular septal defect is usually situated below the infundibular or conal septum, and above the membranous septum. As with other ventricular septal defects, it may close spontaneously and is a common cause of worsening cyanosis and deterioration in a previously stable patient. In a minority of patients, usually those with valvular or Ebstein's type of tricuspid atresia, there may be a true sinus portion of a right ventricle, in potential communication with the right atrium.

In tricuspid atresia patients with transposition, the right ventricle is usually longer and most often is a single smooth-walled cavity without a proximal trabeculated portion. The ventricular septal defect is usually large and may be nearly subaortic in location.

CLASSIFICATION/VARIABLE FEATURES

Tricuspid atresia is normally classified according to two variables, the relationship of the great arteries and status of pulmonary blood flow. Kuhne in 1906 first classified tricuspid atresia into two groups, with and without transposition of the great vessels.[18] Edwards and Burchell subsequently divided each group into two subgroups according to the degree of restriction, if any, of pulmonary blood flow.[19]

The most popular classification is that of Keith and associates, which adds a third group, those with L-transposition, and has eight types all together (Fig. 1).[20,21] Types I (normally related arteries) and II (D-transposition of the great arteries) are further subdivided according to the status of the pulmonary arteries into (a) pulmonary atresia, (b) pulmonary hypoplasia, and (c) no pulmonary artery hypoplasia. In Type I cases the ventricular septal defect is absent in subgroup a (intact ventricular septum), small in subgroup b, and large in subgroup c. In Type II, a large ventricular septal defect is found in all groups, but the degree of subpulmonic stenosis is variable. Type III (L-transposition of the great arteries) is subdivided into two groups: (a) pulmonary or subpulmonary stenosis and (b) aortic stenosis.

Tandon and Edwards proposed an alternative classification in 1974, which added another type for tricuspid atresia associated with truncus arteriosus.[22] Most recently, Rao in 1980 proposed a classification that takes all types of malpositions of the great arteries into account, and has 24 types in all (Table 2).[14]

Tricuspid Atresia with Normally Related Great Arteries

Approximately 70% of patients with tricuspid atresia will have normally related arteries (Table 3).[5,21] In approximately 85% of patients there will be restriction of pulmonary blood flow. Type Ib is most common and constitutes over 50% of all types of tricuspid atresia. In approximately 10% of Type I patients the pulmonary valve is atretic, while in another 15% there is a large ventricular septal defect with no restriction to pulmonary blood flow (Type Ic).

The atria are nearly always situs solitus.[9] The right atrium is hypertrophied and often enlarged, and always contains an interatrial septal defect that is restrictive in less than 5% of patients. A left superior vena cava draining into the coronary sinus was found in 15% of Type I patients by Bharati et al.,[5] which is important to exclude should a Glenn shunt be contemplated. They also found aneurysm of the fossa ovalis in 10% of Type I patients. The eustachian valve is often hypertrophied, and in approximately 5% of patients becomes a superiorly-extending veil that divides the right atrium into two chambers, the so-called cor triatriatum dexter, which can be quite confusing at operation.

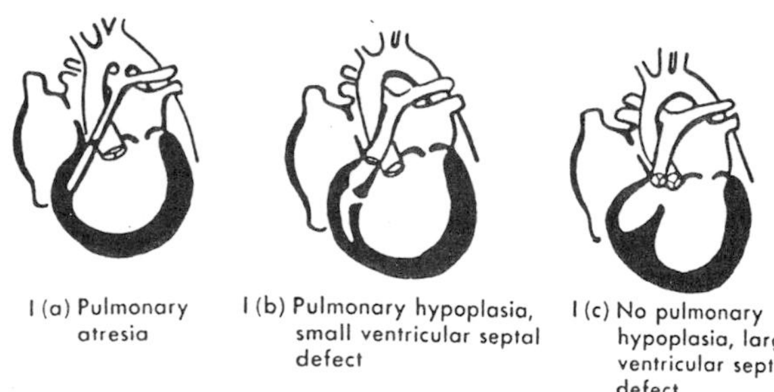

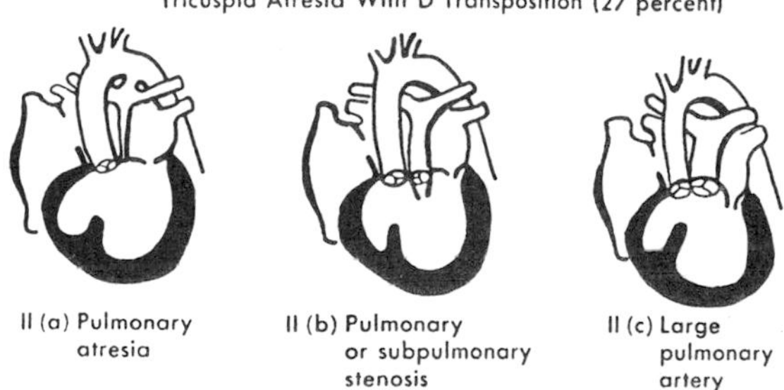

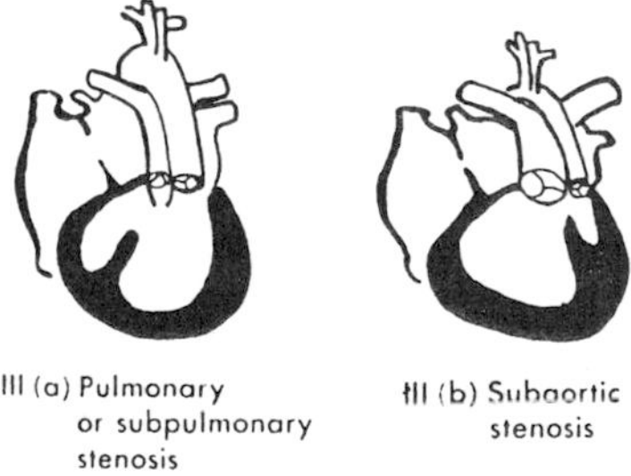

FIGURE 1. Classification of tricuspid atresia according to relationship of great arteries and degree of restriction to pulmonary blood flow, with relative incidences in parentheses. (From Keith JD, Rowe RD, Vlad P: Heart Disease in Infancy and Childhood. New York, MacMillan, 1978, p. 518, with permission.)

The left atrium, mitral valve, and left ventricle are hypertrophied. The severity of right ventricular hypoplasia depends upon the size of the ventricular septal defect. In cases of pulmonary atresia (Type Ia), it is extremely small and may be apparent only at microscopic examination. More commonly, as in Type Ib, it is a small, two-compartment (infundibular and trabecular) ventricle with the features described above. The obstruction to pulmonary blood flow occurring in Type Ib patients may be at the ventricular septal defect, more commonly at the os infundibulum (junction of trabecular and infundibular ventricular compartments), or throughout the entire infundibulum. In Type Ic patients the

TABLE 2. A New Classification of Tricuspid Atresia

Type I: Normally related great arteries

Type II: D-transposition of the great arteries

Type III: Malpositions of the great arteries other than D transposition
- Subtype 1. L-transposition of the great arteries
- Subtype 2. Double-outlet right ventricle
- Subtype 3. Double-outlet left ventricle
- Subtype 4. D-malposition of the great arteries (anatomically corrected malposition)
- Subtype 5. L-malposition of the great arteries (anatomically corrected malposition)

Type IV: Persistent truncus arteriosus

Each Type and Subtype are divided
- Subgroup a. Pulmonary atresia
- Subgroup b. Pulmonary stenosis or hypoplasia
- Subgroup c. Normal pulmonary arteries (no pulmonary stenosis)

Am Heart J 99:799, 1980, with permission.

ventricular septal defect is larger than normal, the right ventricle is less hypoplastic, and there is no infundibular stenosis.

Pulmonary valve and pulmonary artery anatomy also depend on the type. In most Type Ib cases the pulmonary valve is smaller than normal but larger than most cases of tetralogy of Fallot.[5] Bharati et al. found it to be bicuspid and markedly thickened in 48% of Type Ib patients, diaphragm-like in 1%, and absent in 1%.[5] Although somewhat smaller than normal, the valve is usually not obstructive to pulmonary blood flow. Likewise, the main, left, and right pulmonary arteries are slightly smaller than normal but hypoplastic and restrictive

TABLE 3. Relative Frequency of the Anatomic Types—143 Anatomic Specimens

	Literature	The Hospital for Sick Children	Total
I. Without transposition of the great arteries	61	38	99 (69%)
a. Pulmonary atresia	9	4	13
b. Pulmonary hypoplasia Small ventricular septal defect	43	30	73
c. No pulmonary hypoplasia Left ventricular septal defect	9	4	13
II. With D-transposition of the great arteries	31	9	40 (27%)
a. Pulmonary atresia	1	2	3
b. Pulmonary or subpulmonary stenosis	10	1	11
c. Large pulmonary artery	20	6	26
III. With L-transposition of the great arteries	—	4	4 (3%)
a. Pulmonary or subpulmonary stenosis	—	1	1
b. Subaortic stenosis	—	3	3

From Keith JD, Rowe RD, Vlad R: Heart Disease in Infancy and Childhood. New York, MacMillan, 1967, p. 644, with permission.

to flow in less than 5% of patients. In Type Ia patients, the pulmonary valve by definition is atretic and the main, left, and right pulmonary arteries are small, perfused by either a patent ductus arteriosus or aortopulmonary collateral artery. In Type Ic, by definition, there is no pulmonary hypoplasia.

The coronary arteries are normally distributed, typically right-dominant, with the left anterior descending deviated rightward. The conduction system is affected by the atretic tricuspid valve but approaches normal.[6,23] The atrioventricular node is situated adjacent to the central fibrous body in the floor of the right atrium, indicated by the "dimple" previously mentioned, between the coronary sinus and tendon of Todaro. The node then pierces the abnormal central fibrous body to form the bundle of His on the left ventricular side of the septum, coursing on the posterior leftward side of the ventricular septal defect. The more anterior the ventricular septal defect, the further to the left and away from the defect is the His bundle. The left bundle comes off the main His bundle proximally, while the right bundle is elongated, crossing back to the right on the inferior aspect of the ventricular septal defect where it is vulnerable to injury, then descending almost perpendicularly from a subendocardial position toward the apex of the right ventricle.[24]

One other anomaly with surgical significance, particularly since the advent of Fontan repair, is the association of coronary sinus septal defects (unroofed coronary sinus). Rumisek and coworkers found a 3.6% incidence of coronary sinus septal defects, two of which were discovered postoperatively following a Fontan procedure, in which a previously unrecognized and innocent defect allowed significant postoperative right-to-left shunting as a result of the normally increased right atrial pressures occurring after Fontan repair.[25]

The importance of recognizing tricuspid atresia with Ebstein's malformation has been discussed. With this type of tricuspid atresia the right ventricle, although still hypoplastic, is in potential communication with the right atrium and may be large enough to function satisfactorily following prosthetic replacement of the atretic tricuspid valve.[26]

Tricuspid Atresia with D-Transposition of the Great Arteries

D-transposition of the great arteries with tricuspid atresia (Type II), in which the aorta is anterior and to the right with the pulmonary artery posterior and to the left, occurred in 27% of Keith and associates' patients (Table 3).[20,21] The transposition was complete in approximately two-thirds of patients and partial in the remainder (the latter most often with the aorta overriding the ventricular septum and arising partially from the left ventricle).

As already noted, the right ventricle tends to be larger and thicker than in Type I, and instead of two compartments it is normally one compartment with smooth lining, which may appear as a mere diverticulum of the large left ventricle. The ventricular septal defect is large, more anterior than in Type I and may be nearly subaortic. The atria are normally situs solitus, but Bharati and coworkers noted juxtaposition of the atrial appendages in 12.8% of transposition patients.[5] The atrial septal defect is more frequently restrictive—nearly 50% of patients in Weinberg's experience.[12]

Unlike that in Type I patients, pulmonary blood flow in Type II is normally unrestricted and often excessive, with relative percentages of atretic, stenotic, or normal pulmonary annuli of 7.5% (IIa), 27.5% (IIb), and 65% (IIc).[20,21] In Type IIc, the pulmonary artery is large while the aorta may be relatively hypoplastic. The pulmonary valve may be bicuspid, but not as frequently as in Type Ib.

In Type IIa, the pulmonary arteries are small, usually perfused by a patent ductus arteriosus. For the more common Type IIb patients, the pulmonary stenosis may be valvar, subvalvar, or a combination of the two. Isolated subpulmonary stenosis is most common.[20,21] Overriding of the ventricular septum by the aorta is occasionally present in Type IIb and may contribute to pulmonary stenosis.

Abnormalities of the aortic arch are the most common associated anomalies in Type II. Bharati and coworkers found aortic coarctation in 34% of patients with tricuspid atresia with transposition, interrupted arch in 4.3%, and right aortic arch in 6.4%.[5] Aneurysm of the fossa ovalis was also common, being present in 17%. The coronary arteries most often originate from the posterior sinus of Valsalva.

Tricuspid Atresia with L-Transposition of the Great Arteries

L-transposition of the great arteries associated with tricuspid atresia (Type III), in which the aorta arises anterior and to the left of the pulmonary artery, is uncommon and was found in only 3% by Keith and associates,[20,21] and in 8.8% by Tandon and coworkers.[27] Of the two types in this category, that with subaortic stenosis (IIIb) is more common than with pulmonary or subpulmonary stenosis (IIIa). Consequently cyanosis is an uncommon feature in Type III.

The most common ventricular arrangement in Type III is without ventricular inversion, but the latter (corrected transposition) may occur, in which the anatomic right ventricle lies on the left and the anatomic left ventricle lies on the right.[20,21,27] This latter arrangement makes the description "tricuspid atresia" confusing, since it involves the left atrioventricular valve.[27]

Miscellaneous Anatomical Variations

Truncus arteriosus is rarely associated with tricuspid atresia.[22,28] Absent pulmonary valve with tricuspid atresia and intact ventricular septum has been reported and usually presents with cyanosis.[29-32] Unlike absent pulmonary valve and tetralogy of Fallot, bronchial compression and pulmonary dysfunction do not occur. Tricuspid atresia with double-inlet left atrium (duplicated mitral valve) has also been reported.[33]

CLINICAL FEATURES

The most common presenting feature of tricuspid atresia is cyanosis, since over 70% of patients have diminished pulmonary blood flow. The cyanosis is present on the first day of life in 50% of patients,[34] and the age at which cyanosis becomes apparent is prognostically important. Keith and associates found that cyanosis occurring in the first 30 days has an 80% mortality by age 6 months, whereas onset after 1 month of age resulted in an average life span of over 4 years.[21] When cyanosis appears at an older age, it generally means closure of the ventricular septal defect and/or os infundibulum, which may lead to a relatively rapid deterioration from diminished pulmonary blood flow.

Clubbing is very common, being apparent in most cyanotic patients by 2 years of age, and may be present as early as 3 months. Squatting may occur but is infrequent. Dyspnea and exercise intolerance are very frequent, apparent in babies with crying or feeding.

Most patients with tricuspid atresia (over 80%) have a murmur, usually a loud, harsh precordial systolic murmur but occasionally soft.[21] It arises from the ventricular septal defect and may lessen in intensity as the defect closes or right ventricular outflow tract obstruction develops. A thrill is palpable in approximately 20% of patients. A continuous murmur suggests associated patent ductus arteriosus, which in turn suggests pulmonary atresia. As with early onset of cyanosis, an absent murmur with tricuspid atresia is a poor prognostic sign, with few survivors over 1 year of age.

Apical, mid-diastolic rumbles across the mitral valve are usually indicative of increased pulmonary flow, and consequently most commonly indicate tricuspid atresia with transposition of the great arteries. Disappearance of this murmur suggests spontaneous ventricular septal defect closure in a patient without transposition. The pulmonary second sound varies with the amount of pulmonary blood flow, being single with diminished flow and split with increased flow.

Symptoms of right heart failure, such as hepatomegaly with pulsatile liver, distended neck veins, and peripheral edema, suggest restriction of the interatrial septal defect. Taussig recognized that liver pulsations occurring in conjunction with a diminutive right ventricle suggested tricuspid atresia with restrictive atrial septal defect.[35] These symptoms are more common in transposition patients, since the atrial septal defect is more frequently restrictive.[12]

Congestive failure with pulmonary plethora occurs most commonly in tricuspid atresia patients with transposition of the great arteries. It may be severe and associated with the above symptoms of right heart failure. An apical, mid-diastolic rumble and fixed splitting of the second heart sound may be audible. When associated with subaortic obstruction, a particularly lethal situation is present.

DIAGNOSTIC METHODS

Chest X-Ray

The chest x-ray varies according to the amount of pulmonary blood flow and relationship of the great arteries. Keith and associates described five patterns for heart size and configuration:[21]

1. *Characteristic.* Most common for Type Ib, as described by Taussig,[35] there is flattening of the right heart border with a normal-sized heart, and concave upper left heart border due to pulmonary artery hypoplasia (Fig. 2). The lower left heart border is enlarged, consistent with left ventricular hypertrophy. The vascular pedicle is narrow. The lung fields are oligemic. In the left anterior oblique view, the small size of the right ventricle is indicated by the absence of cardiac shadow anterior to that of the aorta.[35]

2. *"Coeur en Sabot."* The apex is less blunt and high, the upper left concavity more prominent, and the right heart border more convex and prominent, resembling tetralogy of Fallot.

3. *"Egg on its Side."* For patients with transposition of the great arteries, the heart has the characteristic "egg on its side" appearance with a very narrow vascular pedicle, and may be indistinguishable from transposition of the great arteries without tricuspid atresia. In cases with L-transposition, the upper left border is formed by the ascending aorta.

4. *Variable.* In some cases, for example in cases with dextrocardia, the x-ray may be abnormal but not fit into any of the above three categories.

5. *Normal.* Occasionally, patients with tricuspid atresia have absolutely normal chest x-rays. These are usually patients with balanced pulmonary and systemic circulations.

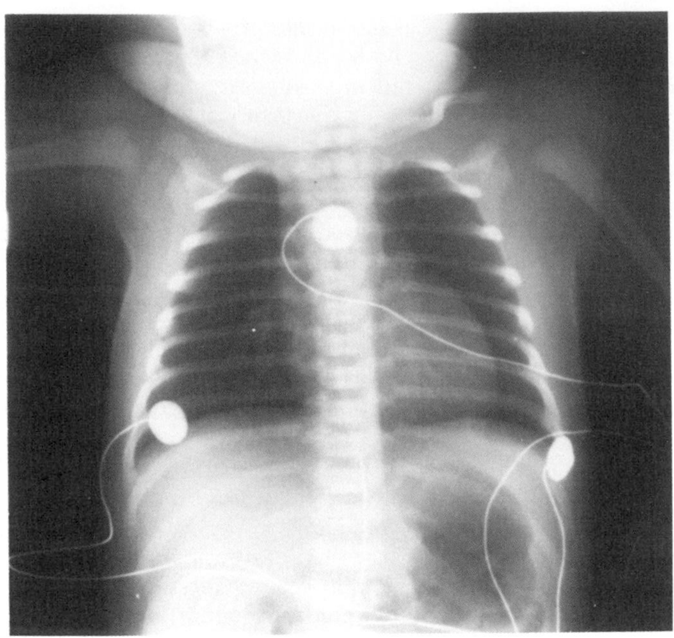

FIGURE 2. Characteristic chest x-ray of infant with Type Ib tricuspid atresia.

In most patients, the lung fields are oligemic, and it may be impossible to identify hilar shadows, especially in small infants. The lung fields may have more markings if and when the child grows due to development of bronchial collaterals. Plethoric lung fields and congestive failure have been discussed, and usually indicate associated transposition of the great arteries. A right aortic arch is present in approximately 8% of patients.[21]

Electrocardiogram

Left axis deviation will be present in over 80% of patients with tricuspid atresia and normally related arteries, and in a cyanotic patient has great diagnostic value.[35] The QRS axis is between 0° and –90° with a superior, counterclockwise frontal vector loop. Left ventricular hypertrophy is virtually always present. The P waves are abnormally high in infants (reflecting right atrial hypertrophy), and with growth evidence of combined atrial hypertrophy develops with prominent, notched P waves with a taller initial peak (P tricuspidale). Vectorcardiography most commonly shows a narrow loop in the horizontal plane with a figure-of-eight contour and small QRS forces.

Patients with associated transposition of the great arteries less commonly show left axis deviation, and normal QRS axis between 0° and +90° is present in more than half of patients. Vectorcardiograms in these patients show a wide QRS loop with large vector forces directed posterior and to the left. Right axis deviation occurs rarely, and strongly suggests transposition of the great arteries.

Echocardiography

The characteristic features in tricuspid atresia by M-mode echocardiogram include a minute right ventricle, large left ventricle, and absence of tricuspid valve

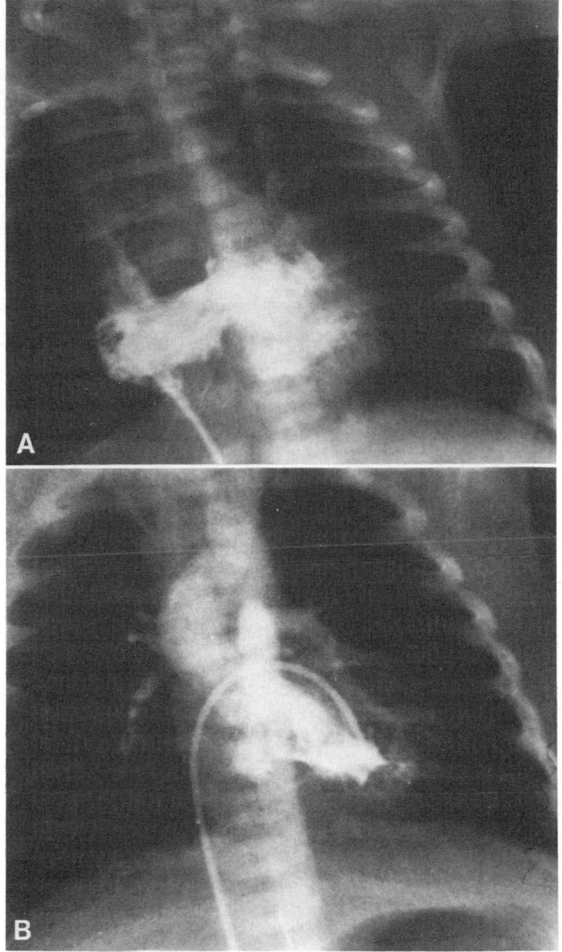

FIGURE 3. *A,* Cineangiogram of Type Ib patient whose chest x-ray is shown in Figure 2. Both major angiograpahic findings are apparent here: (1) the sequence of opacification of the right atrium, left atrium, and left ventricle with (2) the "right ventricular window" showing the nonopacified right ventricle in early films. *B,* Left ventriculogram of same patient, demonstrating the ventricular septal defect and filling of the hypoplastic right ventricle and pulmonary arteries. Following an initial systemic–pulmonary artery shunt, this patient eventually had successful incorporation of the right ventricle into a modified Fontan repair using atrioventricular anastomosis and VSD closure.

echo.[36-38] Two dimensional echocardiography is more definitive, and demonstrates a thick tricuspid area echo without diastolic opening motion and an anterior leaflet of the mitral valve attached to the interatrial septum.[39-42] The latter can also be used to distinguish the more common muscular variety of tricuspid atresia from the membranous type in which potential, direct communication between the right atrium and right ventricle is possible.[41,42]

Angiography and Cardiac Catheterization

The two major cineangiographic signs of tricuspid atresia are the typical sequence of opacification of the heart chambers and the nonopacified area cast by the right ventricle (Fig. 3A), as described by Campbell and Hills[43] and Cooley and associates.[44] The typical "tricuspid atresia sequence" shows contrast filling the right atrium, left atrium, left ventricle and then the great arteries. This sequence is not specific for tricuspid atresia, however, and can be seen with pulmonary atresia with intact ventricular septum, tricuspid hypoplasia, severe pulmonic stenosis with patent foramen ovale, and occasionally tetralogy of Fallot with atrial septal defect (pentalogy).

The nonopacified right ventricle ("right ventricular window") presents as a triangular zone on the frontal view with the base of the triangle being the diaphragm, the right side outlined by the right atrium or inferior vena cava and the left side outlined by the left ventricle. This triangular zone may fill on later films.

In addition to demonstrating the septal defects and size of right ventricle, cine angiography reveals the relationship of the great arteries as well as the degree, if any, of pulmonary hypoplasia. The side of the arch will be apparent, as well as associated coarctation of the aorta if present. Ebstein's anomaly causing tricuspid atresia has a characteristic appearance, with a blind smooth pouch (the atrialized right ventricle) extending downward from the floor of the right atrium, and the left border of the opacified right atrium extending more to the left than is usual for tricuspid atresia.[3,26] In patients with the rarely associated absent pulmonary valve syndrome, late visualization of the right ventricle occurs due to absence of the pulmonic valve.[32]

The left ventriculogram is very important to assess left ventricular contractility and mitral valve function (Fig. 3B). Elevated end-diastolic volume is characteristic, and diminished ejection fraction is frequently noted. Nishioka and coworkers found that 12 of 13 patients with tricuspid atresia had significant elevations of left ventricular end-diastolic pressure (LVEDP) and left ventricular mass, and ejection fractions diminished on average to 56% (compared to normal controls with 69% ejection fraction).[45] LaCorte and coworkers also found that patients with tricuspid atresia commonly experienced significant left ventricular dysfunction as a consequence of longstanding volume overload and chronic hypoxemia, which was most severe in patients with systemic to pulmonary artery shunts for more than 10 years.[46]

Cardiac catheterization often shows a prominent A-wave, and may demonstrate an interatrial pressure gradient if the atrial septal defect is restrictive. Because of the obligatory right-to-left shunt, similar oxygen saturations are often found in the left atrium, left ventricle, pulmonary artery, and aorta.

Other Diagnostic Maneuvers

Radionuclide angiography is useful to evaluate ventricular function in patients with tricuspid atresia. Horwitz and associates found an average ejection fraction of 54% in patients with tricuspid atresia prior to corrective surgery, nearly identical to that found above with contrast ventriculography.[47] Baker and coworkers also found significant depression of ejection fraction by radionuclide measurement (average ejection fraction 51%). Patients with tricuspid atresia with prior shunt or pulmonary artery band procedures had significantly lower ejection fraction (47%) compared to patients with tricuspid atresia who had no prior surgery (56% average ejection fraction).[48] There was no significant correlation between ejection fraction and age, arterial oxygen saturation, or hemoglobin concentration. Magnetic resonance imaging has recently been used to differentiate the classical form of tricuspid atresia, in which atrioventricular connection is absent, from the rare type in which the tricuspid valve is imperforate.[49]

NATURAL HISTORY

Tricuspid atresia is one of the most serious congenital cardiac diseases, and most patients without the benefit of surgical treatment die early in life. Keith and coworkers found that, for all types, 66% of untreated patients died by age 1 year and 90% by 10 years of age.[21]

The prognosis depends on the degree of obstruction to pulmonary blood flow. Dick and coworkers found that 90% of untreated Type Ia and Ib patients died by 1 year of age.[34] The correlation of early cyanosis with bad prognosis was discussed above. As would be expected, patients with pulmonary atresia (Ia), even with a patent ductus arteriosus, have a shorter average life span ($2^2/_3$ months) than those with pulmonary stenosis (Ib—average 11 months). In patients who are not initially cyanotic but become so with growth, spontaneous closure of the ventricular septal defect is the usual reason for deterioration. Rao found that spontaneous ventricular septal defect closure occurred in 42% of patients, most commonly Type I, and was a common reason for deterioration in a previously stable patient.[50,51]

Patients with normally related arteries without restricted pulmonary blood flow (Ic) have the best prognosis, their life expectancy averaging 8 years.[21] However, these patients may occasionally die in infancy from congestive failure, and likewise may deteriorate with cyanosis in later life due to spontaneous closure of the ventricular septal defect.

Most patients with associated transposition of the great arteries have severely increased pulmonary blood flow, and the majority die by the age of 1 year (IIc). Any tendency to closure of the ventricular septal defect in these patients only worsens the pulmonary plethora. Warnes and Somerville reviewed long-term survivors with Type II tricuspid atresia, and found that the development of subaortic stenosis and arrhythmias were common causes of late mortality and morbidity.[52]

Along with Type Ic, the other group with a relatively good prognosis is that with transposition of the great vessels with pulmonary or subpulmonary stenosis (Type IIb). Their average life span is approximately 7 years. Regardless of type, virtually all reports of long-term survivors with tricuspid atresia without surgery are those with a natural balance between pulmonary and systemic blood flow.[53-56] Additionally, for long-term survivors the development of left ventricular dysfunction secondary to chronic hypoxia and volume overload, as discussed above, becomes an important function in late morbidity and mortality.

TREATMENT

Initial therapy for most patients with tricuspid atresia will be a systemic-pulmonary artery shunt. As noted, in 50% of patients cyanosis is present on the first day of life, and in these patients improving pulmonary blood flow is urgent.[34]

For infants, institution of prostaglandin (PGE_1) to maintain ductal patency is very useful to stabilize the patient and allow cardiac catheterization. If catheterization demonstrates a gradient across the atrial septum, or if there are signs of a restrictive foramen including large "a" waves, pulsatile liver, or distended neck veins, balloon atrial septostomy (Rashkind procedure) should be performed at the time of the initial catheterization. Most have found that atrial septostomy is infrequently needed, and Dick and coworkers found a mean interatrial gradient greater than 3 mm Hg in only 6% of patients with tricuspid atresia.[34] Others have noted a more frequent need for atrial septostomy or septectomy,[57,58] with Deverall and associates finding a 20% incidence of obstruction at the atrial septal level.[58]

The choice of systemic-pulmonary artery shunts is discussed in Chapter 3. The modified Blalock-Taussig shunt using 5-mm polytetrafluoroethylene (PTFE) prosthesis on the side of the aortic arch has emerged as the shunt of choice for most groups for infants. It is essential that shunts not only provide adequate oxygenation but also preserve the patency, size, and shape of the pulmonary arteries, and maintain normal pulmonary vascular resistance. For babies over 3 months of age and older children, the classic Blalock-Taussig or the modified Blalock-Taussig shunt is preferred, with the latter having, as principal late advantages, the preservation of normal arm blood flow and better accommodation of natural growth of the arteries.

The Glenn shunt (side of ligated superior vena cava to distal end of right pulmonary artery) has been used most successfully for tricuspid atresia, and compared to systemic artery-pulmonary artery shunts has as advantages no added volume-loading on the left ventricle and no association with pulmonary vascular obstructive disease. This shunt has a high mortality and is contraindicated in patients under 6 months of age. Other disadvantages are creation of pulmonary artery discontinuity and late failures, the latter usually due to development of venous collaterals around the ligated superior vena cava to the inferior vena cava, polycythemia (elevating blood viscosity and pulmonary vascular resistance), and spontaneous closure of the ventricular septal defect reducing left lung blood flow.[59–62] As noted in Chapter 3, the indications for Glenn shunt have declined considerably but it may still be helpful as a staged procedure in selected instances prior to Fontan correction, or in patients with tricuspid atresia otherwise deemed inoperable.

The mortality from shunting procedures varies according to age but has declined steadily. Taussig and associates reported in 1973 a 23.2% mortality in patients with tricuspid atresia receiving shunts (mostly Blalock-Taussig),[63] and Dick and coworkers reported a virtually identical 23% operative mortality in 1976.[34] More recently, shunt mortality has declined to under 10%, and has been reported to be as low as 3.3% in 30 neonates receiving modified Blalock-Taussig shunts for various cyanotic lesions.[64]

Regarding prognosis with benefit of a shunt, Dick and coworkers found that patients who without treatment had only a 10% chance of survival beyond 1 year of age (Type Ia and Ib) had a 50% chance of surviving to 15 years of age when shunted.[34] Crupi and associates also found systemic-pulmonary artery shunts to be effective, with 83% of patients stable and without requirement for other procedures 4 years after the initial shunt.[65] For the infant, usually Type Ia, whose pulmonary arteries appear too small to shunt successfully, long-term administration of prostaglandins may be used to enlarge pulmonary arteries and permit subsequent shunting.[66–70]

Enlargement of the ventricular septal defect, as described by Brock,[71] and/or right ventricular outflow tract reconstruction can be used to palliate tricuspid atresia. They have the theoretic but unproven advantage of stimulating growth of the right ventricle for inclusion in subsequent Fontan repair. The operation is performed on cardiopulmonary bypass avoiding right atrial cannulation, existing shunts are temporarily occluded, and the defect is enlarged on its anterior and superior borders to avoid conduction tissue. It is worth noting that Brock's patient died, at least partly due to inadequate resection of septal tissue,[71] and all obstructive tissue from the left ventricular side of the defect, across the os infundibulum, to and including the pulmonary valve, should be relieved for a successful result, if necessary using a transannular patch. Gersbach and coworkers reported good results in all seven Type Ib patients receiving this palliative operation,[72] as did Annecchino and associates in four of five patients with tricuspid atresia.[73] Santalla and coworkers created a ventricular septal defect in the infundibular septum using a specially designed instrument as a closed (without cardiopulmonary bypass) procedure in dogs, but this has not been reported in humans.[74] Presently, the Brock procedure or its modification is infrequently performed, primarily owing to its magnitude and the success of the Fontan procedure as a more corrective operation. It may, nevertheless, have an occasional role in patients not suitable for the Fontan procedure, especially when bilateral shunts have already been performed, and when performed properly can give lasting relief of cyanosis.[72,73]

For patients with excessive pulmonary blood flow, medical management of congestive failure with digitalis and diuretics is preferred. Pulmonary artery banding may be necessary if congestive failure is severe in spite of medical measures, most commonly those with transposed arteries.[75] In these patients, subsequent narrowing of the infundibulum associated with ventricular septal defect closure may lead to subaortic stenosis, which may require correction at the time of Fontan repair. Pulmonary artery banding should be avoided if possible in patients with tricuspid atresia with normally related arteries, as spontaneous closure of the ventricular septal defect may convert them fairly suddenly into patients with inadequate pulmonary blood flow.[75]

The length of palliation from an initial systemic-pulmonary artery shunt varies according to age at time of procedure, type of shunt, and size of pulmonary arteries. Even for those performed in infancy, adequate palliation is usually achieved for 18 months to 3 years. When palliation becomes inadequate as manifested by recurrent cyanosis, rising hemoglobin, or decreasing exercise tolerance, the patient should be recatheterized and the cause of the deterioration determined. If criteria are met for a successful Fontan procedure, that should now be performed. Otherwise another palliative procedure, e.g., contralateral systemic-pulmonary artery shunt, Glenn shunt, or right ventricular outflow tract reconstruction, is performed.

Because of the importance of the Fontan repair for other forms of cyanotic heart disease, as well as the complexity and scope of issues pertinent to its discussion, its role for tricuspid atresia is discussed separately. It seems appropriate to conclude this section with the consideration that the palliative procedures discussed above will generally be preparatory for subsequent Fontan repair. Once the patient has a systemic-pulmonary artery shunt, close follow-up is very important in order to properly time "corrective" repair, lest pulmonary artery damage, left ventricular decompensation, sudden pulmonary oligemia, and a variety of other problems prevent a smooth transition between procedures.

REFERENCES

1. Kreysig FL: Die Krankheiten des Herzens. Berlin, Maurer, 1817, vol 3.
2. Vlad P: Tricuspid atresia. In Keith JD, Rowe RD, Vlad P (eds): Heart Disease in Infancy and Childhood. New York, MacMillan, 1978, pp 518–541.
3. Van Praagh RV, Ando M, Dungan WT: Anatomic types of tricuspid atresia: Clinical and developmental implications. Circulation 44(Suppl 2):115, 1971.
4. Rosenquist GC, Levy RJ, Rowe RD: Right atrial-left ventricular relationships in tricuspid atresia—position of the presumed site of the atretic valve as determined by transillumination. Am Heart J 80:493, 1970.
5. Bharati S, McAllister HA Jr, Tatooles CH, et al: Anatomic variations in underdeveloped right ventricle related to tricuspid atresia and stenosis. J Thorac Cardiovasc Surg 72:383, 1976.

6. Bharati S, Lev M: The conduction system in tricuspid atresia with and without regular (D-) transposition. Circulation 56:423, 1977.
7. Anderson RH, Wilkins JL, Gerlis LM, et al: Atresia of the right atrioventricular orifice. Br Heart J 39:414, 1977.
8. Dickinson DF, Wilkinson JL, Smith A, Anderson RH: Atresia of the right atrioventricular orifice with atrioventricular concordance. Br Heart J 42:9, 1979.
9. Deanfield JE, Tommasini G, Anderson RH, Macartney FJ: Tricuspid atresia: Analysis of coronary artery distribution and ventricular morphology. Br Heart J 48:485, 1982.
10. Anderson RH, Becker AE, Tynan M, et al: The univentricular atrioventricular connection: Getting to the root of a thorny problem. Am J Cardiol 54:822, 1984.
11. Van Praagh R: In Barratt-Boyes BG, Neutze JM, Harris EA (eds): Heart Disease in Infancy: Diagnosis and Surgical Treatment. London, Churchill Livingstone, 1973, p 246.
12. Weinberg PM: Anatomy of tricuspid atresia and its relevance to current forms of surgical therapy. Ann Thorac Surg 29:306, 1980.
13. Rao PS, Jue KL, Isabel-Jones J, Ruttenberg HD: Ebstein's malformation of the tricuspid valve with atresia. Differentiation from isolated tricuspid atresia. Am J Cardiol 32:1004, 1973.
14. Rao PS: A unified classification for tricuspid atresia. Am Heart J 99:799, 1980.
15. Lev M: Autopsy Diagnosis of Congenitally Malformed Hearts. Springfield, IL, Charles C Thomas, 1953, p 22.
16. Freedom RM, Rowe RD: Aneurysm of the atrial septum in tricuspid atresia. Am J Cardiol 38:265, 1976.
17. Reder RF, Yeh H-C, Steinfeld L: Aneurysm of the interatrial septum causing pulmonary venous obstruction in an infant with tricuspid atresia. Am Heart J 102:786, 1981.
18. Kuhne M: Uber zwei Falle kongenitaler atresie des ostium venosum dextrum. Jahrbuch Kinderheildkunde Physiche Erziehung 63:235, 1906.
19. Edwards JE, Burchell HB: Congenital tricuspid atresia: A classification. Med Clin North Am (1949):1177, 1949.
20. Keith JD, Rowe RD, Vlad P: Heart Disease in Infancy and Childhood. New York, Macmillan, 1958, pp 434–470.
21. Keith JD, Rowe RD, Vlad R: Tricuspid atresia. In Keith JD, Rowe RD, Vlad P (eds): Heart Disease in Infancy and Childhood, 2nd ed. New York, Macmillan, 1967, p 644.
22. Tandon R, Edwards JE: Tricuspid atresia. A re-evaluation and classification. J Thorac Cardiovasc Surg 67:530, 1974.
23. Guller B, DuShane JW, Titus JL: The atrioventricular conduction system in two cases of tricuspid atresia. Circulation 40:217, 1969.
24. Bharati S, Lev M, Kirklin JW: Cardiac Surgery and the Conduction System. New York, John Wiley & Sons, 1983.
25. Rumisek JD, Pigott JD, Weinberg PM, Norwood WI: Coronary sinus septal defect associated with tricuspid atresia. J Thorac Cardiovasc Surg 92:142, 1986.
26. Rao PS, Jue KL, Isabel-Jones J, Ruttenberg HD: Ebstein's malformation of tricuspid atresia. Am J Cardiol 32:1004, 1956.
27. Tandon R, Marin-Garcia J, Moller JM, Edwards JE: Tricuspid atresia with L-transposition. Am Heart J 88:417, 1974.
28. Sharma D, Mehta AB, Bharati S, Lev M: Tricuspid atresia with persistent truncus arteriosus. Chest 79:363, 1981.
29. Marin-Garcia J, Roca J, Bleiden LC, et al: Congenital absence of the pulmonary valve associated with tricuspid atresia and intact ventricular septum. Chest 64:658, 1973.
30. Cox JN, De Siegneux R, Bolens M, et al: Tricuspid atresa, hypoplastic right ventricle, intact ventricular septum and absence of the pulmonary valve. Helv Paediatr Acta 30:389, 1975.
31. Freedom RM, Patel RG, Bloom KR, et al: Congenital absence of the pulmonary valve associated with imperforate membrane type of tricuspid atresia, right ventricular tensor apparatus and intact ventricular septum: A curious developmental complex. Eur J Cardiol 3:171, 1979.
32. Forrest P, Bini RM, Wilkinson JL, et al: Congenital absence of the pulmonic valve and tricuspid valve atresia with intact ventricular septum. Am J Cardiol 59:482, 1987.
33. Bini RM, Pellegrino PA, Mazzucco A, et al: Tricuspid atresia with double-outlet left atrium. Chest 78:109, 1980.
34. Dick M, Fyler DC, Nadas AS: Tricuspid atresia. Clinical course in 101 patients. Am J Cardiol 36:327, 1975.
35. Taussig HB: The clinical and pathological findings in congenital malformations of the heart due to defective development of the right ventricle associated with tricuspid atresia or hypoplasia. Bull Johns Hopkins Hosp 59:435, 1936.

36. Chesler E, Joffe HS, Vecht R, et al: Ultrasound cardiography in single ventricle and the hypoplastic left and right heart syndromes. Circulation 42:123, 1970.
37. Meyer RA, Kaplan S: Echocardiography in the diagnosis of hypoplasia of the left or right ventricles in the neonate. Circulation 46:55, 1972.
38. Godman MJ, Tham P, Kidd BSL: Echocardiography in the evaluation of the cyanotic newborn infant. Br Heart J 36:154, 1974.
39. Beppu S, Nimura Y, Tamai M, et al: Two-dimensional echocardiography in diagnosing tricuspid atresia: Differentiation from other hypoplastic right heart syndromes and common atrioventricular canal. Br Heart J 40:1174, 1978.
40. Rigby ML, Gibson DG, Joseph ML, et al: Recognition of imperforate atrioventricular valves by two dimensional echocardiography. Br Heart J 47:329, 1982.
41. Koiwaya Y, Watanabe K, Orita Y, et al: Contrast two-dimensional echocardiography in diagnosis of tricuspid atresia. Am Heart J 101:507, 1981.
42. Rigby ML, Gibson DG, Joseph MC, et al: Recognition of imperforate atrioventricular valves by two dimensional echocardiography. Br Heart J 47:329, 1982.
43. Campbell M, Hills TH: Angiocardiography in cyanotic congenital heart disease. Br Heart J 12:65, 1950.
44. Cooley RN, Sloan RD, Hanlon CR, et al: Angiocardiography in congenital heart disease of cyanotic type. II. Observations on tricuspid stenosis or atresia with hypoplasia of right ventricle. Radiology 54:848, 1950.
45. Nishioka K, Kamiya T, Ueda T, et al: Left ventricular volume characteristics in children with tricuspid atresia before and after surgery. Am J Cardiol 47:1105, 1981.
46. La Corte MA, Dick M, Scheer G, et al: Left ventricular function in tricuspid atresia. Angiographic analysis in 28 patients. Circulation 52:996, 1975.
47. Hurwitz RA, Caldwell RL, Girod DA, et al: Left ventricular function in tricuspid atresia: A radionuclide study. J Am Coll Cardiol 8:916, 1986.
48. Baker EJ, Jones ODH, Joseph MC, et al: Radionuclide measurement of left ventricular ejection fraction in tricuspid atresia. Br Heart J 52:572, 1984.
49. Fletcher BD, Jacobstein MD, Abramowsky CR, et al: Right atriovenricular valve atresia: Anatomic evaluation with MR imaging. Am J Roentgenol 148:671, 1987.
50. Rao PS: Further observations on the spontaneous closure of physiologically advantageous ventricular septal defect in tricuspid atresia: Surgical implications. Ann Thorac Surg 35:121, 1983.
51. Rao PS: Natural history of the ventricular septal defect in tricuspid atresia and its surgical implications. Br Heart J 39:276, 1977.
52. Warnes CA, Somerville J: Tricuspid atresia with transposition of the great arteries in adolescents and adults: Current state and late complications. Br Heart J 57:543, 1987.
53. Patterson W, Baxley WA, Karp RB, et al: Tricuspid atresia in adults. Am J Cardiol 49:141, 1982.
54. Patel MM, Overy DC, Kozonis MC, et al: Long-term survival in tricuspid atresia. J Am Coll Cardiol 9:338, 1987.
55. Breisch EA, Wilson DB, Laurenson RD, et al: Tricuspid atresia (type Ia): Survival to 21 years of age. Am Heart J 106:149, 1983.
56. Tazelaar HD, Moore W, Hutchins GM: Ventricular inversion and tricuspid atresia (VITA complex): Long survival without surgical treatment. Pediatr Cardiol 6:187, 1986.
57. Kyger ER III, Reul GJ Jr, Sandiford FM, et al: Surgical palliation of tricuspid atresia. Circulation 52:685, 1975.
58. Deverall PD, Lincoln JCR, Aberdeen E, et al: Surgical management of tricuspid atresia. Thorax 24:239, 1969.
59. Williams WG, Rubis L, Fowler RS, et al: Tricuspid atresia: Results of treatment in 160 children. Am J Cardiol 38:225, 1976.
60. Trusler GA, Williams WG: Long-term results of shunt procedures for tricuspid atresia. Ann Thorac Surg 29:312, 1980.
61. Laks H, Mudd JG, Standeven JW, et al: Long term effect of the superior vena cava-pulmonary artery anastomosis on pulmonary blood flow. J Thorac Cardiovasc Surg 74:253, 1977.
62. Pennington DG, Nouri S, Ho J, et al: Glenn shunt: Long-term results and current role in congenital heart operations. Ann Thorac Surg 31:532, 1981.
63. Taussig HB, Keinonen R, Momberger N, Kirk H: Long-time observations on the Blalock-Taussig operation. IV. Tricuspid atresia. Johns Hopkins Med J 132:135, 1973.
64. Ilbawi MN, Grieco J, DeLeon SY, et al: Modified Blalock-Taussig shunt in newborn infants. J Thorac Cardiovasc Surg 88:770, 1984.
65. Crupi G, Alfieri O, Locatelli G, et al: Results of systemic-to-pulmonary artery anastomosis for tricuspid atresia with reduced pulmonary blood flow. Thorax 34:290, 1979.

66. Lewis AB, Lurie PR: Prolonged prostaglandin E_1 infusion in an infant with cyanotic congenital heart disease. Pediatrics 61:534, 1978.
67. Coe JY, Silove ED: Oral prostaglandin E_1 in pulmonary atresia. Lancet 1:1297, 1979.
68. Silove ED, Coe JY, Shiu MF, et al: Oral prostaglandin E_1 in ductus-dependent pulmonary circulation. Circulation 63:682, 1981.
69. Pitlick P, French JW, Maze A, et al: Long-term low-dose prostaglandin E_1 administration. J Pediatr 96:318, 1980.
70. Coe JY, Radley-Smith R, Yacoub M: Management of tricuspid atresia with orally administered prostaglandin E_2. J Pediatr 100:496, 1982.
71. Brock R: Tricuspid atresia: A step toward corrective treatment. J Thorac Cardiovasc Surg 47:17, 1964.
72. Gersbach PH, Freidli B, Hahn C: Treatment of tricuspid atresia with small pulmonary flow (type Ib) by surgical enlargement of the ventricular septal defect. Thorac Cardiovasc Surg 29:82, 1981.
73. Annecchino FP, Fontan F, Chauve A, et al: Palliative reconstruction of the right ventricular outflow tract in tricuspid atresia: A report of five patients. Ann Thorac Surg 29:317, 1980.
74. Santalla A, Quero M, Yen-Ho S, et al: New surgical approach to palliate tricuspid atresia in infants. Ann Thorac Surg 33:297, 1982.
75. Marcano BA, Reimenschneider TA, Ruttenberg HD, et al: Tricuspid atresia with increased pulmonary blood flow. Analysis of 13 cases. Circulation 40:399, 1969.

L. DOUGLAS COWGILL, MD

TRICUSPID ATRESIA

B. Fontan Repair

From the Department of Surgery
Dean Clinic
Madison, Wisconisn

Reprint requests to:
L. Douglas Cowgill, MD
Department of Surgery
Dean Clinic
1313 Fish Hatchery Rd.
Madison, WI 53715

HISTORY

The first reported bypass of the right ventricle clinically was in 1954 by Hurwitt and colleagues[1] in a 4-month-old intensely cyanotic boy with tricuspid atresia. This was preceded by considerable experimental work suggesting that the right ventricle could be bypassed. Starr and associates[2] demonstrated in 1943 that the canine right ventricle could be destroyed without causing systemic venous hypertension. Rodbard and Wagner[3] showed that the right ventricle could be bypassed in 1949, and Warden and colleagues[4] demonstrated the feasibility of right ventricular bypass in dogs using a direct anastomosis of the right atrial appendage to the main pulmonary artery with suture obliteration of the tricuspid valve orifice. Hurwitt's patient died intraoperatively of low cardiac output, and they postulated several potential problems with right ventricular bypass.[1] These included persistence of interatrial shunting if any atrial defects were not securely closed, ineffectual atrial pumping action if atrial arrhythmias occurred, reversal of pressure gradient if left ventricular or mitral valvular dysfunction developed, obliteration of the necessary right atrial-pulmonary artery pressure gradient if acute or chronic pulmonary disease arose, and unacceptable pressure gradients with any significant degree of pulmonary artery hypoplasia.

Fontan and Baudet[5,6] first successfully bypassed the right ventricle in 1968. Three tricuspid atresia patients were operated on with two survivors (aged 12 and 33 years). The third patient (aged 23 years) died from low cardiac

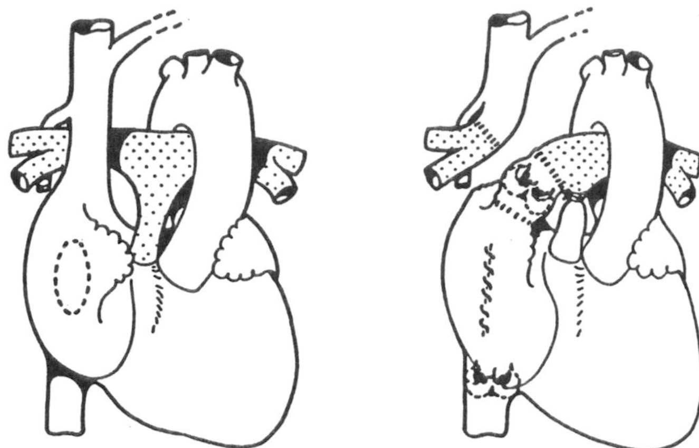

FIGURE 1. Fontan's original repair. (Reprinted with permission from Thorax 26:240–248, 1971.)

output 6 hours postoperatively, which at autopsy appeared to be due to mitral valve insufficiency. The procedure consisted of a cavopulmonary (Glenn) anastomosis, a direct anastomosis between the right atrial appendage and the proximal end of the divided right pulmonary artery, closure of the atrial septal defect, ligation of the main pulmonary artery, and the insertion of an aortic homograft valve into the inferior vena cava (IVC) ostium (Fig. 1). In the last two patients, an aortic homograft valve-conduit was inserted between the right atrial appendage and the proximal right pulmonary artery. They emphasized that the procedure was not an anatomic correction, since that would require creation of a right ventricle, "but a procedure of physiological pulmonary blood flow restoration, with suppression of right and left blood mixing (shunting)." They also emphasized that the procedure applied only to well-developed children without pulmonary hypertension, and recognized the need to provide a large amount of fluid postoperatively to maintain satisfactory pulmonary blood flow, the detrimental effect of positive pressure ventilation on central venous return, and the frequency of pleural effusions postoperatively.

Kreutzer and colleagues[7] reported in 1973 a modification of Fontan's operation, whereby the pulmonary valve with main pulmonary artery was disinserted from the outflow tract of the right ventricle and anastomosed to the right atrial appendage (Fig. 2). The septal defects and ventriculotomies were closed, but unlike Fontan's repair neither a Glenn shunt nor IVC valve was used. Ross and Somerville[8] reported in 1973 two tricuspid atresia repairs similar to Fontan's, with the exception that Glenn shunts were not performed. They believed that the arterial desaturation and mild cyanosis Fontan observed in his patients were probably due to intrapulmonary shunts secondary to the Glenn procedure, and like Kreutzer's group demonstrated that a Glenn shunt was unnecessary for survival. Other early reports of successful Fontan-type repairs were those of Stanford and colleagues[9] in 1973, and Henry and associates in 1974,[10] the latter group using porcine xenograft valves with and without Dacron conduits. Problems with valves and conduits led to growing concern about their

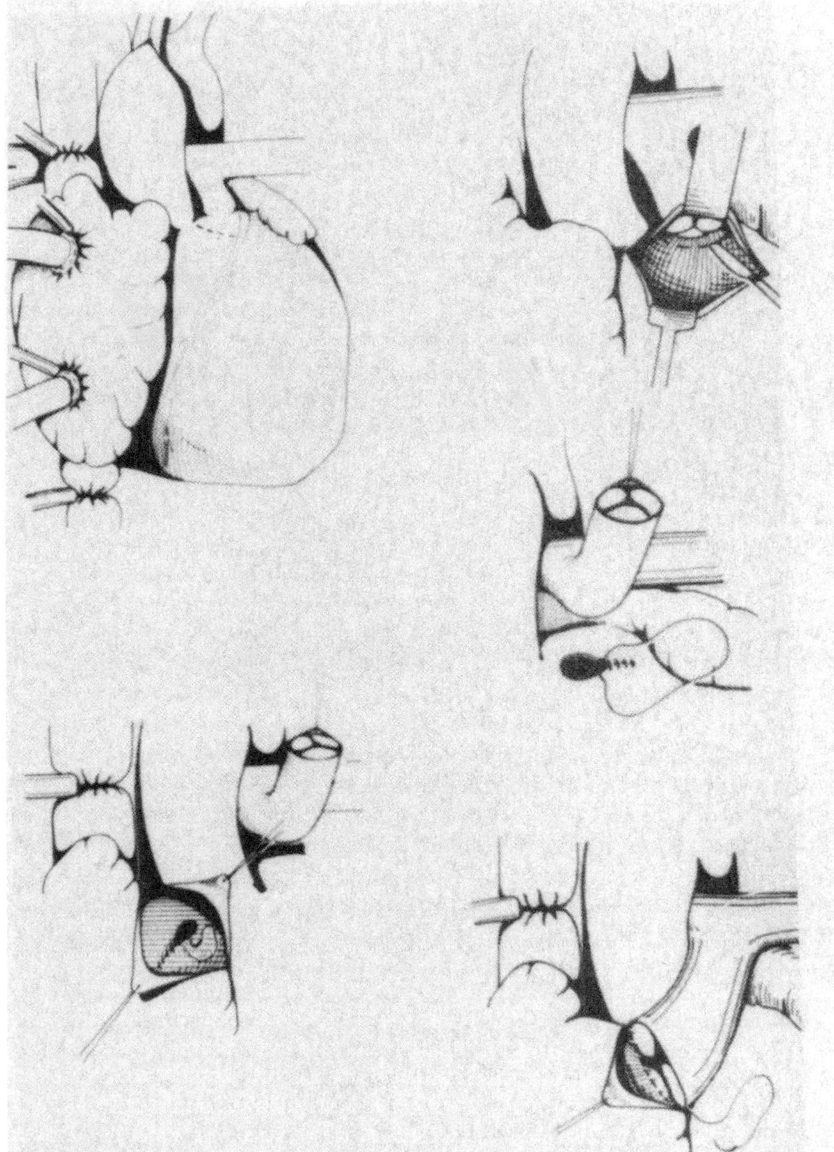

FIGURE 2. The Kreutzer modification of the Fontan procedure, with disinsertion of the pulmonary valve and anastomosis to the right atrial appendage. (Reprinted with permission from J Thorac Cardiovasc Surg 66:613–621, 1973.)

usefulness, with Tatooles and associates reporting late ascites and hepatomegaly resulting from fibrous stenosis of an IVC valve.[11]

An important modification was that of Bjork and colleagues[12] in 1979, in which they reported three successful right atrial-right ventricular anastomoses in tricuspid atresia Type I patients using a roof of autologous pericardium (Fig. 3).

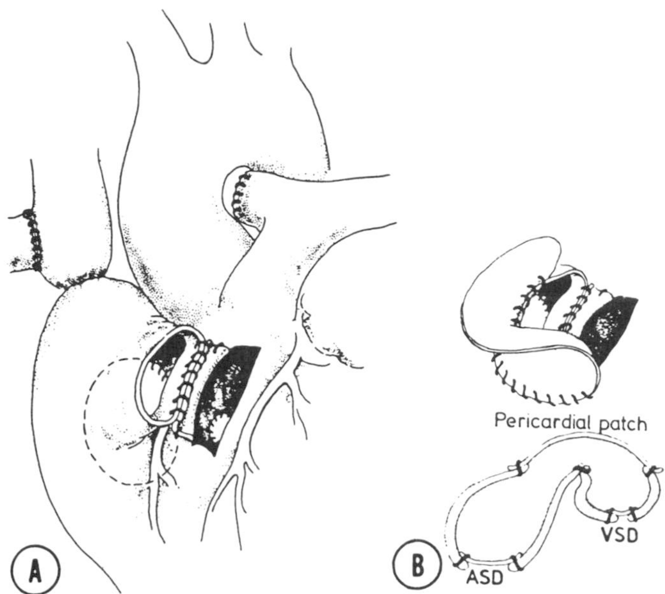

FIGURE 3. The Bjork modification of the Fontan procedure. (Reprinted with permission from J Thorac Cardiovasc Surg 77:452–458, 1979.)

Advantages of this technique were no foreign material, either valve or conduit, was used, the right ventricle was incorporated into the repair with the potential of augmenting right heart function if the right ventricle developed, and the native pulmonary valve was preserved, which should reduce if not eliminate pulmonary regurgitation. Numerous subsequent reports[13–17] of the problems with foreign valves and conduits, the latter with tendency to be outgrown when placed in small children, be compressed by the sternum, or form neointimal obstructive "peel," emphasize the importance of Bjork's use of only native tissue.

The importance of incorporating the right ventricle into the repair is still debated. Bowman and associates[18] in 1978 reported incorporation of the right ventricle into Fontan repair using porcine-valved Dacron conduits from the right atrium to right ventricle in nine patients. Subsequent cardiac catheterization in five patients showed significant enlargement of a pulsatile right ventricular chamber with "ventricularized" pressure tracings recorded in the right ventricle. With this type of repair, they concluded that a four-chambered, four-valved heart was feasible, both anatomically and physiologically.

An important group of modifications, which have been increasingly used recently, involves direct right atrial–pulmonary artery connection similar to that used by Fontan in his first case.[13,29–21] The report by Doty and coworkers[19] is most comprehensive, describing six different techniques of right atrial–pulmonary artery reconstruction, depending on relationship of the great arteries, status of atrial appendages, and presence of prior Glenn shunt (Fig. 4). Advantages of this technique include no foreign tissue, usually no pericardial tissue externally, no valves, no potential for right ventricular outflow tract or pulmonary valve obstruction, and no risk of conduction tissue injury or insecure ventricular septal

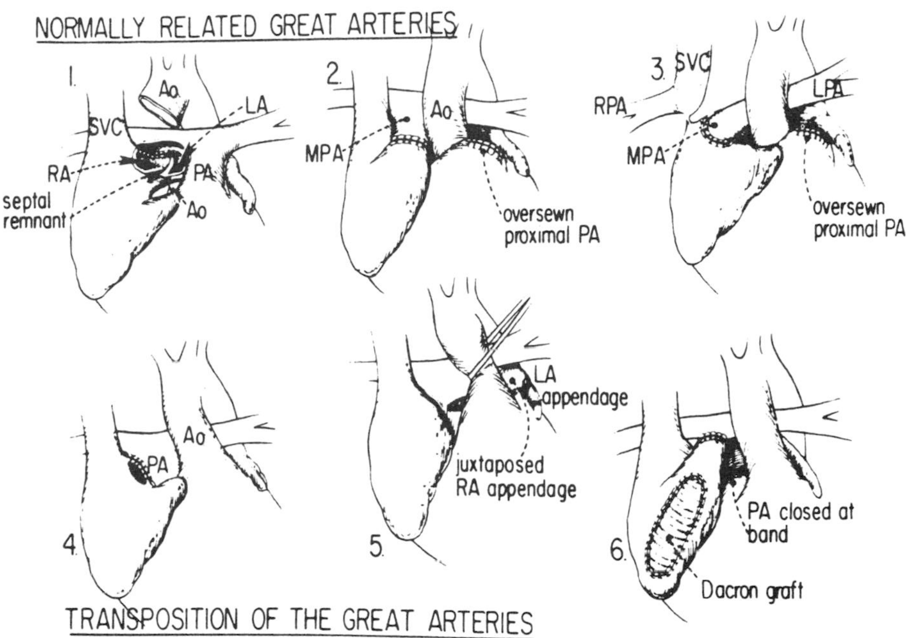

FIGURE 4. Modified Fontan operation. Shown are the options available to achieve direct anastomosis of the right atrium to the pulmonary artery with normally related great arteries (top row, 1–3) and transposition of the great arteries (bottom row, 4–6). (1) The opening into the superior aspect of the right and left atria across the excised atrial septum, which may be anastomosed to a side opening in the pulmonary artery posterior to the aorta. The aorta is shown cut away for clarity even though in the actual operation the aorta is simply retracted. (2) Direct anastomosis of the main pulmonary artery to the right atrial appendage after mobilization and division of the pulmonary artery just above the valve. The proximal pulmonary artery is oversewn. (3) This is similar to 2, except that there has been a previous superior vena cava-right pulmonary artery anastomosis. (4) Simple side-to-side anastomosis of the pulmonary artery to the right atrium when the pulmonary artery assumes a posterior position in transposition of the great arteries. (5) The fortuitous situation of transposition of the great arteries and juxtaposition of the right atrial appendage to the left, which brings it into direct posterior relation with the pulmonary artery for side-to-side anastomosis. (6) The right atrial appendage advances to the bifurcation of the pulmonary artery for anastomosis after the pulmonary artery band has been removed and the proximal end closed. The right atrial defect is filled with Dacron patch. SVC = superior vena cava. Ao = aorta. RA = right atrium. LA = left atrium. PA = pulmonary artery. MPA = main pulmonary artery. RPA = right pulmonary artery. LPA = left pulmonary artery. (Reprinted with permission from J Thorac Cardiovasc Surg 81:47–475, 1981.)

defect closure from suturing in the right ventricle. The value of incorporating the right ventricle into a repair, as described by Bjork, was questioned by Doty since only one of Bjork's three patients had significant postoperative right ventricular contractile wave forms, and this patient also had an estimated 25% regurgitation into the right atrium.[12]

CHOICE OF OPERATION

It should not be surprising, with all of the modifications of Fontan's original operation, that no single form of repair is universally favored or uniformly applicable. Considering the substantial anatomical variations of tricuspid atresia, single ventricle and other entities, the importance of flexibility is apparent. Basic maxims for successful results are careful selection of patients preoperatively (see Indications), meticulous closure of atrial and, when the right ventricle is incorporated, ventricular septal defects, creation of a right atrial–pulmonary artery or right atrial–right ventricular anastomosis with no gradient, and excellent intra- and postoperative care. In addition, foreign material should be avoided whenever possible, excepting perhaps use of the newer homograft valve–conduits (see last chapter).

Important technical questions presently are which reconstruction, right atrial–pulmonary artery versus right atrial–right ventricle, is preferable and should a valve(s) be incorporated into the repair? The arguments for and against incorporation of the right ventricle were discussed above, with a question as to whether the hypoplastic right ventricle can grow and augment cardiac output. The Mayo Clinic group compared 60 patients with atriopulmonary connections against 24 patients with atrioventricular connections, without the addition of valves (all with ventriculoarterial concordance), and found the former group had a slightly higher mean right atrial pressure postoperatively (18 vs. 16 mm Hg) but there was no difference in operative mortality or late survival.[22] They concluded that for patients with tricuspid atresia with normally related arteries, the choice of connection should be dictated by the anatomy (e.g., presence of pulmonary valve or pulmonary artery stenoses, size of outlet chamber, and presence of anomalous coronary arteries) with no important differences in clinical outcome between the two techniques. Since no valve was incorporated in the right ventricle (or subpulmonary ventricular chamber by their terminology), it could be argued that regurgitation from right ventricle to right atrium might negate any hemodynamic benefit of right ventricular pumping capacity. This latter issue was addressed by the Great Ormond Street group,[23] who provided detailed hemodynamic analysis of atriopulmonary and atrioventricular connections. They found that in the immediate postoperative period mean pulmonary artery pressure was no higher than mean superior vena cava pressure, regardless of whether the right ventricle was incorporated or not. As 15 of 17 atrioventricular connections had valves in this series, there was no early hemodynamic evidence of ventricular augmentation of pulmonary blood flow with the atrioventricular connection even when a subpulmonary valve was inserted. Nevertheless, since late evaluation demonstrated substantial growth of the right ventricle in three patients (Fig. 5), they concluded that a right ventricle should be incorporated, provided an obstruction-free atrioventricular connection could be established. In discussing this paper, Bowman[24] reported "definite evidence of augmentation of blood flow by right ventricular contraction" in 14 of 16 valved atrioventricular connections studied from one to five years postoperatively, and supported this method of repair in patients with a trabeculated as well as infundibular subpulmonic chamber. DiSessa and colleagues[25] evaluated Doppler pulmonary artery and superior vena cava profiles in 15 Fontan repairs with various atriopulmonary or atrioventricular connections and found that neither pulmonary artery nor superior vena cava flow patterns postoperatively were dependent on the preoperative anomaly or type of communication used at surgery. However, only one

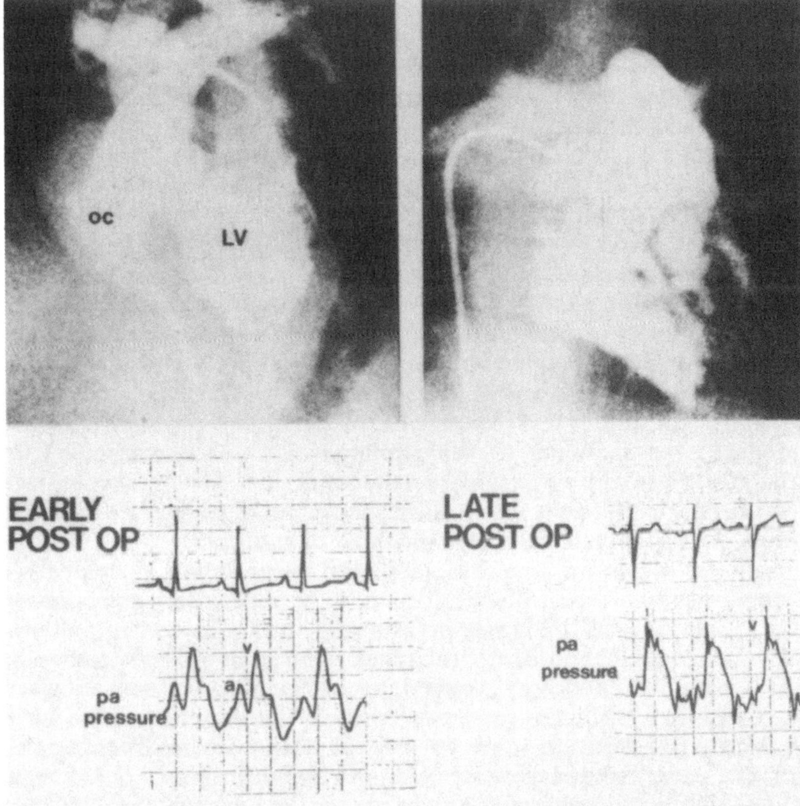

FIGURE 5. Outlet chamber growth. Angiograms showing the outlet chamber preoperatively and 1 year postoperatively in a patient with tricuspid atresia who underwent an atrioventricular connection. The right atrium-dependent circulation became right ventricle-dependent. pa = pulmonary artery. (Reprinted with permission from J Thorac Cardiovasc Surg 85:21–31, 1983.)

of these patients had a valved right atrial– right ventricular connection. Certainly, as with the Great Ormond Street and Bowman's experiences, growth and function of the right ventricle have been demonstrated late postoperatively with use of a valved atrioventricular connection.[26,27]

The need for incorporation of the native pulmonary valve or incorporation of additional valves has been addressed by a number of investigators. Regarding the native pulmonary valve, Ishikawa and coworkers[28] followed patients with tricuspid atresia undergoing the Kreutzer procedure (disinsertion of native pulmonary valve with atriopulmonary connection) using echocardiography, and found that these valves did not close under normal conditions but remained in a permanently open position. Kreutzer's own group[20] found no advantage for his original technique in his follow-up report and, in a comparison of four atriopulmonary connections (none of which were valved atrioventricular connections), found the posterior non-valved atriopulmonary anastomosis to be consistently superior. Neveux and associates,[29] describing a technique of pulmonary valve preservation with right ventricle exclusion, report good long-term clinical results in all 10 operative survivors, but no hemodynamic data are provided. In a widely quoted experimental canine study, Shemin and coworkers[30] evaluated atriopulmonary conduit connections with and without valves, and found that early postoperative blood flow was not significantly altered by the presence of a valve, presence of ventricular rhythm, or tachycardia. The most important factor influencing conduit blood flow was right atrial pressure.

Presently, the debate as to the preferred method of Fontan repair for tricuspid atresia is typified by no less authorities than Kirklin and Barratt-Boyes[31] in their comprehensive text, the former using direct non-valved right atrial–pulmonary artery anastomosis as a routine procedure, whereas the latter prefers, for normally related arteries, right atrial–right ventricular connection using homograft valve–conduit. Fontan's own group[32,33] has demonstrated better exercise tolerance and better preservation of right atrial contractions in patients with valve–conduits than without. They recommend a homograft valve–conduit right atrial–right ventricular connection in patients with ventriculoarterial concordance, and a homograft valve–conduit right atrial–pulmonary artery connection in those with ventriculoarterial discordance. Fontan cautions against non-valved right atrial–right ventricular connections because of development of significant regurgitation from right ventricle to right atrium.

As for use of inferior vena cava valves and Glenn shunts as originally used by Fontan, both have repeatedly been proven to be unnecessary and occasionally harmful. There may still be a role occasionally for a Glenn shunt, either as a staged or concomitant procedure, to reduce right atrial volume loading in the early postoperative period (see Chapter 3), recognizing that a disadvantage of the Glenn procedure is the diversion of two-thirds of venous return to the left lung, which normally constitutes only 40–45% of lung volume. Pennington and coworkers[34] have found staged Glenn shunts useful prior to Fontan repair in situations such as a small volume right atrium or proximal right pulmonary artery stenosis from prior Waterston shunt.

With these considerations the following principles guide a necessarily flexible approach to reconstruction:

1. The "connection" must be without gradient.

2. Inferior vena cava valves and Glenn shunts are unnecessary, although the latter may have a role in selected patients.

3. Tricuspid atresia with transposition (Type II) is well suited to direct atriopulmonary connection, whereas tricuspid atresia with normally related arteries (Type I) lends itself to atrioventricular connection.

4. The atrioventricular connection has not been shown to be hemodynamically superior to the atriopulmonary connection in the immediate postoperative period, and carries risk of anastomotic or outflow tract gradient, conduction injury, and recurrent ventricular septal defect.

5. A valveless atrioventricular connection has not been shown to be hemodynamically superior to the atriopulmonary connection over the long term, and may be associated with detrimental regurgitation during ventricular contraction.

6. A valved atrioventricular connection for Type I tricuspid atresia has demonstrated right ventricular growth and function over the long term, with limited evidence of superior hemodynamic and exercise performance.

7. Insertion of a valve into a direct atriopulmonary connection has not been shown to confer late hemodynamic or exercise performance advantage in the experience of most, with the very notable exception of Fontan's group.[32,33]

TECHNIQUE OF OPERATION

Direct Right Atrial–Pulmonary Artery Anastomosis

Through a median sternotomy, the pericardium is opened. Dacron, if it is to be used, is preclotted, and the patient is heparinized and cannulated. Cannulae are placed directly into the superior vena cava and right atrial/inferior vena cava junction to preserve right atrial volume and function as much as possible. Any patent systemic–pulmonary arterial shunts are dissected and closed immediately after institution of cardiopulmonary bypass (CPB) to prevent pulmonary congestion. The superior vena cava cannula is placed at or above the pericardial reflection with a tourniquet inferiorly for total cardiopulmonary bypass. If a Glenn shunt is already present, the cava is cannulated directly without a tourniquet, using a Cooley caval clamp if necessary to limit pulmonary blood flow. The patient is placed on total CPB and cooled to 22–25° C, during which time the main pulmonary artery is dissected away from the ascending aorta, and the right and left pulmonary arteries mobilized several centimeters beyond the bifurcation. The ligamentum arteriosum may be divided for increased mobility. A left ventricular vent may be placed during cooling via the right superior pulmonary vein, or following cross-clamp across the atrial septal defect.

The ascending aorta is cross-clamped, and cold blood–cardioplegic solution is infused (10 cc/kg) into the aortic root with cold saline applied topically for external cooling, and repeated intermittently during cross-clamp to maintain myocardial temperatures less than 15° C. The right atrium is incised obliquely parallel to the atrioventricular groove, and the right atrium, atrial septal defect, pulmonary venous drainage, and mitral valve are inspected. The coronary sinus is inspected with a right-angle clamp to exclude unroofed coronary sinus, and excess eustachian valve tissue (cor triatriatum dexter) identified and excised. Any preexisting mitral valve pathology must be corrected. The anatomic relationship of the right atrium and pulmonary artery is visualized, and the most appropriate method of anastomosis determined, preferably posterior to the aorta to avoid compression (Fig. 4).

The most important goal at this point is the largest possible, gradient-free opening between the right atrium and pulmonary artery. Prior to closure of the atrial septal defect, the need for removal of superior atrial septal tissue with leftward realignment of the atrial septum to enlarge the right atrial–pulmonary artery anastomosis is determined. The superior aspect of the right atrium is tented upward with a right-angle clamp within the right atrium, and opened opposite the pulmonary artery. The incision is carried rightward to the superior vena cava (avoiding the sinoatrial node artery) and leftward well beneath the great arteries. Additional atrial tissue is excised anteriorly and at the corners to create a large, essentially circular opening in the right atrium. The atrial septal defect is closed meticulously with a pre-clotted knitted Dacron velour patch, aligning it superiorly to the left if necessary.

For Type I (normally related arteries) patients, the main pulmonary artery is now divided near its origin and the proximal end oversewn with a double-row of 4–0 or 5–0 polypropylene suture. The mobilized pulmonary artery is brought behind the aorta and aligned opposite the right atrial opening. Both right and left pulmonary arteries are inspected within to exclude any stenosis. If present this is corrected with an onlay patch of either pericardium or polytetrafluoroethylene (PTFE). Generally to ensure a widely patent anastomosis, the pulmonary artery

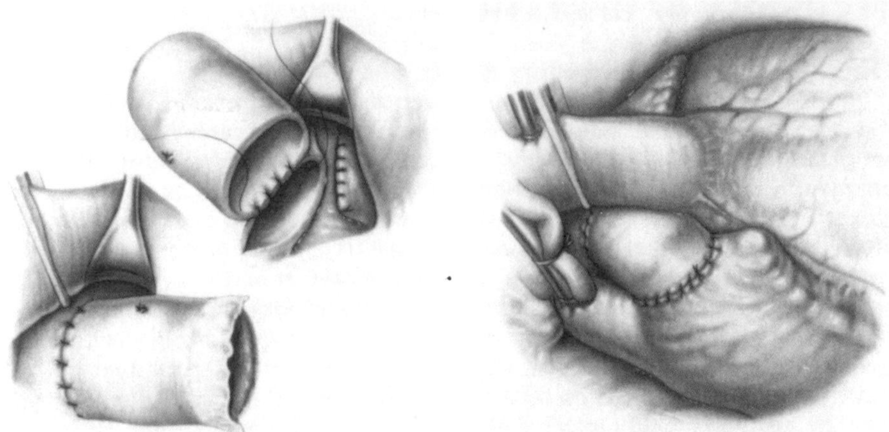

FIGURE 6. Atriopulmonary anastomosis with use of interposed homograft valve-conduit. (Reprinted with permission from de Leval M: Surgery for Congenital Heart Defects. New York. Grune & Stratton, 1983, pp. 453–466.)

is opened laterally along the inferior aspect of the right pulmonary artery, and the right atrial–pulmonary artery connection is now performed with polypropylene, optimally using interrupted sutures anteriorly. If a homograft right atrial–pulmonary artery connection is to be performed, it is interposed at this time (Fig. 6). Occasionally to ensure a large, tension free right atrial–pulmonary artery communication, the anastomosis must be supplemented with a convex roof of pericardial or prosthetic material anteriorly.

For Type II patients, the transposed pulmonary artery is already posterior to the aorta, opposite the right atrium. Consequently the right atrial incision need not cross the atrial septum, and direct right atrial–pulmonary artery anastomosis, again with extension of the pulmonary artery incision along the inferior aspect of the right pulmonary artery to enlarge the communication, is performed. For patients with prior Glenn shunt, the left pulmonary artery is mobilized, brought behind the aorta, and sutured either to a large opening in the roof of the right atrium or directly to the right atrial appendage (Fig. 4). Direct right atrial–pulmonary artery anastomosis is also appropriate for leftward juxtaposition of the atrial appendages.

The right atriotomy is closed, the heart carefully de-aired, and the cross-clamp released. With the aid of left atrial, pulmonary artery, and right atrial monitoring lines, the patient is weaned from bypass using right atrial filling pressures of 15–18 as a guide for fluid administration. Vasopressor may be used as needed to augment cardiac output, but has the potential disadvantage of increasing pulmonary as well as systemic afterload. A right atrial–pulmonary artery gradient should be excluded with pressure measurement, and if present requires anastomotic correction. The mean right atrial/left atrial pressure ratio is usually less than 2 mm Hg.[31] Mean airway pressure is kept low to facilitate pulmonary blood flow.

When hemostasis and hemodynamics are satisfactory, temporary atrial and ventricular pacing wires are placed (if not already being utilized), both chests as well as the mediastinum are drained, and the wound closed.

Non-Valved Right Atrial–Right Ventricular Connection

This operation, which is the Bjork modification of the Fontan procedure, may be used for patients with Type I tricuspid atresia when the right ventricle is of some size and the pulmonary valve nonrestrictive. The initial steps of the procedure are the same as those for direct right atrial–pulmonary artery anastomosis, with the exception that extensive pulmonary artery mobilization is unnecessary.

Once blood cardioplegia solution is administered, the right atrium is opened with an incision parallel to the long axis of the right atrial appendage and about 1 cm to its right, extending the incision anteriorly at each corner to form a "trap door" (Fig. 3). Internal trabeculations in this area are excised. The atrial inspection is the same as outlined above, and the atrial septal defect is carefully closed with a Dacron velour patch. The hypoplastic right ventricle is then opened with a vertical incision, between the atrioventricular groove to the right and the left anterior descending coronary artery to the left, ending the incision just proximal to the pulmonary valve. The anterior free wall is usually rather thin, and the ventricular septal defect will be identified inferiorly. The ventricular septal defect is then closed with a small patch or excluded altogether with a large patch by the method of Nevcux.[29] (The conduction tissue runs on the posteroinferior, leftward aspect of the ventricular septal defect.)

The pulmonary valve and ring are internally calibrated to be sure they are nonstenotic, and any valvar stenosis is corrected. The ventriculotomy incision can be widened by excising the free wall on the right side if necessary, which brings the edge of the ventriculotomy incision into closer proximity with the incised right atrial appendage. The incised appendage is now unfolded to the left, suturing its edge to the rightward edge of the ventriculotomy to form the posterior wall of the right atrial–right ventricular anastomosis. An appropriately tailored piece of pericardium is now sutured over the remaining defect to form a generous convex roof (Fig. 7). The remaining steps of the operation are as described previously.

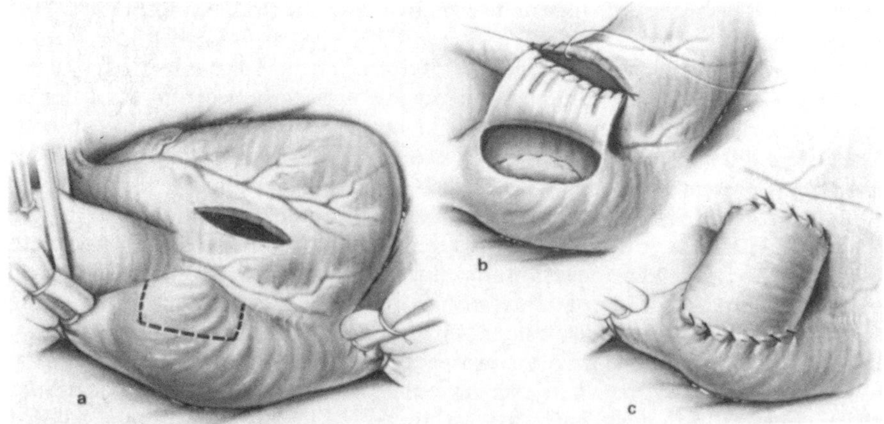

FIGURE 7. Illustration of non-valved atrioventricular connection. (Reprinted with permission from de Leval M: Surgery for Congenital Heart Defects. New York, Grune & Stratton, 1983, pp. 453–466.)

Valved Right Atrial–Right Ventricular Connection

This operation is indicated in the same patients as those in the preceding section, and carries a lower risk of significant regurgitation late postoperatively compared to a valveless connection. Because of the limited longevity of porcine valves, fresh antibiotic-preserved aortic or pulmonary valve homografts are preferred, recognizing their limited availability and still uncertain durability. The initial operative steps are as those discussed above.

Following aortic cross-clamp and cardioplegic arrest, the right atrium is opened across the top of the right atrial appendage, and the atrial inspection and atrial septal defect closure done through this generous opening. The right ventricle is vertically opened in similar fashion to that described in the preceding section, excising enough anterior right ventricle free wall to accommodate the homograft. The VSD is closed with a Dacron patch, and any muscular infundibular restriction excised. A homograft is selected which will be nonrestrictive, usually 22–24 mm for child and 26–28 mm for an adult.[31] The homograft is cut obliquely on the aortic (or pulmonary) side to within several millimeters of the valve, and transversely just below the valve. The subvalvular homograft is sutured to the opening in the right atrial appendage, after which the obliquely trimmed distal end is sewn to the opening in the right ventricle, with the longer side sutured to the left edge of the ventriculotomy (Fig. 8). Air is evacuated from the heart, the cross-clamp released, and the remaining steps are as those described in the preceding sections.

SPECIAL OPERATIVE PROBLEMS

Unroofed Coronary Sinus. Any residual atrial septal defect following Fontan repair is poorly tolerated, with excessive right-to-left shunting being the rule due to the high right atrial pressures. A number of reports of unroofed coronary sinus being recognized postoperatively emphasize the importance of inspection of the coronary sinus intraoperatively.[35–38] Unfortunately, this defect is not always identifiable pre- or intraoperatively, and if discovered postoperatively immediate repair is warranted. Its incidence is variable, with Rumisek and associates[38] discovering it in 4/159 tricuspid atresia specimens. It is most common with persistent left superior vena cava, and should be carefully searched for when that is present.

Options for surgical repair include direct closure with pledgetted sutures, reroofing with a patch, or complete unroofing with closure of the atrial septal defect to the right of the coronary sinus. The latter is well tolerated in the absence of persistent left superior vena cava, but cannot be performed when left superior vena cava is present unless the LSVC can be ligated or rerouted.

Absent Atrial Septum (Common Atrium). Although common atrium is rare with tricuspid atresia, it may occur with tricuspid atresia or more frequently with other complex anomalies occasionally requiring Fontan repair. Di Carlo and coworkers[39] reported four patients with common atrium undergoing Fontan correction for complex cardiac lesions, three of whom died. They concluded that the excess amount of pericardial or prosthetic material necessary for creation of an atrial septum could result in excessive loss of contractile atrial myocardium and/or complex intra-atrial pathways with potential for obstruction, and advised caution for Fontan repair associated with this entity. A large, mobile, septal patch may deviate away from high pressure, which for Fontan repair may result in leftward shift with obstruction to pulmonary venous return.

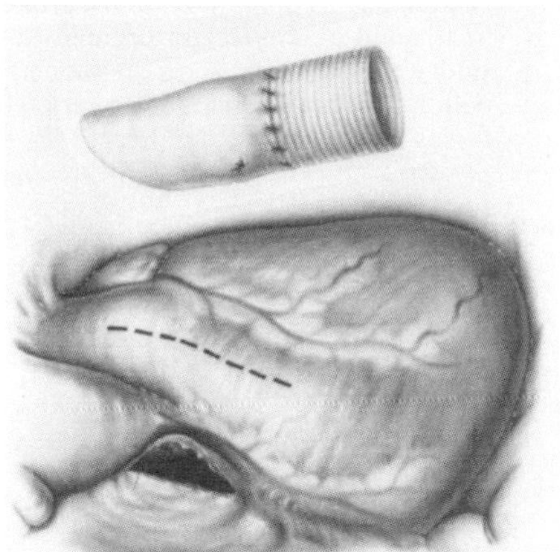
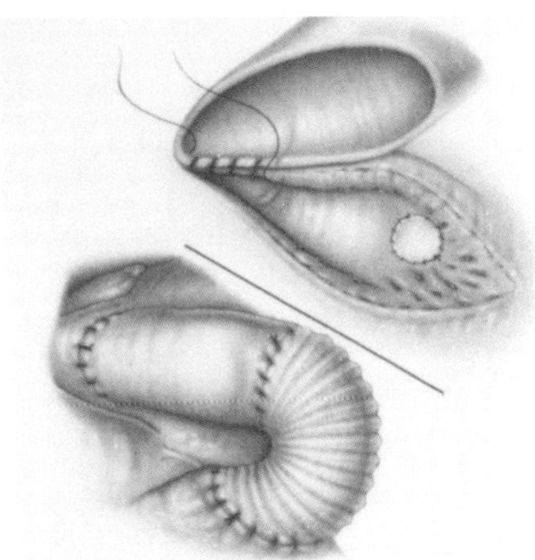

FIGURE 8. Homograft-valved right atrial-right ventricular connection in patient with hypoplastic pulmonary valve annulus requiring transannular incision. Preferably, as described in the text, for patients without hypoplastic pulmonary annulus the interposed Dacron would be deleted, and a direct atrial to ventricular anastomosis made with interposition of the homograft valve, ending the ventricular incision below the pulmonary valve annulus. (Reprinted with permission from de Leval M: Surgery for Congenital Heart Defects. New York, Grune & Stratton, 1983, pp. 453–466.)

Outlet Chamber/Pulmonary Valve Stenosis. When the right ventricle or outlet chamber is incorporated into the repair, the experience of Fontan's group is worth noting.[40] They found that in 15 patients with Type I tricuspid atresia, eight had anterior deviation of the outlet septum relative to the primary septum which functioned as infundibular pulmonary stenosis. Conversely, for patients with Type II tricuspid atresia, five of 13 patients had posterior deviation of the outlet septum which restricted pulmonary blood flow. In those Type II patients without restricted pulmonary blood flow, the outlet chamber was restrictive, causing subaortic stenosis. The Great Ormond Street Group[41] has also reported early mortality related to obstruction within an outlet chamber. The importance of gradient-free connection cannot be overemphasized, and Fontan's group recommends resection of the lower, anterior part of the outlet septum to enlarge the outlet chamber and allow incorporation of the trabecular portion of this chamber with its capacity for growth.

The frequency of pulmonary wave stenosis was assessed by Weinberg.[42] He found that two-thirds of patients with tricuspid atresia with normally related arteries had significant pulmonary valvular stenosis, which would not have been alleviated with a typical right atrial/right ventricular connection. Again, this must either be corrected at time of surgery (preferably by valvotomy but, if necessary, valvectomy with or without transannular patch)[43] or avoided altogether by direct right atrial–pulmonary artery reconstruction.

Subaortic Obstruction. A particularly vexsome problem, and one associated with a high mortality, is that of subaortic obstruction associated with tricuspid atresia, ventriculoarterial discordance, and closing ventricular septal defect.[33,44,45] This problem is more commonly seen with univentricular heart, and is associated with pulmonary artery bands to control excessive pulmonary blood flow. This

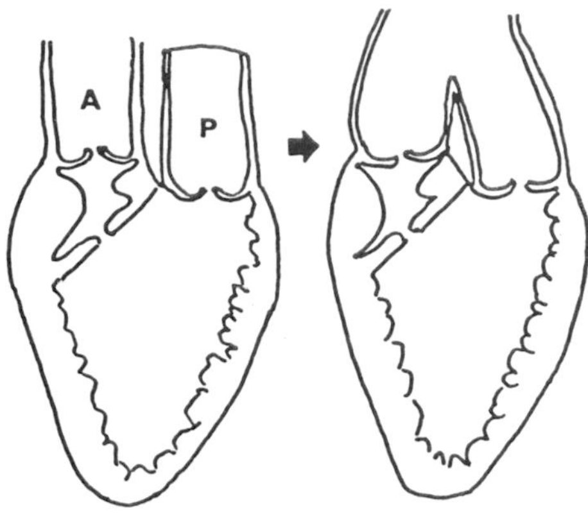

FIGURE 9. Anastomosis of the proximal main pulmonary artery end-to-side to the ascending aorta for patients with subaortic obstruction and various forms of univentricular heart. (Reprinted with permission from Circulation 54(Suppl III):63–70, 1976.)

latter point deserves emphasis, as patients with pulmonary artery bands should be followed closely for development of subaortic stenosis, and referred for corrective surgery before it becomes severe. Since their pulmonary resistances may also be relatively high due to previous excessive pulmonary blood flow, they are formidable challenges for Fontan repair.

Surgical options are resection of subaortic tissue through the aorta or through the right ventricular outflow tract with concomitant enlargement of the ventricular septal defect, apical-aortic conduit, and anastomosis of the proximal main pulmonary artery directly or with conduit end-to-side to the ascending aorta by the method of Yacoub (Fig. 9).[46] Castaneda's group[44] found an overall 58% operative mortality for subaortic stenosis associated with either univentricular heart or tricuspid atresia using the three surgical options just cited, with no survivors when the gradient was over 75 mm Hg. The best procedure in their hands was the pulmonary artery to ascending aorta anastomosis, even though 7 of 13 patients died with that technique. Fontan[33] prefers resection of subaortic tissue because of its simplicity, and avoidance of using the pulmonary valve as systemic valve. This technique does carry a significant hazard of conduction injury and residual gradient.

Miscellaneous Operative Problems. Previous pulmonary artery bands may increase the difficulty of Fontan correction. One solution to this problem, which also corrected ventriculoarterial discordance, was proposed by Freedom and coworkers,[47] who performed arterial switch, coronary artery reimplantation, and valved right atrioventricular conduit for a 14-year-old boy with Type II tricuspid atresia and previous pulmonary artery band. This technique was also used successfully in a similar patient subsequently with associated subaortic obstruction.

Previous Waterston shunts may also pose difficulty, particularly from distortion and stenosis of the right pulmonary artery. The Mayo Clinic group[48] successfully repaired four such patients by transsecting the right pulmonary artery at the site of anastomosis, sewing the distal end to the side of the superior vena cava to construct a modified Glenn shunt (the superior vena cava is not ligated), completing the repair with a right atrial–right ventricular or right atrial–main pulmonary artery anastomosis. Alternatively, the stenotic right pulmonary artery must be enlarged with patch graft angioplasty if pulmonary artery continuity is desired.

Three other reports are worth citing. Two deal with corrective procedures for unusual anomalies rarely associated with tricuspid atresia, one the Wolff-Parkinson-White syndrome,[49] the other dextrotransposition, dextrocardia, and mitral insufficiency.[50] The third report[51] evaluated techniques of ventricular exclusion by closure of the right atrioventricular ostium during Fontan correction for entities such as univentricular heart, and found that suturing the patch above the valve into the atrial wall gave superior results to a patch sutured into the valve leaflets.

POSTOPERATIVE CARE

Emphasis postoperatively is on maintenance of adequate pulmonary blood flow, cardiac output, and urine output, for which right atrial, pulmonary artery, and left atrial monitoring lines are helpful. Because pulmonary blood flow following Fontan repair is effected primarily by right atrial volume, maintenance of right atrial pressure from 10–15 mm Hg and occasionally higher is necessary for adequate cardiac output. In the event oliguria, constricted extremities, hepatomegaly, peripheral edema, and other signs of poor perfusion appear in the face of elevated right atrial pressures, the pulmonary artery and left atrial lines provide critical information.

If left atrial pressure is also elevated, ventricular dysfunction or mitral incompetence or stenosis is present, and dopamine is instituted. Williams and associates[52] found that when dopamine was administered following Fontan repair at 7.5 μg/kg/min four important hemodynamic responses were observed: (1) an increase in cardiac index, (2) an increase in heart rate, (3) a decrease in pulmonary vascular resistance (PVR), and (4) no change in right atrial pressure. When nitroprusside (NTP) was administered at a rate of 4.5 μg/kg/min, cardiac index increases significantly while right atrial pressure, PVR, left atrial pressure, systemic vascular resistance, and blood pressure all decreased.

If right atrial pressure is more than 5 mm Hg above left atrial pressure, the pulmonary artery pressure is used to determine site of the pathway resistance. If pulmonary artery pressure is also elevated, either increased PVR or small size of the pulmonary arteries is likely. The principles of reducing PVR are to optimize blood gases (specifically correct hypoxia, hypercardia, and acidosis, all of which promote pulmonary vasoconstriction), avoid vasoconstrictors at high doses, use NTP or nitroglycerin (NTG) as much as allowable by blood pressure, and keep mean airway pressures as low as possible. Positive end-expiratory pressure (PEEP) is not used, and extubation is performed as early as possible, assuming the patient is otherwise stable. Whether NTP or NTG is preferable as initial pulmonary vasodilator is debatable. Ilbawi and coworkers[53] found high dose NTG (5 μg/kg/min) to be very effective at lowering pulmonary artery pressure after heart surgery and concluded that it was the vasodilator of choice for the pulmonary vascular bed (although NTP was not compared in a comparable group of patients).

If pulmonary artery pressure is low and the right atrial pressure is more than 1–2 mm Hg higher, then significant stenosis is present somewhere along the right atrial–pulmonary artery connection. In this situation, if the right atrial pressure is greater than 18 mm Hg or there is evidence of hemodynamic instability, reoperation with revision of the right atrial–pulmonary artery connection should be seriously considered. In this setting, a Glenn shunt has been used to reduce right atrial volume loading (which, if performed to the side of the right pulmonary artery, maintains pulmonary artery continuity).[54]

Use of an external compression (MAST) suit on the lower body has been advocated as a "venous assist device" to improve low cardiac output caused by venous congestion and inadequate preload.[55,56] The suit is attached to a pneumatic pressure–volume cycled extremity pump (Jobst Institute) inflated to a pressure of 45–50 mm Hg for 45 seconds, then deflated to O mm Hg for 15 seconds, and cycled repeatedly. This assists in moving extravascular fluid back into the vascular space, augmenting central venous pressure to overcome pulmonary resistance.

The tendency to collect fluid in the pleural, peritoneal, pericardial, and tissue spaces has been noted, and chest tubes are routinely placed at surgery and left in until drainage is minimal. Use of colloid as opposed to crystalloid solutions may be helpful to retain the fluid intravascularly. Additionally, sodium restriction, digitalis, and diuretic therapy are generally indicated. The effusions frequently become chylous, escaping from the vascular system at multiple points rather than an isolated thoracic duct site.[31] Although chylous effusions may occasionally be serious and persistent after Fontan repair, in most cases they will subside with appropriate therapy as outlined above.

When all supportive measures are failing with a technically satisfactory repair, De Leon and colleagues[45] suggest that takedown of the repair should be considered. They report two of four survivors of takedown (closure of atriopulmonary anastomosis, creation of both atrial septal defect, and systemic-pulmonary artery shunts) from 6 to 65 hours postoperatively and suggest its usefulness in persistent low cardiac output states following Fontan operation.

OPERATIVE MORTALITY

Initial operative mortality for the Fontan operation was appreciable, varying from 15–30%.[21,35,57–62] With a better understanding of both preoperative and technical risk factors, however, it has now declined to less than 10%.[21,35,56,57,63,64] Recent mortality for the Fontan procedure in patients with tricuspid atresia has been reported as 7% by Kirklin's group,[57] 4.5% at the Mayor Clinic,[21] and a remarkable 3.7% by Fontan.[35]

A number of important risk factors have been identified which carry higher operative mortality. Conditions other than tricuspid atresia such as univentricular heart and other complex malformations have consistently had a higher operative mortality.[13,21,56,57,61,65] Young age (< 4 years) also carries higher risk,[21,35,57] as does older age, by which time left ventricular function may be compromised by chronic volume overload.[52,64] Significant preoperative pulmonary vascular disease and mitral valve disease are universally recognized as being associated with higher operative mortality. Fontan[35] also noted a slightly higher operative mortality in patients with associated transposition (Type II) versus Type I patients (partly due to subaortic obstruction as discussed above), but the type of right atrial–pulmonary artery connection did not significantly influence operative mortality. Laks and associates[65] found that valveless right atrial–pulmonary artery connections fared worse than those with valves in the early postoperative period, but this has not been observed by most groups, provided the connection is without gradient.

PROGNOSIS

Most survivors of the Fontan procedure have done well. Premature late death is uncommon, with Fontan[35] reporting an actuarial 14-year survival rate of over 90% once operative deaths were excluded. Ninety-four percent of the survivors were in New York Heart Association (NYHA) Class I or II. Although the type of connection did not significantly influence the operative mortality in Fontan's experience, those patients receiving homograft valves fared better (more asymptomatic patients, better postoperative exercise capacity) over the long term than did those patients receiving valveless connections. In a separate report, Fontan's group[66] noted five late deaths—one was during arrhythmia, one was sudden and unexplained, and the other three were after reoperation. Of these five patients, four had evidence of obstruction of the atriopulmonary or atrioventricular conduit.

Excellent long-term results have also been consistently reported by other groups as well.[21,57,58,61,63,67] De Brux and associates[58] reported that 88% of Fontan survivors led a normal life, two-thirds requiring no treatment. De Vivie and Rupprath[67] found that 75% of survivors had excellent results at late catheterization. Gale and colleagues[21] reported that 17/19 (89.5%) patients had either no or only mild restriction during exercise. Kirklin's experience[57,61] was that 96% of Fontan survivors were in NYHA Class I or II.

The most common reasons for late problems, occasionally requiring reoperation, in these various experiences were anastomotic or conduit obstruction, deterioration of homograft or porcine valves, mitral or left ventricular dysfunction, and occasionally residual atrial septal defects.

LATE COMPLICATIONS

The problem of neointimal "peel formation" inside Dacron conduits obstructing Fontan repairs has been noted by several observers.[14,21,68] It may be fatal, and has led to widespread discontinuation of cloth conduits for Fontan repair. Similar problems with porcine valve degeneration has decreased enthusiasm for their incorporation into Fontan repair,[14,15,21,30] with increasing use of homograft valves.[35] Mitral valvular or left ventricular dysfunction may cause late morbidity and mortality, as can residual atrial septal defects as already noted.

Protein-losing enteropathy has been noted following Fontan repair.[69,70] Presumably it is similar in etiology to other conditions with elevated right atrial pressure which may cause it, even though patients developing protein-losing enteropathy may not have obvious differences in right atrial pressure compared to those without. Hess and associates[69] did note higher diastolic right atrial pressure in patients with protein-losing enteropathy, although mean right atrial pressures did not differ between those with and without it. Crupi and colleagues[70] noted it in a patient with marked regurgitation through a valveless Dacron conduit, and successfully corrected it with subsequent insertion of a right atrial valve. Cirrhosis of the liver from chronic passive congestion in a patient 5.5 years after Fontan repair with mild conduit stenosis has also been reported.[71]

Development of late heart block is uncommon, occurring only once in the experience of Gale et al.[21] Likewise, susceptibility to late infection has not been found to be very common in Fontan's experience.[35] An increased susceptibility to cerebrovascular accident has been reported.[78]

Two other reports deserve comment regarding late complications. Juaneda and Haworth[72] found that patients with increased pulmonary blood flow prior to Fontan repair, even when protected by a pulmonary artery band and with PVR < 4 units/m^2, had a significant increase in pulmonary vascular smooth muscle and poorer long-term result than patients with diminished pulmonary blood flow. Warnes and Somerville[51] also found pulmonary vascular disease and subaortic stenosis to be difficult problems in adolescents and adults with Type II tricuspid atresia, and recommend Fontan repair only in older patients who met all selection criteria for the operation preoperatively. A shunt was the preferred option when any of the criteria were not met.

POSTOPERATIVE RIGHT HEART/PULMONARY ARTERY FLOW PATTERNS

Postoperative right atrial pressure is the most important variable influencing pulmonary artery flow in the experience of most authorities, assuming the right atrial–pulmonary artery connection is nonobstructive and pulmonary artery size and pressure are reasonable. This was the finding of Shemin and colleagues[30] in the experimental study previously described, which also found that the absence of a valve, ventricular rhythm, and tachycardia did not significantly alter flow. The observation that right atrial contraction is not critical to maintenance of pulmonary blood flow was also supported by separate clinical studies by Matsuda et al.[73] and Nakazawa et al.[74]

Studies of actual right atrial pressure, not surprisingly, have shown variation. Serratto and associates[15] found that right atrial pressure increased to an average of 17 mm Hg late postoperatively, with all patients showing good atrial transport function regardless of rhythm. Castaneda's group[59] found mean right atrial pressure studied late after Fontan procedure for tricuspid atresia to be only 8 mm Hg, with mean pulmonary artery pressure only 7 mm Hg. In their experience, early postoperative right atrial pressure of 17 or greater was invariably associated with serious morbidity and mortality. Laks et al.[56] found that postoperative exercise testing resulted in marked rise in right atrial pressure and reduced (compared to normal) rise in cardiac index, even in patients without functional limitations.

Pulmonary artery flow is biphasic following Fontan repair, being influenced by right atrial contraction and relaxation, and by left atrial emptying.[25,65,73,75] In the experience of DiSessa et al.,[25] the most common biphasic pattern following Fontan repair is one flow period beginning in early ventricular diastole and peaking at or before atrial systole, followed by a second phase peaking during ventricular systole. Sharatt and associates[76] found pulmonary blood flow to be pulsatile, with atrial systole an important factor. Nakazawa and colleagues[77] found the size of pulmonary arteries to be important factors in flow patterns, with right atrial contraction more important in patients with smaller pulmonary arteries. Average right atrial and pulmonary artery pressures in patients with tricuspid atresia after Fontan repair were 16 and 16 respectively, with pulmonary artery size an important determinant of postoperative hemodynamics.

As noted, controversy still exists as to the importance of valves and/or preservation of the right ventricle in augmenting pulmonary blood flow. Certainly numerous survivors of direct, nonvalved right atrial–pulmonary artery connections attest to the feasibility of valveless right heart bypass for many patients. Laks and colleagues[56] found pulmonary blood flow to be biphasic in all without distinction between the type of connection or presence of a valve, whereas Nakazawa et al.[74] found that pulmonary regurgitation was not significant after Fontan repair, even when valves were not inserted. However, Bull and coworkers[23,41] have demonstrated incorporation of the right ventricle, while conferring no early advantage postoperatively, may perform useful work subsequently with growth. Catheterization in these patients has frequently shown mean right atrial pressures to be less than mean pulmonary artery pressures, suggesting a right ventricle-dependent pulmonary circulation with more normal hemodynamic pattern. This was also the conclusion of Bowman et al.,[18] as discussed earlier.

The leading advocate of valve incorporation is Fontan, who has consistently demonstrated less regurgitation and better postoperative exercise capacity in patients receiving homografts.[32,35] In discussing the experience of Laks and associates,[56] Fontan noted exercise to 75%–100% of normal capacity postoperatively in patients receiving valved connection. In concluding discussion of his paper, Laks[56] agrees that although valves are not usually necessary in right atrial–right ventricular connections, "in the borderline patient with somewhat elevated venous pressure, [they] may make a critical difference."

LEFT VENTRICULAR FUNCTION

Left ventricular function following Fontan repair for tricuspid atresia is often abnormal, even though most patients will be in NYHA Class I or Class II.[79-84] Graham and associates[79] found that Fontan repair for tricuspid atresia resulted in less volume overload and left ventricular hypertrophy than palliation only, but increased afterload and abnormal contractile function persisted in a significant number of patients. Schachar and colleagues[80] noted that cardiac index was low at rest (average 2.3 ± 0.6 L/min/m^2) and during exercise (4.9 ± 1.1 L/min/m^2) due to low stroke index, even though all exercised patients were in NYHA Class I. They also noted that exercise increased mean conduit gradients to 8 mm Hg, and found this "functional conduit obstruction" partly causative of the abnormal exercise response.

Tarso and associates[81] also found that left ventricular contraction at rest and after exercise were abnormal after Fontan repair, even though patients were asymptomatic. Hurwitz and associates[82] evaluated patients receiving Fontan repair after the age of 5 years, and noted that these patients may not have an increase in ejection fraction over preoperative values and may have a decrease. Ejection fraction averaged 0.56 ± 0.14 in 14 postoperative patients. Nakue et al.[83] found an average 24% reduction in postoperative left ventricular end-diastolic volume (LVEDV), but only 8% reduction in postoperative left ventricular end-systolic volume (LVESV). Because of the small change in LVESV, the ejection fraction decreased from an average 0.61 preoperatively to 0.48 postoperatively. This study suggests that one reason for the slightly reduced ejection fraction in Fontan repairs may be development of a somewhat stiff, noncompliant left ventricle preoperatively which does not return completely to normal after removal of the chronic volume overload.

Improved ventricular function following Fontan repair has been noted by others.[32,35,64,75,85,86] Peterson and associates[85] found mean cardiac index following Fontan repair to be 5.2 ± 2.0 L/min/m^2 at rest, increasing to 9.4 ± 3.5 L/min/m^2 during exercise. Although ejection fractions were significantly less than those in normal children, the ability of the left ventricle to generate a large and acceptable exercise cardiac output, without a functioning right ventricle, was clearly demonstrated. Driscoll and coworkers[86] also noted substantial increase in exercise capacity following Fontan repair, again noting cardiac output and stroke volume response to exercise were still subnormal compared to control values. Hagler and associates[75] demonstrated normal or only mildly reduced ventricular function (ejection fraction > 40%) in two-thirds of Fontan patients, but also noted mitral valve insufficiency in varying severity in 30% of the total group. Mair and colleagues[64] found 77% of 65 operative survivors to be in excellent condition late after Fontan repair. Late catheterization in 25 of these patients demonstrated significant decline in LVEDP (from mean 16.5 preoperatively to 8.5 mm Hg postoperatively), with the mean volume load on the left ventricle after operation decreased to less than one-third of the preoperative level. Seven late deaths occurred from 0.5 to 6 years after surgery, with progressive left ventricular deterioration and failure the cause of death in four. As two of these four had the operation performed in adulthood, the Mayo Clinic group recommends the Fontan operation by age 6 years to protect myocardial function.

To summarize, left ventricular function, at rest and during exercise, following Fontan repair for tricuspid atresia will be improved in over 75%, due primarily to removal of the chronic volume overload. Postoperative stroke volume and ejection fraction will usually be reduced compared to normal controls, however, partly due to development of a less than normally compliant ventricle. Conduit gradients developing with exercise may also diminish exercise capacity. Offering the Fontan repair too late (after 6 years) may result in a poor result due to irreversible left ventricular dysfunction acquired preoperatively.

INDICATIONS

The appropriate selection of patients for the Fontan procedure, along with meticulous surgical technique and excellent postoperative care, are the most important factors to ensure a successful outcome.[32,35] Once tricuspid atresia is diagnosed, the timing of ultimate Fontan correction should be considered. Assuming a systemic–pulmonary artery shunt is necessary initially, close follow-up is important to recognize the optimal age for Fontan repair, with the knowledge that the higher risk of operating at an early age at some point becomes offset by the added risk of left ventricular dysfunction developing from chronic volume overload. Certainly, when patients outgrow their initial palliative shunt, as evidenced by increasing cyanosis, rising hemoglobin, or progressive exercise intolerance, their eligibility for Fontan repair should be evaluated. A subset of patients with tricuspid atresia in whom close follow-up is especially important are those with transposition of the great arteries (Type II) with increased pulmonary blood flow in whom pulmonary artery bands are placed. As discussed earlier, the subsequent development of subaortic stenosis in these patients is associated with a high mortality with Fontan repair, and correction should be performed before it becomes severe.

Based upon their extensive experience, Fontan's group has suggested a set of rules, the "ten commandments," to be followed for optimal results (Table 1). Of the 10 criteria, a few deserve special comment. Small pulmonary arteries or pulmonary vascular resistance above 4 units/m^2 are strict contraindications. If pulmonary artery pressure is elevated as a result of a systemic–pulmonary artery shunt that will be closed at the time of correction, it is not a contraindication. Mitral incompetence is a contraindication, unless it can be corrected at the time of repair.[31,87] Significant left ventricular dysfunction portends a bad result, with Kreutzer et al.[20] obtaining the best results when left ventricular end-diastolic and right atrial pressures were low preoperatively. This also emphasizes the importance of not delaying repair too long. Finally young age still carries a higher mortality, although recently good results have been reported with Fontan repairs performed

TABLE 1. Selection of Patients for Fontan Procedure: The Ten Commandments

1. Minimum age of 4 years
2. Sinus rhythm
3. Normal caval drainage
4. Right atrium of normal volume
5. Mean pulmonary artery pressure $\leq$ 15 mm Hg
6. Pulmonary arteriolar resistance $<$ 4 units.m^2
7. Pulmonary artery to aorta diameter ratio $\geq$ 0.75
8. Normal ventricular function (ejection fraction $\geq$ 0.6
9. Competent left atrioventricular valve
10. No impairing effects of previous shunt

From Fontan I, Choussat A, Besse P: Pediatric Cardiology 1977. Edinburgh, Churchill Livingstone, 1978, Ch. 64, with permission.

under 4 years of age using otherwise strict criteria and meticulous surgical technique.[31]

More recently good operative results have been achieved outside these criteria, but with increased operative risk.[21,88] Whether one should accept a higher risk with a better result for most survivors, or a lower operative risk but less corrective procedure by performing another systemic–pulmonary artery shunt, requires considerable judgment. Fontan still stresses the importance of strict preoperative guidelines, denying the repair to patients not meeting them.[33]

REFERENCES

1. Hurwitt ES, Young D, Escher DJW: The rationale of anastomosis of the right auricular appendage to the pulmonary artery in the treatment of tricuspid atresia. J Thorac Surg 30:503, 1955.
2. Starr I, Jeffers WA, Meade RH: The absence of conspicuous increments of venous pressure after severe damage to the right ventricle of the dog, with a discussion of the relation between clinical congestive failure and heart disease. Am Heart J 26:291, 1943.
3. Rodbard S, Wagner D: Bypassing the right ventricle. Proc Soc Exp Biol Med 71:69, 1949.
4. Warden HE, DeWall RA, Varco RL: Use of the right auricle as a pump for the pulmonary conduit. Surg Forum 5:16, 1954.
5. Fontan F, Mounicot F-B, Baudet E, et al: "Correction" de l'atresie tricuspidienne. Rapport de deux cas "corriges" par l'utilisation d'une technique chirurgicale nouvelle. Ann Chir Thorac Cardiovasc 10:39, 1971.
6. Fontan F, Baudet E: Surgical repair of tricuspid atresia. Thorax 26:240, 1971.
7. Kreutzer G, Galindez E, Bono H, et al: An operation for the correction of tricuspid atresia. J Thorac Cardiovasc Surg 66:613, 1973.
8. Ross DN, Somerville J: Surgical correction of tricuspid atresia. Lancet 1:845, 1973.
9. Stanford W, Armstrong RG, Cline RE, King TD: Right atrium–pulmonary artery allograft for correction of tricuspid atresia. J Thorac Cardiovasc Surg 66:105, 1973.
10. Henry JH, Devloo RAE, Ritter DG, et al: Tricuspid atresia. Successful surgical "correction" in two patients using porcine xenograft valves. Mayo Clin Proc 49:803, 1974.
11. Tatooles CJ, Ardekani RG, Miller RA, et al: Results following physiological repair for tricuspid atresia. Ann Thorac Surg 22:578, 1976.
12. Bjork VO, Olin CL, Bjarke BB, Thoren CA: Right atrial–right ventricular anastomosis for correction of tricuspid atresia. J Thorac Cardiovasc Surg 77:452, 1979.
13. Gale AW, Danielson GK, McGoon DC, Mair DD: Modified Fontan operation for univentricular heart and complicated congenital lesions. J Thorac Cardiovasc Surg 78:831, 1979.
14. Behrendt DM, Rosenthal A: Cardiovascular status after repair by Fontan procedure. Ann Thorac Surg 29:322, 1980.
15. Seratto M, Miller RA, Tatooles C, Ardekani R: Hemodynamic evaluation of Fontan operation in tricuspid atresia. Circulation 54(Suppl 3):99, 1976.
16. Heck HA Jr, Schieken RM, Lauer RM, Doty DB: Conduit repair for complex congenital heart disease. Late follow-up. J Thorac Cardiovasc Surg 75:806, 1978.

17. Bailey WW, Kirklin JW, Bargeron LM, et al: Late results with synthetic valved external conduits from venous ventricle to pulmonary arteries. Circulation 56(Suppl 2):73, 1979.
18. Bowman FO, Malm JR, Hayes CJ, Gersony WM: Physiological approach to surgery for tricuspid atresia. Circulation 58(Suppl I):I-83, 1978.
19. Doty DB, Marvin WW Jr, Lauer RM: Modified Fontan procedure. J Thorac Cardiovasc Surg 81:470, 1981.
20. Kreutzer GO, Vargas FJ, Schlichter AJ, et al: Atriopulmonary anastomosis. J Thorac Cardiovasc Surg 83:427, 1982.
21. Gale AW, Danielson GK, McGoon DC, et al: Fontan procedure for tricuspid atresia. Circulation 62:91, 1980.
22. Lee C-N, Schaff HV, Danielson GK, et al: Comparison of atriopulmonary versus atrioventricular connections for modified Fontan/Kreutzer repair of tricuspid valve atresia. J Thorac Cardiovasc Surg 92:1038, 1986.
23. Bull C, de Leval MR, Stark J, et al: Use of a subpulmonary ventricular chamber in Fontan circulation. J Thorac Cardiovasc Surg 85:21, 1983.
24. Bowman F Jr, in discussion, Bull C, de Leval MR, Stark J, et al: Use of a subpulmonary ventricular chamber in the Fontan circulation. J Thorac Cardiovasc Surg 85:21, 1983.
25. DiSessa TG, Child JS, Perloff JK, et al: Systemic venous and pulmonary arterial flow patterns after Fontan's procedure for tricuspid atresia or single ventricle. Circulation 70:898, 1984.
26. Gussenhoven WJ, The JK, Schippers L, et al: Growth and function of the right ventricular outflow tract after Fontan's procedure for tricuspid atresia: A two-dimensional echocardiographic study. Thorac Cardiovasc Surg 34:236, 1986.
27. de Vivie ER, Weber H, Kirchhoff PG, et al: Fontan procedure and surgical modification in tricuspid atresia. Thorac Cardiovasc Surg 28:162, 1980.
28. Ishikawa T, Neutze JM, Brandt PWT, Barratt-Boyes BG: Hemodynamics following the Kreutzer procedure for tricuspid atresia in patients under 2 years of age. J Thorac Cardiovasc Surg 88:373, 1984.
29. Neveux J-Y, Dreyfus G, Leca F, et al: Modified technique for correction of tricuspid atresia. J Thorac Cardiovasc Surg 82:457, 1981.
30. Shemin RJ, Merrill WH, Pfeifer JS, et al: Evaluation of right atrial pulmonary conduits for tricuspid atresia. J Thorac Cardiovasc Surg 77:685, 1979.
31. Kirklin JW, Barratt-Boyes BG: Tricuspid atresia. In Kirklin JW, Barratt-Boyes BG (eds): Cardiac Surgery. New York, John Wiley and Sons, 1986, pp. 857–888.
32. Ottenkamp J, Rohmer J, Quaegebeur JM, et al: Nine years' experience of physiological correction of tricuspid atresia: long-term results and current surgical approach. Thorax 37:718, 1982.
33. Fontan FM, in discussion, Lee C-N, Schaff HV, Danielson GK, et al: Comparison of atriopulmonary versus atrioventricular connections for modified Fontan/Kreutzer repair of tricuspid valve atresia. J Thorac Cardiovasc Surg 92:1038, 1986.
34. Pennington DG, Nouri S, Ho J, et al: Glenn shunt: Long-term results and current role in congenital heart operations. Ann Thorac Surg 31:532, 1981.
35. Fontan F, Deville C, Quaegebeur J, et al: Repair of tricuspid atresia in 100 patients. J Thorac Cardiovasc Surg 85:647, 1983.
36. Quaegebeur J, Kirklin JW, Pacifico AD, et al: Surgical experience with unroofed coronary sinus. Ann Thorac Surg 27:418, 1979.
37. Kurosawa H, Yagi Y, Imamura E, et al: A problem in Fontan's operation: Sinus septal defect complicating tricuspid atresia. Heart and Vessels 1:48, 1985.
38. Rumisek JD, Pigott JD, Weinberg PM, et al: Coronary sinus septal defect associated with tricuspid atresia. J Thorac Cardiovasc Surg 92:142, 1986.
39. Di Carlo D, Marcelletti C, Nijveld A, et al: The Fontan procedure in the absence of the interatrial septum. J Thorac Cardiovasc Surg 85:923, 1983.
40. Ottenkamp J, Wenink ACG, Quaegebeur JM, et al: Tricuspid atresia: Morphology of the outlet chamber with special emphasis on surgical implications. J Thorac Cardiovasc Surg 89:597, 1985.
41. Bull C, Stark J, de Leval M: The Fontan procedure: Which modification? J Am Coll Cardiol 5:478, 1985.
42. Weinberg PM: Anatomy of tricuspid atresia and its relevance to current forms of surgical therapy. Ann Thorac Surg 29:306, 1980.
43. Ishizawa E, Horiuchi T, Sato S, et al: Successful surgical correction in two patients with tricuspid atresia using autologous pericardial valve-bearing tube graft. J Cardiovasc Surg 21:11, 1980.
44. Rothman A, Lang P, Lock JE, et al: Surgical management of subaortic obstruction in single left ventricle and tricuspid atresia. J Am Coll Cardiol 10:421, 1987.

45. DeLeon SY, Ilbawi MN, Idriss FS, et al: Persistent low cardiac output after the Fontan operation. Should takedown be considered? J Thorac Cardiovasc Surg 92:402, 1986.
46. Yacoub MH, Radley-Smith R: Use of a valved conduit from right atrium to pulmonary artery for "correction" of a single ventricle. Circulation 54(Suppl III):III-63, 1976.
47. Freedom RM, Williams WG, Fowler RS, et al: Tricuspid atresia, transposition of the great arteries, and banded pulmonary artery. Repair by arterial switch, coronary artery reimplantation, and right atrioventricular valved conduit. J Thorac Cardiovasc Surg 80:621, 1980.
48. Uretzky G, Puga FJ, Danielson GK: Modified Fontan procedure in patients with previous ascending aorta-pulmonary artery anastomosis. J Thorac Cardiovasc Surg 85:447, 1983.
49. Dick M II, Behrendt DM, Byrum CJ, et al: Tricuspid atresia and the Wolff-Parkinson-White syndrome: Evaluation methodology and successful surgical treatment of the combined disorders. Am Heart J 101:496, 1981.
50. Jennings RB Jr, Crisler C, Johnson DH, et al: Tricuspid atresia with dextrotransposition, dextrocardia, and mitral insufficiency: Successful circulatory correction. Ann Thorac Surg 29:369, 1980.
51. DiDonato R, Becker AE, Nijveld A, et al: Ventricular exclusion during Fontan operation: An evolving technique. Ann Thorac Surg 39:283, 1985.
52. Williams DB, Keirman PD, Schaff HV, et al: The hemodynamic response to dopamine and nitroprusside following right atrium–pulmonary artery bypass (Fontan procedure). Ann Thorac Surg 34:51, 1982.
53. Ilbawi MN, Idriss FS, DeLeon SY, et al: Hemodynamic effects of intravenous nitroglycerin in pediatric patients after heart surgery. Circulation 72(Suppl II):II–101, 1985.
54. DeLeon SY, Idriss FS, Ilbawi MN, et al: The role of the Glenn shunt in patients undergoing the Fontan operation. J Thorac Cardiovasc Surg 85:669, 1983.
55. Heck H, Doty D: Assisted circulation by phasic external lower body compression. Circulation 64(Suppl II):118, 1981.
56. Laks H, Milliken JC, Perloff JK, Hellenbrand WE, et al: Experience with the Fontan procedure. J Thorac Cardiovasc Surg 88:939, 1984.
57. Cleveland DC, Kirklin JK, Naftel DC, et al: Surgical treatment of tricuspid atresia. Ann Thorac Surg 38:447, 1984.
58. Brux JL, Zannini L, Binet JP, et al: Tricuspid atresia. Results of treatment in 115 children. J Thorac Cardiovasc Surg 85:440, 1983.
59. Sanders SP, Wright GB, Keane JF, et al: Clinical and hemodynamic results of the Fontan operation for tricuspid atresia. Am J Cardiol 49:1733, 1982.
60. Tatooles CJ, Ardekani RG, Miller RA, Serrato M: Operative repair for tricuspid atresia. Ann Thorac Surg 21:499, 1976.
61. Stefanelli G, Kirklin JW, Naftel DC, et al: Early and intermediate term (10-year) results of surgery for single ventricle. Am J Cardiol 54:811, 1984.
62. de Vivie ER, Ruschewski W, Koveker G, et al: Fontan procedure—indication and clinical results. Thorac Cardiovasc Surg 29:348, 1981.
63. Stanton RE, Lurie PR, Lindesmith GG, Meyer BW: The Fontan procedure for tricuspid atresia. Circulation 64(Suppl II):II-140, 1981.
64. Mair DG, Rice MJ, Hagler DJ, et al: Outcome of the Fontan procedure in patients with tricuspid atresia. Circulation 72(Suppl II):88, 1985.
65. Laks H, Williams WG, Hellenbrand WE, et al: Results of right atrial to right ventricular and right atrial to pulmonary artery conduits for complex congenital heart disease. Ann Surg 192:382, 1980.
66. Girod DA, Fontan F, DeVille C, et al: Long-term results after the Fontan operation for tricuspid atresia. Circulation 75:605, 1987.
67. de Vivie E-R, Rupparth G: Long-term results after Fontan procedure and its modifications. J Thorac Cardiovasc Surg 91:690, 1986.
68. Ben-Shachar G, Nicoloff DM, Edwards JE: Separation of neointima from Dacron graft causing obstruction. Case following Fontan procedure for tricuspid atresia. J Thorac Cardiovasc Surg 82:268, 1981.
69. Hess J, Kruizinga K, Bijleveld CMA, et al: Protein-losing enteropathy after Fontan operation. J Thorac Cardiovasc Surg 88:606, 1984.
70. Crupi G, Locatelli G, Tiraboschi R, et al: Protein-losing enteropathy after Fontan operation for tricuspid atresia (imperforate tricupsid valve). Thorac Cardiovasc Surg 28:359, 1980.
71. Lemmer JH, Coran AG, Behrendt DM, et al: Liver fibrosis (cardiac cirrhosis) five years after modified Fontan operation for tricuspid atresia. J Thorac Cardiovasc Surg 86:757, 1983.
72. Juaneda E, Haworth SG: Pulmonary vascular structure in patients dying after a Fontan procedure. The lung as a risk factor. Br Heart J 52:575, 1984.

73. Matsuda H, Kawashima T, Takano H, et al: Experimental evaluation of atrial function in right atrium-pulmonary artery conduit operation for tricuspid atresia. J Thorac Cardiovasc Surg 81:762, 1981.
74. Nakazawa M, Nakanishi T, Okuda H, et al: Dynamics of right heart flow in patients after Fontan procedure. Circulation 69:306, 1984.
75. Hagler DJ, Seward JB, Tajik AK, Ritter DG: Functional assessment of Fontan operation: Combined M-mode, two-dimensional and doppler echocardiographic studies. J Am Coll Cardiol 4:756, 1984.
76. Sharratt GP, Johnson AM, Monro R: Persistence and effect of sinus rhythm after Fontan procedure for tricuspid atresia. Br Heart J 42:78, 1979.
77. Nakazawa M, Nojima K, Okuda H, et al: Flow dynamics in the main pulmonary artery after the Fontan procedure in patients with tricuspid atresia or single ventricle. Circulation 75:1117, 1987.
78. Mathews K, Bale JF Jr, Clark EB, et al: Cerebral infarction complicating Fontan surgery for cyanotic congenital heart disease. Pediatr Cardiol 7:161, 1986.
79. Graham TP, Franklin RCG, Wyse RKH, et al: Left ventricular wall stress and contractile function in childhood: normal valves and comparison of Fontan repair versus palliation only in patients with tricuspid atresia. Circulation 74(Suppl I):I-61, 1986.
80. Shacher GB, Furhman BP, Wang Y, et al: Rest and exercise hemodynamics after the Fontan procedure. Circulation 65:1043, 1982.
81. Torso SD, Kelly MK, Kalff V, et al: Radionuclide assessment of ventricular contraction at rest and during exercise following the Fontan procedure for either tricuspid atresia or single ventricle. Am J Cardiol 55:1127, 1985.
82. Hurwitz RA, Caldwell RL, Girod DA, et al: Left ventricular function in tricuspid atresia: A radionuclide study. J Am Coll Cardiol 8:916, 1986.
83. Nakue S, Imai Y, Harada Y, et al: Assessment of left ventricular function before and after Fontan's operation for the correction of tricuspid atresia. Heart and Vessels 1:83, 1985.
84. Gidding SS, Rosenthal A, Rocchini A, et al: Response to the Valsalva maneuver after the Fontan procedure for tricuspid valve atresia, single ventricle or pulmonic valve atresia. Am J Cardiol 56:905, 1985.
85. Peterson RJ, Franch RH, Fajman WA: Noninvasive determination of exercise cardiac function following Fontan operation. J Thorac Cardiovasc Surg 88:263, 1984.
86. Driscoll DJ, Danielson GK, Puga FJ, et al: Exercise tolerance and cardiorespiratory response to exercise after the Fontan operation for tricuspid atresia or functional single ventricle. JACC 77:1087, 1986.
87. Choussat A, Fontan F, Besse P, et al: Selection criteria for Fontan's procedure. In RH Anderson, EA Shinebourne (eds): Pediatric Cardiology 1977. Edinburgh, Churchill Livingstone 1978, ch. 64.
88. Marcelletti C, Mazzera E, Olthof H, et al: Fontan's operation: An expanded horizon. J Thorac Cardiovasc Surg 80:764, 1980.

H. ASHRAF, MD
S. SUBRAMANIAN, MD

THE UNIVENTRICULAR HEART

From the Division of
Cardiovascular Surgery
Miami Children's Hospital
Miami, Florida

Reprint requests to:
H. Ashraf, MD
3200 S.W. 60th Court
Miami, FL 33155

The description of a univentricular heart has been a matter of controversy for a long time. The designations included single ventricle with a rudimentary outlet chamber,[1-3] common ventricle,[4] and double-inlet ventricle.[5,6] In the last decade, Anderson has made a major contribution toward simplifying the understanding of the univentricular heart.[6]

MORPHOGENESIS

The important concept in the embryology of univentricular heart is that the entire atrioventricular junction is connected to the inlet part of the primary heart tube and the arterial segments are supported by the outlet component (Fig. 1, center).[7] Normally the left ventricular trabecular component is derived from the inlet part, whereas the right ventricular apical component develops from the outlet part of the primary heart tube, which at the same time undergoes division by an apical trabecular septum. Failure to develop two separate pouches results in the formation of a ventricle with indeterminate morphology (Fig. 1, top). When the pouches form normally but the atrioventricular junction remains connected to the inlet portion, a double-inlet left ventricle results (Fig. 1, lower right). Hypoplasia of the trabecular part of outlet component would result in a rudimentary right ventricle or an outlet chamber of right ventricular morphology.

Transfer of the entire inlet part of the primary heart tube to the outlet component is responsible for a double-inlet right ventricle with rudimentary left ventricular chamber or an outlet chamber of left ventricular morphology (Fig. 1, lower left).

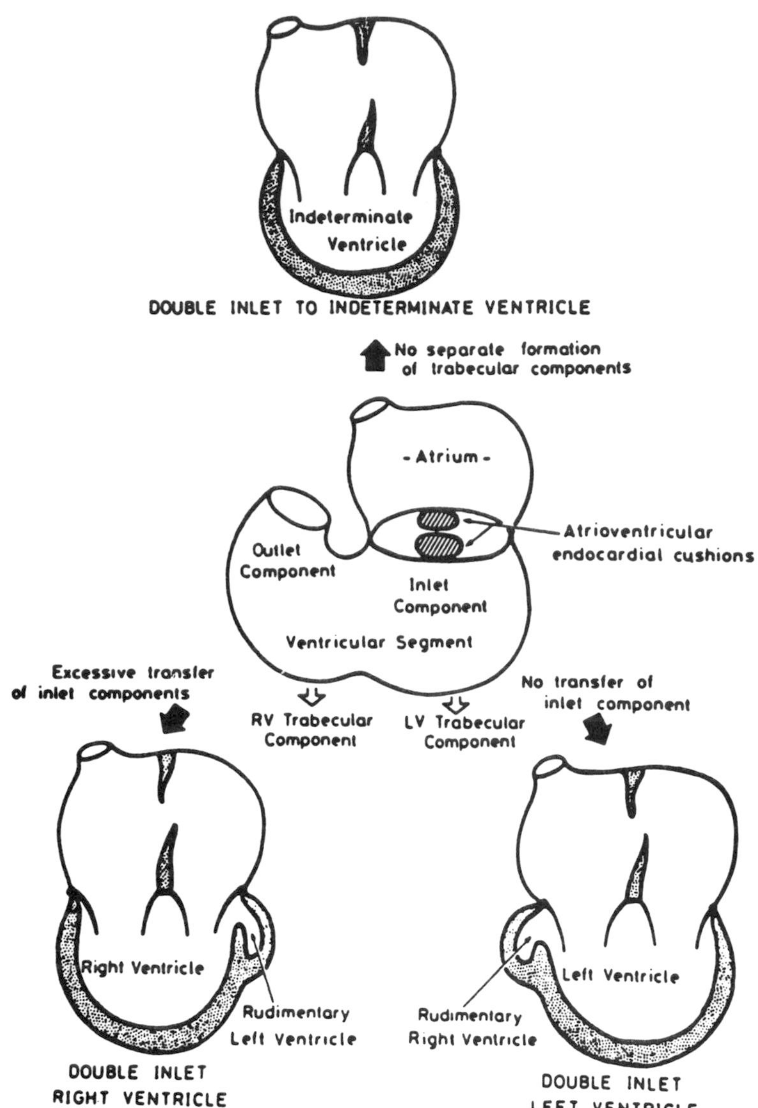

FIGURE 1. Possible mode of development of the different types of univentricular heart. (From Anderson RH, et al (eds): Pediatric Cardiology, Vol 2. New York, Churchill Livingstone, 1987, p. 653, with permission.)

ANATOMY

A univentricular heart is a cardiac malformation in which the two atria communicate with a single ventricle through two atrioventricular valves; less frequently, a common atrioventricular valve leads from the two atria into the

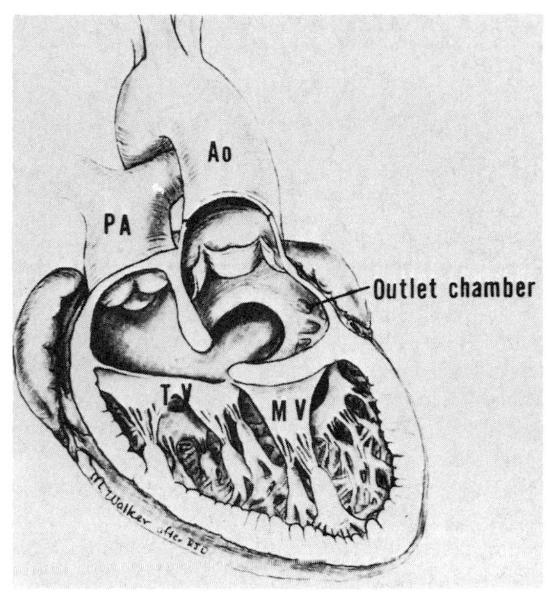

FIGURE 2. Schematic representation of univentricular heart with an outlet chamber and L-transposition of the great arteries. (From Graham TP Jr, Friesinger GG: Cardiovasc Clin 10:385, 1979, with permission.)

common ventricle. Mitral and tricuspid atresia are thus excluded from this definition.[8]

For a chamber to be characterized as a ventricle, it must receive at least 50% of an inlet valve; the chamber not receiving an inlet portion but supporting the greater part of an arterial valve is called an outlet or rudimentary chamber rather than a ventricle.[9–11] Therefore, a univentricular connection includes the heart with a sole ventricular chamber as well as that with two chambers, one of which is a ventricle, and the other, without an inlet portion, is an outlet chamber. Approximately 80% of univentricular hearts have an outlet chamber giving rise to one or both great arteries.[3,12] A typical univentricular heart of left ventricular morphology has an outlet chamber of right ventricular morphology and vice versa. Most commonly the ventricular morphology is of left ventricular type (78%), much less frequently right ventricular (18%), and occasionally of indeterminate type (4%).[3,13] The great arteries in a univentricular heart may be normally related but are transposed in approximately 85% of cases, with half of these being D-transposition and the other half L-transposition. In the common type of univentricular heart, a chamber with left ventricular morphology receives both atrioventricular valves, and the aorta is located anterior and leftward, arising from an outlet chamber of right ventricular morphology (Fig. 2).[5] In clinical practice, a univentricular heart with an outlet chamber is classified as A, and without an outlet chamber as C. When the aorta and pulmonary artery are normally related, it is further subdivided as I, with a dextroposed aorta as II, and with a levoposed aorta as III. Type A III univentricular heart is more common (Table 1).[14] In a small number of univentricular hearts, the great arteries are normally related and the pulmonary artery arises from an outflow chamber of right ventricular morphology; this condition is designated Holmes heart.[15]

Conduction System. A univentricular heart has an abnormal atrioventricular conduction axis,[16,17] which is of major surgical importance. The regular

TABLE 1. Anatomic Types in Clinical Practice (n = 145)

Type	% of Total	Pulmonic Stenosis % of Type
A-I	6	44
A-II	10	50
A-III	47	45
C-I	4	68
C-II	20	76
C-III	13	94

From Ritter DG, et al: Univentricular heart (common ventricle): Preoperative diagnosis. Herz 4:198, 1979, with permission.

atrioventricular node is unable to make contact with the ventricular conduction tissue. Instead, an anomalous atrioventricular node is located in the anterior quadrant of the atrioventricular orifice. From this node, the conduction axis penetrates the atrioventricular fibrous plane and ramifies as the ventricular conduction tissues. The precise course of the bundle depends upon the position of the rudimentary right ventricle. When the rudimentary right ventricle is right-sided, the bundle descends directly onto the septum and is unrelated to pulmonary outflow tract (Fig. 3A). When the rudimentary right ventricle is left-sided, the bundle extends anterosuperiorly around the pulmonary valve ring to reach the septum (Fig. 3B).

Coronary Arteries. Keeton and associates[18] studied the coronary artery anatomy in 26 univentricular hearts and determined their relationship to the ventricle and outlet chamber. Twenty-one univentricular hearts had a left ventricular type of main chamber and an anterior outlet chamber. Right and left delimiting arteries outlined the outlet chamber in 16 (76%) hearts. In 20 hearts, large, delimiting, parallel branches of the right coronary artery crossed over the anterior wall of the heart. These arteries are vulnerable to surgical injury at the time of conventional septation procedure.

NATURAL HISTORY

The incidence of univentricular heart is approximately 3% of all congenital cardiac malformations, with a male to female ratio of 2.5 to 1. As a general rule, these patients seem to be at a lesser risk of dying during the neonatal period and infancy than patients with total anomalous pulmonary venous connection, pulmonary atresia with intact septum, severe tetralogy of Fallot, or hypoplastic left heart syndrome.[19] In one series, only 15% of patients required surgical palliation within the first month of life, but 33% in the first 6 months and 40% by the first year required surgical treatment.[19] Moodie et al.[20] published the natural history of 122 patients with univentricular heart diagnosed between the ages of 7 days and 38 years (mean 8.4 years). At a mean follow-up period of 9 years, 44 (36%) patients were dead. Of the surviving patients, 62 (79%) had clinical cyanosis and decreased exercise tolerance. These authors subsequently[21] reported the long-term course of 83 unoperated patients; of these, 67 (81%) had type A and 16 (19%) type C univentricular heart. Fourteen years after diagnosis, 50% of patients with type A univentricular heart had died (annual death rate 4.8%), and by 16 years, only 30% of patients were alive (Fig. 4). In this series, 50% of patients with type C defect were dead 4 years after the diagnosis (Fig. 5). The most common cause of death was dysrhythmia, followed by congestive heart

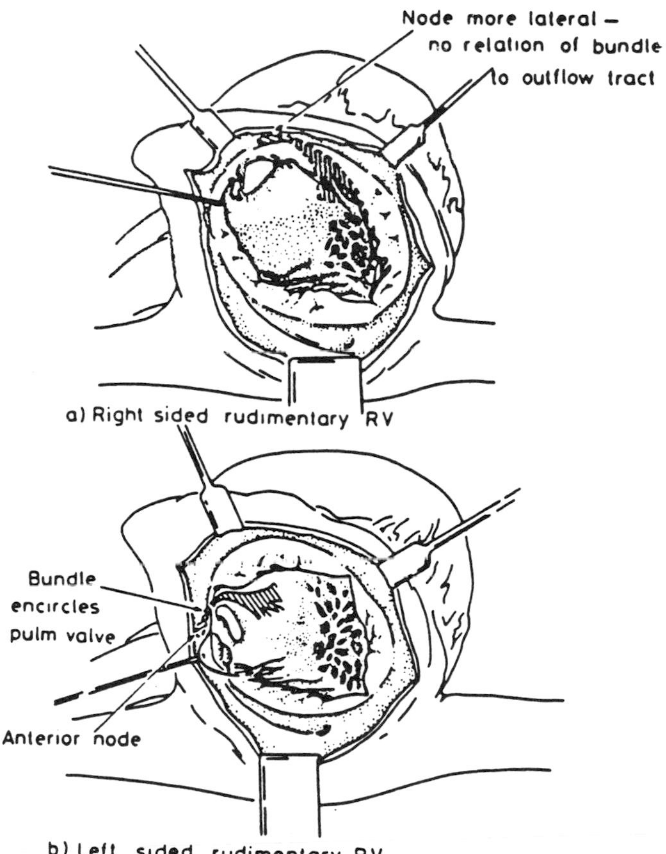

FIGURE 3. The conduction tissue disposition in univentricular heart as would be seen by the surgeon through a right atriotomy. (From Anderson RH, et al (eds): Pediatric Cardiology. New York, Churchill Livingstone, 1987, p. 649, with permission.)

failure, pneumonia, and sudden death. The majority of the surviving patients in the same follow-up period had cyanosis with decreased exercise tolerance.

CLINICAL PRESENTATION AND HEMODYNAMICS

The signs and symptoms of infants with univentricular heart depend upon the status of the pulmonary blood flow.[22] Congestive heart failure is the presenting feature in one group of patients due to excessive pulmonary blood flow, whereas varying degrees of hypoxia and cyanosis are dominant features in another group of patients, depending upon the severity of concomitant pulmonary stenosis.[23-27] Additional associated lesions, such as coarctation of the aorta and outlet chamber obstruction, further worsen the extent of heart failure. Atrioventricular valve anomalies in a univentricular heart can considerably alter the clinical presentation. Obstruction to the left atrioventricular valve in the presence of a restrictive foramen ovale results in severe pulmonary venous hypertension,

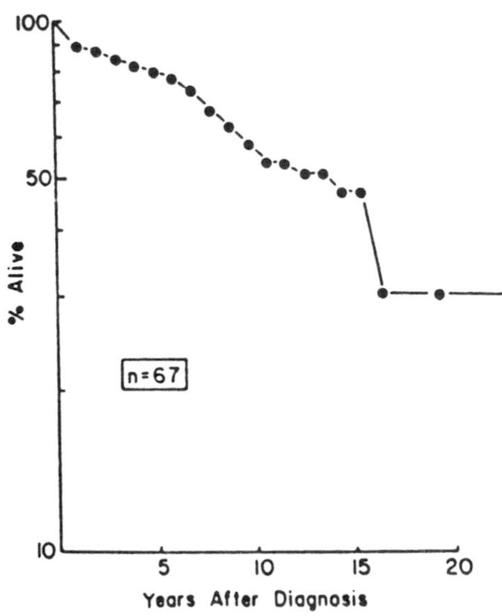

FIGURE 4. Survival curves of 67 patients with type A univentricular heart. (From Moodie DS, et al: Am J Cardiol 53:1127, 1984, with permission.)

causing severe respiratory distress in infancy.[28] Severe incompetence of left atrioventricular valve results in elevated atrial pressure and congestive heart failure.[29]

DIAGNOSIS

Physical findings and electrocardiogram are not pathognomonic of univentricular heart. The x-ray appearance is nonspecific but may show oligemic lung fields and small heart in the presence of pulmonary stenosis, or increase of vascular markings with cardiomegaly when the pulmonary blood flow is increased. Echocardiography is of great value in establishing the diagnosis and

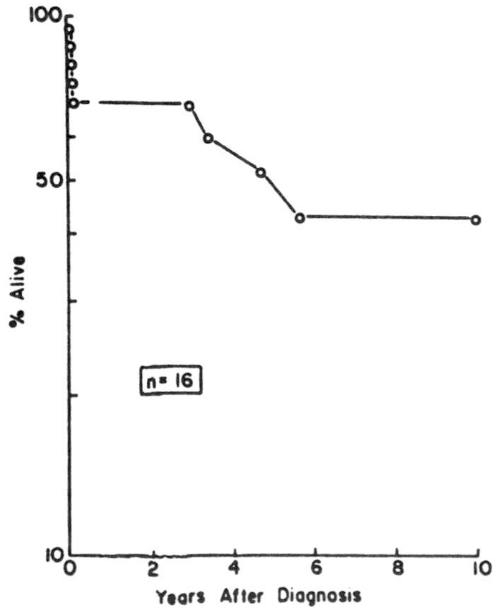

FIGURE 5. Survival curve of 16 patients with type C univentricular heart. (From Moodie DS, et al: Am J Cardiol 53:1127, 1984, with permission.)

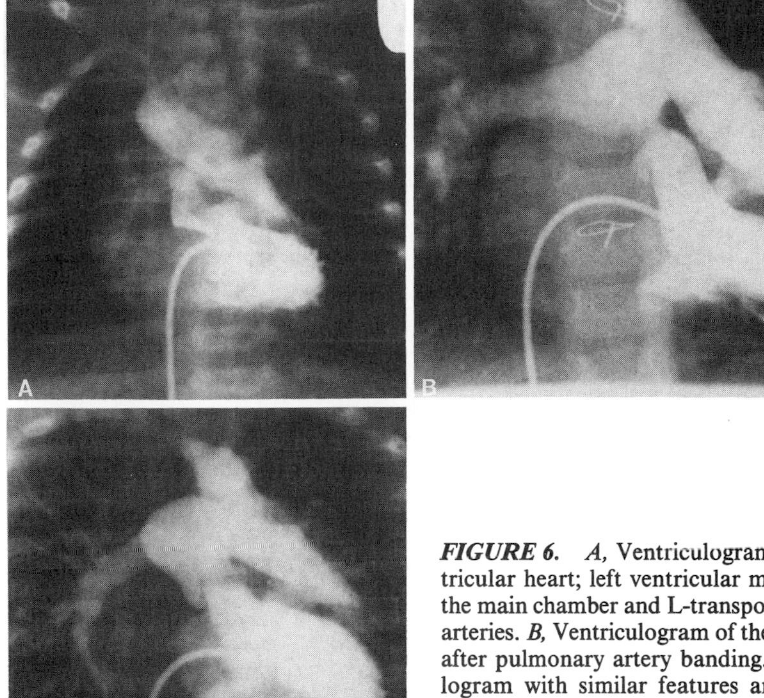

FIGURE 6. *A,* Ventriculogram of a univentricular heart; left ventricular morphology of the main chamber and L-transposition of great arteries. *B,* Ventriculogram of the same patient after pulmonary artery banding. *C,* Ventriculogram with similar features and associated pulmonic stenosis.

can demonstrate the absence of inlet septum between the atrioventricular valves[30] and apposition of unsupported cusps of two atrioventricular valves.[31] Two-dimensional (2-D) echocardiography has recently become an excellent noninvasive means of diagnosing univentricular heart. In most cases, it can accurately delineate atrioventricular and great vessel connections, position of the atrioventricular valves, as well as the morphology of the main chamber and outlet chamber.[32-34] Addition of pulsed Doppler to 2-D echocardiography enhances the ability to define anatomic and hemodynamic characteristics, especially of atrioventricular valves. Angiographic visualization of these valves may on occasion be less accurate because their identification depends upon the negative contrast effect superimposed on a dye-filled ventricle. Quantification of atrioventricular valve regurgitation by ventriculography also has limitations,[35] and unless proper angiographic angulation is obtained, mild degrees of regurgitation may be missed. By comparison, the Doppler sample volume is positioned in the valve orifice to evaluate atrioventricular valve regurgitation.[36] Cardiac catheterization and serial angiography provide the definitive diagnosis. Oximetry shows the shunting and the pressure data reveal the degree of outflow tract obstruction, if present. Flow and resistance are calculated to determine operability, and serial angiography shows the anatomic and functional status of the various segments of the heart, including associated anomalies (Fig. 6).

SURGICAL TREATMENT

The management of the univentricular heart consists of surgical palliation alone, palliation followed by definitive repair, and in occasional suitable patients, primary definitive repair.

Palliative procedure depends upon the hemodynamic situation. Most common procedures are pulmonary artery banding and systemic to pulmonary artery shunts. Pulmonary artery banding is carried out in infants with excessive pulmonary blood flow and pulmonary artery hypertension to reduce the pressure and to prevent pulmonary vascular occlusive disease. Even in the absence of congestive heart failure, patients with a univentricular heart without pulmonary stenosis should undergo pulmonary artery banding within 2–3 months of life to prepare them for a later surgical repair and to prevent pulmonary vascular occlusive disease.[37]

In infants with reduced pulmonary blood flow (due to pulmonic stenosis), a systemic–pulmonary artery shunt procedure is carried out, usually either a standard Blalock-Taussig shunt or a modified Blalock-Taussig shunt.[38,39] We prefer the modified Blalock-Taussig shunt and use prosthetic tube made of polytetrafluoroethylene (Gor-tex) to create a shunt between the subclavian and the pulmonary artery. It has the advantage of regulating a constant pulmonary blood flow because of its fixed diameter and can be used to enlarge the smaller of the two pulmonary arteries, irrespective of the position of the aortic arch. To prevent tenting or kinking of the pulmonary artery, the anastomosis is placed on the superior surface of the pulmonary artery as proximal as possible. This also facilitates takedown of the shunt at the time of definitive repair. The Glenn shunt, which involves an anastomosis of superior vena cava to the right pulmonary artery, is another palliative procedure that has the theoretical advantage of increasing effective pulmonary blood flow without the risk of ventricular volume overload. However, there is the disadvantage of the development of pulmonary arteriovenous fistulas as a late sequela, especially when the shunt is carried out in infancy.[40–42] An atrial septectomy (Blalock-Hanlon procedure) is an additional palliative procedure that is carried out if the atrial septal defect is restrictive and the left artrioventricular valve is obstructed.

Ventricular Septation

The first successful septation of the ventricular chamber into the pulmonary and systemic halves was performed by Kirklin in 1956. Although a logical surgical procedure, the high incidence of operative mortality and heart block limited the use of this procedure during the subsequent decade.[43] Surgical advances and expanded knowledge of anatomy, especially of the various positions of conduction tissue in a univentricular heart, renewed interest in ventricular septation.[44–48] Good results from this procedure are achieved in the subset of univentricular heart of left ventricular type, two atrioventricular valves, an anterior aorta arising from an outflow chamber, a moderate size of ventricular chamber, and no pulmonary hypertension.[48] This anatomic arrangement allows placement of a Dacron patch between the two atrioventricular valves, leaving equal volumes of ventricular chambers on each side (Fig. 7).

Staged Septation. Ebert, in 1984, reported the successful repair of univentricular heart in five patients with no operative mortality using two-staged ventricular septation.[49] This is a promising technique but has not been widely adopted yet. This technique consists of placement of a loose partial septation

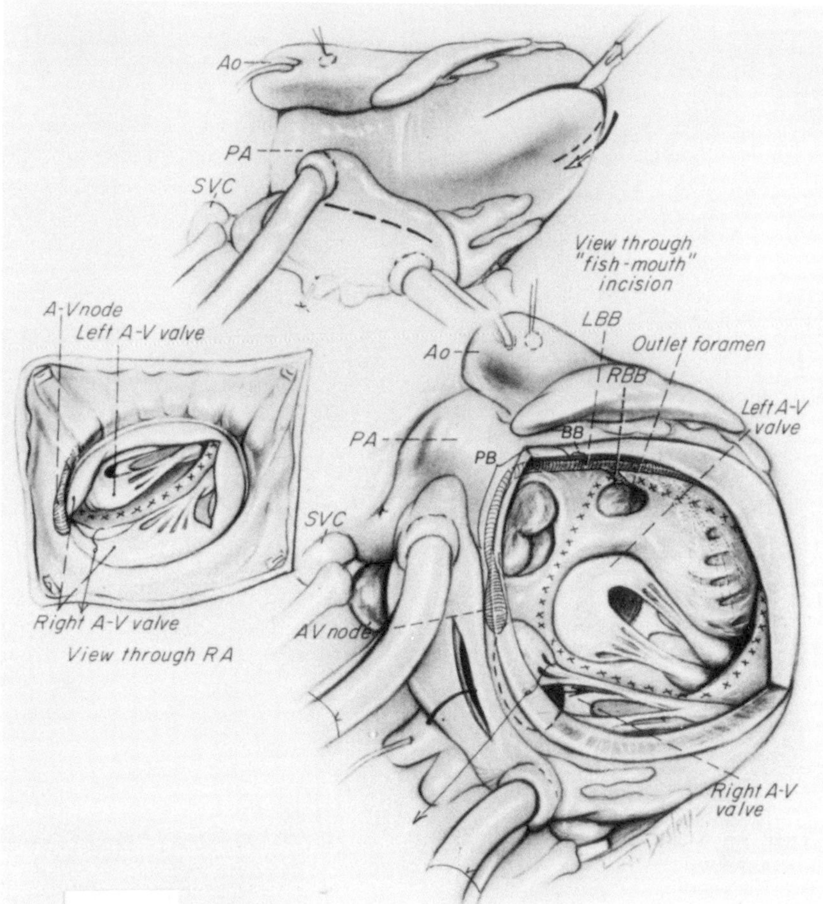

FIGURE 7. The septation operation of a univentricular heart of left ventricular type with subaortic left-sided outlet chamber. The position of atrioventricular node and bundle of His are shown. (From Bharati S, et al: In Cardiac Surgery and the Conduction System. New York, John Wiley & Sons, 1983, p. 93, with permission.)

patch with concomitant pulmonary artery banding followed by debanding and completion of the septation (Fig. 8).

Right Atrial Diversion

In 1971, Fontan and Baudet described an operation for the physiological correction of tricuspid atresia in which the distal right pulmonary artery was anastomosed to the superior vena cava and the proximal right pulmonary artery was connected to the right atrial appendage, using an aortic homograft.[50] The principle of this operation was to bypass the right ventricle by using the right atrium as a unidirectional pumping chamber, delivering blood directly into the pulmonary circuit. This concept was based on earlier experimental work that studied the exclusion of the right ventricle from circulation[51–53] and the effect of using right atrium as a pumping chamber for pulmonary circulation.[54]

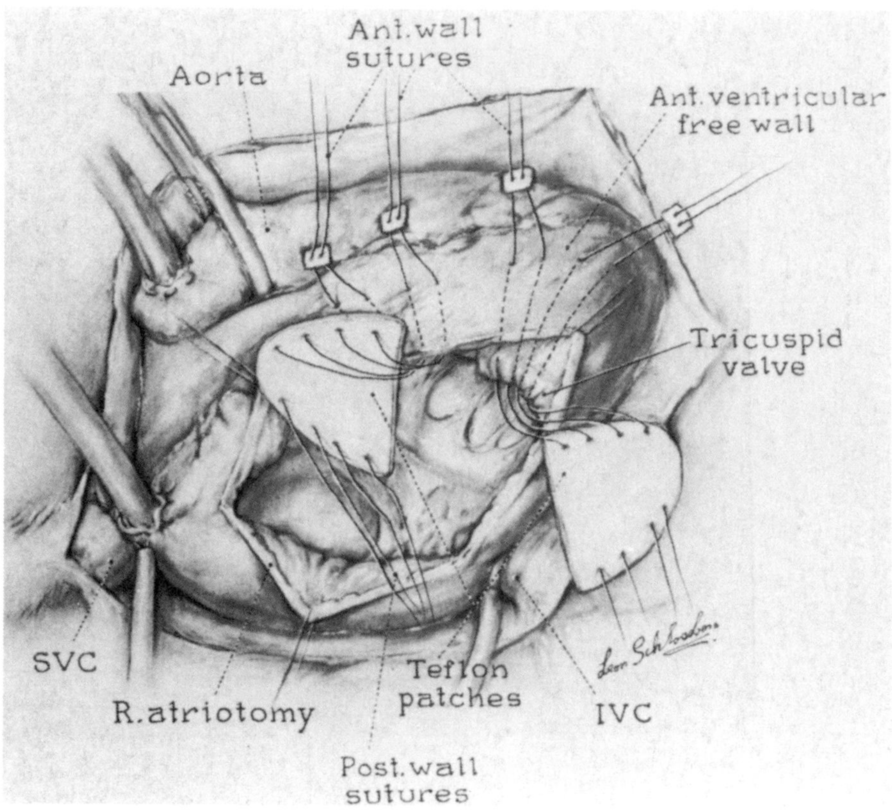

FIGURE 8. Staged septation. (From Ebert PA: Thorac Cardiovasc Surg 88:908, 1984, with permission).

In 1976, Yacoub used right atrial diversion for the surgical correction of univentricular heart by using a valved conduit from right atrium to pulmonary artery.[55] The conduit and homograft or xenograft valves were commonly used but they resulted in late complications of calcification and obstruction.[56–58] Kreutzer[59] in 1973 proposed a direct atrial-pulmonary anastomosis for right atrial diversion for tricuspid atresia. This technique, with some modification, has been widely adopted for the surgical repair of univentricular heart.[60–64]

Current Technique

Our modification[64] has been to use a large, intraatrial baffle to avoid the conduction tissue and divert both atrioventricular valves into the ventricle, maintaining the double inlet so that the size of the left atrioventricular valve is inconsequential (Fig. 9). With this technique, in a univentricular heart with left atrioventricular valve stenosis, the blood would easily flow through the atrial septal defect under the baffle to the right atrioventricular valve into the ventricle. In addition, in the presence of left atrioventricular valve regurgitation, it is possible to close the left valve and redirect the blood as for left atrioventricular valve stenosis.

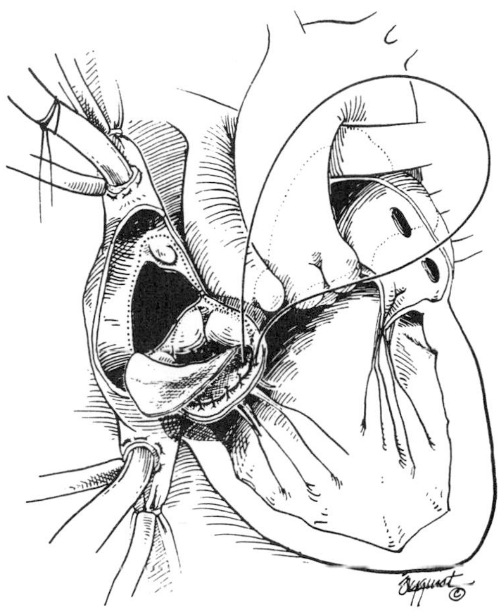

FIGURE 9. Sagittal section of a univentricular heart with L-transposition of great arteries. The interatrial septum is excised widely, coronary sinus is cut back and the Gor-Tex patch for intraatrial baffle is sutured around the atrioventricular node in the anterior superior quadrant.

For the intraatrial baffle, we prefer to use polytetrafluoroethylene (Gor-Tex) cardiovascular patch rather than the natural pericardium. Pericardium has the potential of stretching and ballooning into the left atrium because of the differential in atrial pressure in the postoperative period, which can result in pulmonary venous obstruction (Kreutzer, personal communication). The lack of pliability of Gor-Tex would prevent this possible complication in the postoperative period, when the right atrial pressure rises. The size of the patch is large enough to go around the right atrioventricular valve, well away from the coronary sinus. The coronary sinus is cut back and deliberately positioned on the left atrial side of the patch exposed to a lower pressure to prevent myocardial edema in the postoperative period.

In a univentricular heart with ventriculoarterial discordance with aorta in L-position (Fig. 9), where the dominant atrioventricular node is in the anterosuperior quadrant, the Gor-Tex patch is anastomosed superiorly almost to the junction of the right atrium and superior vena cava cephalad to the area of the node. Prior to the right atrial–pulmonary artery anastomosis, the pulmonary arteries are fully mobilized to the hilar branches for a tension-free anastomosis. The pulmonary valve is closed with a separate patch instead of the direct suture closure, to prevent dehiscence (Fig. 10). The incision in the roof of the right atrium is made as proposed by Doty,[62] and is extended into the superior vena cava to construct a large right atrial–pulmonary artery anastomosis (Fig. 11). In order to achieve this, the superior and inferior vena cava are directly cannulated as distal as possible.

Direct atrio–pulmonary artery anastomosis is also applicable in the presence of normally related great arteries by fully mobilizing both pulmonary arteries, dividing the main pulmonary artery at the level of the valve and moving it behind the aorta toward the roof of the right atrium.[62] To perform the operation accurately, we use profound hypothermia and circulatory arrest. At the completion of operation, temporary atrial and ventricular pacing wires are placed on the heart for the atrioventricular sequential pacing in the postoperative period.

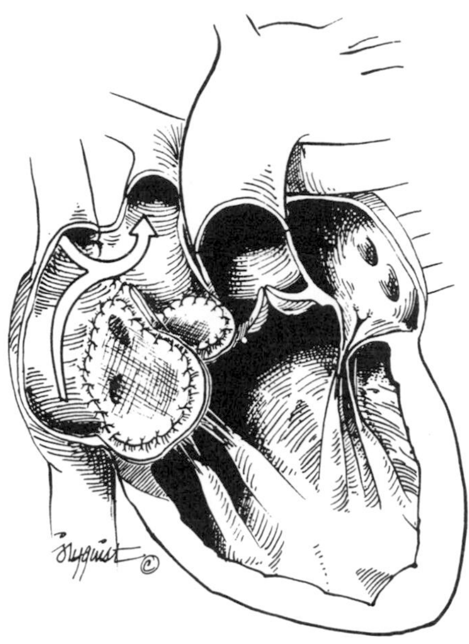

FIGURE 10. The intraatrial baffle is around the atrioventricular node and the coronary sinus. A separate patch is used to close the pulmonary valve.

COMMENTS

The natural history of univentricular heart is generally poor, with a mortality of 30% in restricted pulmonary blood flow and 42% in nonrestricted pulmonary blood flow at a mean follow-up of 9 years.[20] Surgical procedure, therefore, must be considered in children with a univentricular heart. An accurate diagnosis by utilizing pulsed Doppler, 2-D echocardiography, and cardiac catheterization must be made early in infancy, and a strategy for surgical management should be planned. This includes a commitment to early palliation, when indicated, followed by definitive repair in majority of cases. In symptomatic infants, relief of symptoms can be adequately provided by pulmonary artery banding or systemic–pulmonary artery shunts. These measures also prepare the patient for later repair.

Infants with excessive pulmonary blood flow and pulmonary hypertension require pulmonary artery banding to restore normal pulmonary artery pressure and to prevent the development of pulmonary vascular occlusive disease.[65,66] The child is thus prepared for later repair by atrial diversion, for which a normal pulmonary vascular resistance is essential. Undue delay between pulmonary artery banding and definitive repair may cause subaortic obstruction from progressive narrowing of outlet foramen, ventricular hypertrophy, volume reduction, and chronic ischemic changes in the ventricular muscle. Removal of pulmonary artery band and surgical repair have been recommended as early as 6 to 12 months of age,[67] but no data are available to support this opinion. Subclavian to pulmonary artery shunt increases blood flow with minimal risk of causing congestive heart failure or increasing pulmonary vascular resistance. However, it is important to realize that any type of systemic–pulmonary artery shunt creates a volume overload for a single functioning ventricle. Therefore, a large shunt or multiple shunts may be detrimental to the ventricular function. Waiting too long even in the presence of single shunt before the definitive repair

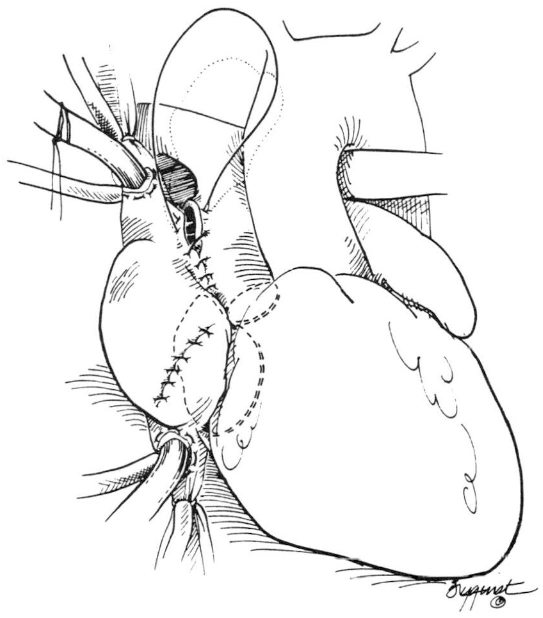

FIGURE 11. Direct atriopulmonary anastomosis. The right atrial incision is extended into the superior vena cava, which is cannulated distally.

may contribute to the onset of ventricular dysfunction. Surgical repair should be performed early after the shunt procedure, usually between 2 and 4 years of age.[67] Atik and colleagues[68] compared the results of Fontan repair in 10 children under the age of 3 years (mean 22.5 months) with that of 16 children above 3 years (mean 8.9 years). The overall hospital mortality was 12% and late mortality was 4%. There was no statistically significant difference in survival between the two groups. The degree of systemic venous congestion in the immediate postoperative period was lower in the former group of patients. Based on our similar observations in the past, we elect to perform definitive repair at 3 years of age.

Septation

Early attempts of septation carried high operative mortality and heart block. Therefore, only a few centers have substantial experience with septation in univentricular heart. In a report from the Mayo Clinic, patients operated upon between 1973 and 1978 had an operative mortality of 47% and a late mortality of 18% when all patients were considered together. However, in a subgroup of patients in the same series who had a leftward subaortic outlet chamber with no additional defect and no previous palliation or history of congestive heart failure, the operative mortality was 18%.[45] In a recent report by Pacifico et al.,[48] septation was performed in 36 patients between 1967 and 1983, with an operative mortality of 36% of the entire series. Surgical heart block developed in 28 of these patients and all required permanent pacemakers. However, 13 patients had "ideal" morphology (atrial situs solitus, double-inlet ventricle with a leftward and anterior rudimentary right ventricle, and a discordant ventriculoarterial connection without associated anomalies). There were no hospital deaths in this subgroup but three patients died later. Septation procedure, therefore, is applicable in only a small subgroup of patients with univentricular heart and, thus far, has not affected the outcome favorably.

The two-stage septation proposed by Ebert[49] for appropriately selected cases is an excellent proposition. The important advantage of this method is the absence of surgically induced heart block. To date, very little experience has been accumulated for the use of this technique.[69]

Right Atrial Diversion

Because of the high incidence of operative death and heart block and the fact that very few patients meet the criteria for septation, a Fontan type of right atrial diversion has become an accepted means of physiological correction of univentricular heart, which is also our choice. The recent results of this procedure have been encouraging. Laks et al.[63] reported 13% hospital deaths and 10% late deaths in 24 patients with univentricular heart who underwent the modified Fontan operation between 1975 and 1984. The late survivors were in New York Heart Association Class I or II. In our own series,[64] there were no early or late deaths in 9 consecutive patients with univentricular heart who underwent direct atriopulmonary anastomosis, maintaining the integrity of both inlets to the ventricle. Using a similar technique, Stellin et al. recently published their experience with the repair of univentricular heart in 10 patients with no operative deaths.[70]

Kreutzer and colleagues in 1986 reported the results of their modification of Fontan procedure in 26 patients with univentricular heart, with 2 early and 4 late deaths.[71] The success of this operation depends upon the normal pulmonary artery pressure, good ventricular function, and a wide, nonrestrictive anastomosis between the right atrium and the pulmonary artery to facilitate free blood flow and to avoid a very high right atrial pressure. The relationship of postoperative right atrial pressure to the outcome was shown in the Mayo Clinic report[60] of 17 patients with univentricular heart who underwent modified Fontan procedure. Of these, 4 patients died, whose postoperative right atrial pressure was more than 19 mm Hg.

Another important factor to be considered is the size of the pulmonary artery. A "pulmonary artery index," which may be a predictor of successful outcome, is calculated by measuring the cross-sectional area of the pulmonary arteries on the preoperative angiogram.[72] In the early postoperative period, a high right atrial pressure (above a mean of 15 mm Hg) is required to maintain an adequate cardiac output, which may necessitate over-transfusion of blood or colloid. To prevent the volume overload, we use a right heart assist device for 24–36 hours by intermittent abdominal compression, similar to that described by Guyton et al.[73] This helps to maintain an improved hemodynamic status and still achieve an overall negative fluid balance. In the experience of others as well as ours, in some patients systemic venous hypertension is associated with bilateral pleural effusion, ascites, and pericardial effusion,[60,62] which usually clear after diuretic therapy during convalescence.

The functional status of most of the survivors of right atrial diversion has been satisfactory; 93% are in NYHA Class I or II, although abnormalities of ventricular systolic function are often evident at rest and on exercise.[74] In a recently published report from the Mayo Clinic,[75] cardiorespiratory response to exercise was compared between the patients who underwent definitive repair and those who had not undergone repair. Cardiorespiratory functions improved after the definitive operations but remained abnormal when compared to normal subjects. Exercise duration and total workload increased significantly after the

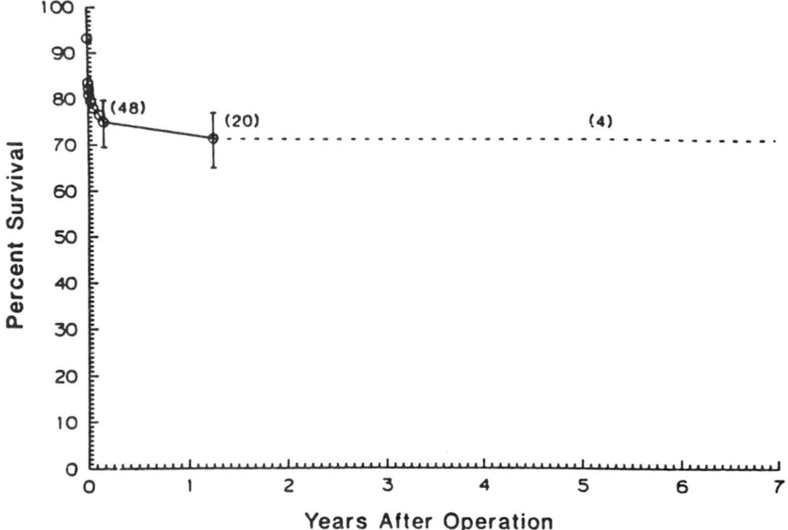

FIGURE 12. Actuarial survival, including hospital death, after Fontan type repair of congenital heart disease. (From Stefanelli A, et al: Am J Cardiol 54:811, 1984, with permission.)

Fontan procedure but not after the septation operation. After discharge from the hospital, death is uncommon after the Fontan procedure. Including hospital deaths, the actuarial survival at 5 years has been 71% (Fig. 12).[76] The major advantages of direct atriopulmonary anastomosis and diversion of both atrioventricular valves into the ventricle are: elimination of conduit and valve-related complications, avoidance of complete heart block, and feasibility of this operation even when the left atrioventricular valve is stenotic or regurgitant. In addition, there is a potential for growth of the anastomosis of autologous tissues.

SUMMARY

In view of the reasonably good intermediate-term results of surgical treatment of univentricular heart, it is appropriate to adopt an aggressive surgical plan for these patients. We believe that detailed anatomical identification, early intervention to reduce pulmonary vascular occlusive disease in unrestricted pulmonary blood flow, and systemic–pulmonary artery shunts when pulmonic stenosis is present, followed by an early surgical repair, can favorably alter the natural history of this disease.

REFERENCES

1. Abbott ME: Atlas of Congenital Cardiac Disease. New York, The American Heart Association, 1936, p 52.
2. Taussig HB: Cardiovascular anomalies: A single ventricle with a diminutive outlet chamber. Journal of Technical Methods 19:120, 1939.
3. Lambert EC: Single ventricle with a rudimentary outlet chamber: Case report. Bull Johns Hopkins Hosp 88:231, 1951.
4. Edwards JE: Congenital malformations of the heart and great vessels. In Gould SE: Pathology of the Heart, 2nd ed. Springfield, IL, Charles C Thomas, 1960, p 335.
5. Van Praagh R, Ongley PA, Swan HJC: Anatomic types of single or common ventricle in man: Morphologic and geometric aspects of 60 necropsied cases. Am J Cardiol 13:367–386, 1964.

6. Anderson RH, Becker AE, Wilkinson JL, Gerlis LM: Morphogenesis of univentricular hearts. Br Heart J 38:558–572, 1976.
7. Anderson RH, Macartney FJ, Shinebourne E, Tynan M: Pediatric Cardiology, Vol. 2. New York, Churchill Livingstone, 1987, p 653.
8. Arey JB: Cardiovascular Pathology in Infants and Children. Philadelphia, W.B. Saunders, 1984, p 104.
9. Anderson RH, Becker AE, Tynan FJ, et al: The univentricular atrioventricular connection: Getting to the root of a thorny problem. Am J Cardiol 54:822, 1984.
10. Girod DA, Lima RC, Anderson RH, et al: Double inlet ventricle: Morphologic analysis and surgical implications in 32 cases. J Thorac Cardiovasc Surg 88:590, 1984.
11. Anderson RH, Tynan MJ, Freedom RM, et al: Ventricular morphology in the univentricular heart. Herz 4:184, 1979.
12. Edwards JE, Carey LS, Neufeld HN, Lester RG: Congenital Heart Disease. Philadelphia, W.B. Saunders, 1965.
13. Kirklin JW, Barratt-Boyes BG: Cardiac Surgery. New York, Wiley Medical, 1986, p 1303.
14. Ritter DG, Seward JB, Moodie D, Danielson GK: Univentricular heart (common ventricle): Preoperative diagnosis. Herz 4:198, 1979.
15. Holmes AF: Case of malformation of the heart. Trans Med Chir Soc Edin 1:252, 1824; republished by Abbott ME: Montreal Med J 30:522, 1901.
16. Anderson RH, Arnold R, Thapar MK, et al: Cardiac specialized tissue in hearts with an apparently single ventricular chamber (double inlet left ventricle). Am J Cardiol 33:95–106, 1974.
17. Bharati S, Lev M: The course of the conduction system in single ventricle with (L-) loop and inverted (L-) transposition. Circulation 51:723–730, 1975.
18. Keeton BR, Lie JT, McGoon DC, et al: Anatomy of coronary arteries in univentricular hearts and its surgical implications. Am J Cardiol 43:569, 1979.
19. Kirklin JW, Barratt-Boyes BG: Cardiac Surgery. New York, Wiley Medical, 1986, p 1307.
20. Moodie DS, Tajik AJ, Ritter DG: The natural history of common (single ventricle) (abstract). Am J Cardiol 39:311, 1977.
21. Moodie DS, Ritter DG, Tajik AJ, O'Fallon WM: Long-term follow-up in the unoperated univentricular heart. Am J Cardiol 53:1124, 1984.
22. Macartney FJ, Anderson RH: Angiocardiography and hemodynamics of the univentricular heart with two atrioventricular valves. In Anderson RH, et al (eds): Pediatric Cardiology. New York, Churchill Livingstone, 1977, pp 345–372.
23. Van Praagh R, Plett JA, Van Praagh S: Single ventricle. Pathology, embryology, terminology and classification. Herz 4:113–150, 1979.
24. Marin-Garcia J, Tendan R, Moller JH, Edwards JE: Common (single) ventricle with normally related great vessels. Circulation 49:565–573, 1974.
25. Marin-Garcia J, Tendan R, Moller JH, Edwards JE: Single ventricle with transposition. Circulation 49:994–1004, 1974.
26. Anselmi G, Armas SM, De La Cruz MV, et al: Diagnosis and classification of single ventricle. Report on 17 cases with an embryologic discussion. Am J Cardiol 21:813–829, 1968.
27. Lev M, Liberthson RR, Kirkpatrick JR, Eckner FAO, Ancilla RA: Single (primitive) ventricle. Circulation 39:577–591, 1969.
28. Rao PS, Kulangara RJ, Moore VH, Strong WB: Syndrome of single ventricle without pulmonary stenosis but with left atrioventricular valve atresia and obstruction. J Thorac Cardiovasc Surg 81:127–130, 1981.
29. Moak JP, Gersony WM: Progressive atrioventricular valvular regurgitation in single ventricle. Am J Cardiol 59:656–658, 1987.
30. Felnar JM, Brewer DB, Franch RH: Echocardiographic manifestation of single ventricle. Am J Cardiol 38:80, 1976.
31. Beardshaw JA, Gibson DG, Peason MC, et al: Echocardiographic diagnosis of primitive ventricle with two atrioventricular valves. Br Heart J 39:266, 1977.
32. Rigby ML, Anderson RH, Gibson D, et al: Two dimensional echocardiographic characterization of the univentricular heart. Ventricular morphology, type and mode of atrioventricular connection. Br Heart J 46:603, 1981.
33. Huhta JC, Seward JB, Tajik AJ, Hager DJ: Two dimensional echocardiographic spectrum of univentricular heart (abstract). Circulation 64(Suppl. IV):IV–166, 1981.
34. Sahn DJ, Harder JR, Freedom R, et al: Cross-sectional echocardiographic diagnosis and subclassification of univentricular hearts: Imaging studies of atrioventricular valves, septal structures and rudimentary outflow chambers. Circulation 66:5,1070–1077, 1982.

35. Sandler H, Dodge HT, Hay RE, Rackley CE: Quantification of valvular insufficiency in man by angiography. Am Heart J 66:501–513, 1963.
36. Bisset GS, Hirschfeld SS: The univentricular heart: Combined two dimensional–pulsed Doppler (duplex) echocardiographic evaluation. Am J Cardiol 51:1149–1154, 1983.
37. Bove EL: Cardiac surgery for the adolescent with univentricular heart. Pediatrician 13:171–179, 1986.
38. Moulton AL, Brenner JI, Ringel R, et al: Classic vs. modified Blalock-Taussig shunts in neonates and infants. Circulation 72(Suppl II):35, 1985.
39. de Leval MR, McKay R, Jones M, et al: Modified Blalock-Taussig shunt: Use of subclavian artery orifice as flow regulator in prosthetic systemic-pulmonary artery shunts. J Thorac Cardiovasc Surg 81:112, 1981.
40. Mathew M, Glenn WWL: Long term evaluation of cava–pulmonary artery anastomosis. Surgery 74:899–916, 1973.
41. VanDenBogaert-VanHessveld AM, Derom F, Kunnen M, et al: Surgery for arteriovenous fistula and dilated vessels in the right lung after the Glenn procedure. J Thorac Cardiovasc Surg 76:195–197, 1978.
42. McFaul RC, Tajik AJ, Mair DD, et al: Development of pulmonary artery venous shunt after superior vena cava–right pulmonary artery (Glenn) anastomosis. Report of 4 cases. Circulation 55:212–216, 1977.
43. Moodie DC, Danielson GK, Ritter DG, et al: Correction of univentricular heart having two atrioventricular valves. J Thorac Cardiovasc Surg 74:218, 1977.
44. Edie RN, Ellis K, Gersony WL, et al: Surgical repair of single ventricle. J Thorac Cardiovasc Surg 66:350, 1973.
45. Feldt RH, Mair DD, Danielson GK, et al: Current status of the septation procedure for univentricular heart. J Thorac Cardiovasc Surg 82:93, 1981.
46. McKay R, Pacifico AD, Blackstone EH, et al: Septation of the univentricular heart with left anterior subaortic outlet chamber. J Thorac Cardiovasc Surg 84:77, 1982.
47. Pacifico AD, McKay R, Kirklin JW, Kirklin JK: Surgical management of the univentricular heart. In Anderson RH, et al: Pediatric Cardiology, Vol. 5. New York, Churchill Livingstone, 1983, pp 276–293.
48. Pacifico AD, Kirklin JK, Kirklin JW: Surgical management of double inlet ventricle. World Surg 9:579–589, 1985.
49. Ebert PA: Staged partitioning of single ventricle. J Thorac Cardiovasc Surg 88:908, 1984.
50. Fontan F, Baudet E: Surgical repair of tricuspid atresia. Thorax 26:240, 1971.
51. Rodbard S, Wagner D: By-passing the right ventricle. Proc Soc Exp Biol Med 71:69, 1949.
52. Glenn WWL: Circulatory bypass of the right side of the heart. IV. Shunt between superior vena cava and distal right pulmonary artery. Report of clinical application. N Engl J Med 259:117, 1958.
53. Robicsek F, Sanger PW, Taylor FH, et al: Complete bypass of the right heart. Am Heart J 66:791, 1963.
54. Warden HE, DeWall RA, Varco RL: Use of the right auricle as a pump for the pulmonary circuit. Surg Forum 5:16, 1954.
55. Yacoub MH, Radley-Smith R: Use of a valved conduit from right atrium to pulmonary artery for "correction" of single ventricle. Circulation 54(Suppl III):63–70, 1976.
56. Gale AW, Danielson GK, McGoon DC, et al: Fontan procedure for tricuspid atresia. Circulation 62:91–96, 1980.
57. Behrendt DM, Rosenthal A: Cardiovascular status of the repair of Fontan procedure. Thorac Surg 29:322–330, 1980.
58. Heck HA Jr, Schieken RM, Lauer RM, Doty DB: Conduit repair for complex congenital heart disease. Late follow-up. J Thorac Cardiovasc Surg 75:806–814, 1978.
59. Kreutzer G, Galindez E, Bono H, et al: An operation for the correction of tricuspid atresia. J Thorac Cardiovasc Surg 66:613, 1973.
60. Gale AW, Danielson GK, McGoon DC, Mair DD: Modified Fontan operation for univentricular heart and complicated congenital lesions. J Thorac Cardiovasc Surg 78:831–838, 1979.
61. Kreutzer GO, Vargas FG, Schlichter AJ, et al: Atrial and pulmonary anastomosis. J Thorac Cardiovasc Surg 83:427, 1982.
62. Doty DB, Marvin W Jr, Lauer RM: Modified Fontan procedure. Methods to achieve direct anastomosis of right atrium to pulmonary artery. J Thorac Cardiovasc Surg 81:470–475, 1981.
63. Laks H, Milliken JC, Perloff JK, et al: Experience with the Fontan procedure. J Thorac Cardiovasc Surg 88:939, 1984.
64. Ashraf H, Cotroneo J, Hans S, et al: Right atrial pulmonary artery diversion for double inlet ventricle (abstract). J Am Coll Cardiol 5:478, 1985.

65. Albus RA, Trusler GA, Izukawa T, Williams WG: Pulmonary artery banding. J Thorac Cardiovasc Surg 88:645, 1984.
66. Stewart S, Harris P, Manning J: Pulmonary artery banding. An analysis of current risks, results and indications. J Thorac Cardiovasc Surg 80:431, 1980.
67. Kirklin JW, Barratt-Boyes BG: Cardiac Surgery. New York, Wiley Medical, 1986, p 1323.
68. Atik E, Marcial BM, Macruz R, et al: Is Fontan operation feasible in patients under three years of age? Pediatric Cardiology: Proceedings of the Second World Congress. New York, Springer-Verlag, 1985, p 553.
69. McKay R, Bine RM, Wright JP: Staged septation of double inlet left ventricle. Br Heart J 56:563–566, 1986.
70. Stellin G, Mazzucco A, Bortolotti U, et al: Tricuspid atresia versus other complex lesions. Comparison of results with a modified Fontan procedure. J Thorac Cardiovasc Surg 96:204–211, 1988.
71. Kreutzer GO, Schlichter AJ, Michelli G, et al: Fontan-Kreutzer atriopulmonary connection. Revista Latina de Cardiologia y Cirugia Cardiovascular Infantil 2:37–56, 1986.
72. Nakata S, Imari Y, Takanashi Y, et al: A new method for the quantitative standardization of cross-sectional areas of the pulmonary arteries in congenital heart diseases with decreased pulmonary blood flow. J Thorac Cardiovasc Surg 88:610–619, 1984.
73. Guyton RA, Davis SC, Michalik RE, et al: Right heart assist by intermittent abdominal compression after surgery for congenital heart disease. Circulation 72(Suppl II):97–100, 1985.
74. Del Torso S, Kelly MJ, Kalff V, Venabels AW: Radionuclide assessment of ventricular contraction at rest and during exercise following the Fontan procedure for either tricuspid atresia or single ventricle. Am J Cardiol 55:1127, 1985.
75. Driscoll DJ, Feldt RH, Mottram CD, et al: Cardiorespiratory response to exercise after definitive repair of univentricular atrioventricular connection. Int J Cardiol 17:73–81, 1987.
76. Stefanelli A, Kirklin JW, Naftel DC, et al: Early and intermediate term (10 year) results of surgery for univentricular atrioventricular connection ("single ventricle"). Am J Cardiol 54:811–821, 1984.

JOHN W.E. DOUGLAS-JONES, MD

EBSTEIN'S ANOMALY

From the Department of Surgery
Division of Cardiovascular and Thoracic Surgery
Marshfield Clinic
Marshfield, Wisconsin

Reprint requests to:
John W.E. Douglas-Jones, MD
Cardiovascular and Thoracic Surgery
Marshfield Clinic
1000 North Oak Avenue
Marshfield, WI 54449-5777

Ebstein's anomaly is a rare congenital malformation of the tricuspid valve first described by Wilhelm Ebstein in 1866. In this original case report he gave an accurate description of the anatomy and pathophysiology of this unusual anomaly.[1,2] In 1927 Alfred Arnstein published a similar case report and recommended that the anomaly be called "Ebstein's disease."[3] In 1937 Yater and Shapiro presented another similar case and reviewed previous cases with reference to the anomaly as Ebstein's disease.[4] Ebstein's anomaly occurs in less than 1% of patients with congenital heart disease.[5]

EMBRYOLOGY

During cardiac embryogenesis the tricuspid valve is formed from the lining of the ventricular inlet by a process of delamination.[6,7] In Ebstein's anomaly this process is obviously significantly altered, and the mechanism producing the deformity of the right ventricular structures is uncertain. Anderson and Lie theorize that the etiology of the malformation is the maldevelopment of the atrioventricular junction.[8]

PATHOLOGY

The characteristic finding in Ebstein's anomaly is the downward displacement of the tricuspid valve into the right ventricle.[9] The septal and posterior leaflets, instead of being attached to the annulus fibrosus, are attached distally in the right ventricle to the septum and posterior ventricular walls.[8] The malformation is not limited to these two leaflets but rather all right ventricular structures are involved.[10] The degree of malformation varies considerably.[11]

The commissure shared by the septal and posterior leaflet is the point of maximal displacement downward into the right ventricle. This commissure is usually located at the crux of the heart.[12] These leaflets also vary markedly in size and range from almost normal to barely discernible ridges or severely dysplastic leaflets fused to the ventricular wall.[13] The septal leaflet is usually the more deformed of the two. The anterior leaflet is attached normally to the tricuspid valve annulus and it too is abnormal. It is usually large, described as being "sail-like," and may have fibrous or muscular bands coursing through it. The free edge may attach normally to the chordae of the papillary muscles or fuse directly to the ventricular endocardium at the inlet portion of the trabeculum. In addition, the leaflet may also be fenestrated or fused to the abnormal chordae and papillary muscles. Occasionally fusion of the commissures occurs, resulting in a stenotic and occasionally an imperforate valve that completely divides the right ventricle into two noncommunicating chambers. The latter occurs in approximately 10% of patients with Ebstein's anomaly.[12] The abnormal tricuspid valve divides the right ventricle into a functional right ventricle and an inlet portion connected to the right atrium commonly referred to as the atrialized right ventricle. This segment is usually thinned out and dilated, with a decrease in muscular fibers, or it may be fibrotic. The functional right ventricle is usually a small chamber but may also be thin-walled and dilated. Also noted is an absolute decrease in muscle fibers.[14] The right atrium varies from normal in size in mild forms of the anomaly to massively dilated in cases with severe tricuspid regurgitation. A patent foramen ovale or an atrial septal defect is usually present.[15] The atrioventricular orifice is enlarged.[14] Coronary artery anatomy is normal; however, displacement of the right coronary artery occurs with massive dilatation of the atrioventricular junction. Anomalies associated with Ebstein's anomaly are pulmonary stenosis, pulmonary atresia, and accessory conduction pathways.

Ebstein's anomaly also occurs in a left-sided form in atrioventricular discordance. This differs somewhat from the right-sided in that the anterior leaflet is somewhat smaller and may be cleft. The atrioventricular valve orifice is normal. Interatrial communication is unusual as opposed to common or almost always present in right-sided Ebstein's, and the conduction tissue in being anterior is away from the left-sided tricuspid valve. Dilatation of the right ventricle is not as prominent in left-sided Ebstein's.[16,17]

The major hemodynamic problem in Ebstein's anomaly is failure of the right heart to function as an efficient pump (i.e., it cannot pass blood from the right atrium into the pulmonary artery). The combination of anomalies in the right ventricle and atrium act in concert to defeat this. The tricuspid valve is usually insufficient or may be stenotic in a minority of patients. The thinned-out right ventricle results in poor contractility. Retrograde transmission into the right atrium in tricuspid insufficiency results in increased right atrial pressures, and, in the presence of a patent foramen ovale or an atrial septal defect, a right-to-left shunt occurs. If the interatrial communication is restrictive, further increase in right atrial pressures occurs, resulting in dilatation of the right atrium, and, in the presence of pulmonary atresia or pulmonary stenosis with tricuspid insufficiency, massive dilatation of the right atrium and atrialized segment occurs, especially with longstanding tricuspid insufficiency. An unrestrictive right-to-left shunt predisposes to congestive heart failure. Further dilation of the right heart only serves to increase the tricuspid incompetence and worsen the hemodynamics.

Patients with Ebstein's anomaly are diagnosed over a rather wide age range—from the neonatal period to late in life.[18] As there is such a wide variation in the pathology, similarly there is a range in the hemodynamics and symptoms based on right ventricular function. Very few patients have favorable hemodynamics consistent with long-term asymptomatic survival. Most patients survive into early adulthood mildly symptomatic, then symptoms progress or the patient deteriorates rapidly.[15,19] During the early neonatal period pulmonary vascular resistance is high and the patent foramen ovale or atrial septal defect is present with tricuspid insufficiency and resulting high right atrial pressures. This results in a right-to-left shunt with systemic desaturation, and cyanosis is a predominant symptom. In the presence of an unrestrictive atrial septal defect or severe tricuspid insufficiency, congestive heart failure and respiratory insufficiency may occur. As the pulmonary vascular resistance decreases with growth and development, pulmonary blood flow increases, the right-to-left shunt decreases, and the neonate significantly improves, sometimes with complete resolution of cyanosis. If the disease is mild and the neonate survives infancy, development tends to be normal, and early adulthood is reached with minimal symptoms. Most patients at this time are in the NYHA Class I–Class II, and the common symptoms are cyanosis, dyspnea, and easy fatigability.[15] Occasionally palpitations occur.

DIAGNOSIS

Physical Findings. In patients with Ebstein's anomaly the precordium is usually quiet. The anterior chest may be mildly deformed and asymmetrical, with slight right-sided prominence. Auscultation reveals a variety of murmurs, the most consistent being that of tricuspid insufficiency: a systolic murmur varying in intensity increasing with inspiration. It is best heard at the left lower sternal border. Both first and second heart sounds are widely split, the latter usually associated with right bundle branch block. Clubbing of the fingers and cyanosis are also common.[20]

Electrocardiogram. The electrocardiogram may be normal; however, several abnormalities are frequently noted. These include peaked P-waves associated with atrial hypertrophy and first and second degree heart block. Several arrhythmias may be present, usually atrial fibrillation, atrial flutter, and paroxysmal atrial tachycardias, usually of the Wolff-Parkinson-White pattern Type B.[19]

Roentgenogram. Chest roentgenograms usually show an enlarged cardiac silhouette with decreased pulmonary vascularity. The shape of the heart is similar to that seen with large pericardial effusions and is commonly described as being globular. In longstanding forms of the anomaly with severe tricuspid insufficiency, massive enlargement may occur and results in the heart radiologically or roentgenographically filling the entire width of the chest.[11,21]

Echocardiogram. Two-dimensional echocardiography (2-D) accurately delineates the anatomy and correlates well with surgical pathology. 2-D may be of use preoperatively in planning the surgical procedure or in determining whether valve replacement or tricuspid valve repair may be necessary.[22,23]

Cardiac Catheterization. Definitive diagnosis is made at cardiac catheterization. right atrial pressures may be normal or increased, or may show tricuspid insufficiency. Usually the right atrial tracing shows a prominent V-wave. An intracardiac electrocardiogram may be diagnostic by revealing a ventricular tracing with the tip of the catheter in the atrialized portion of the right ventricle, while correspondingly monitoring atrial pressures. This finding may be absent in the presence of severe tricuspid insufficiency or if the atrialized segment is fibrotic, thin-walled, and dilated.[24–27] Oximetry reveals desaturation of the left atrium indicative of a right-to-left shunt. Angiocardiography is usually diagnostic. A right ventriculogram is obtained in an anteroposterior and also a lateral view utilizing biplane cine and usually shows the displaced tricuspid valve to the left of the spine, the small functional right ventricle, the dilated right atrium and atrialized segment of the right ventricle between the right atrium and the right ventricle, sometimes appearing as a distinct chamber, the dilated atrioventricular ring, and flow of regurgitant or insufficient tricuspid valve filling the right atrium retrograde, with flow of dye from the right atrium into the left atrium demonstrating the right-to-left shunt.[19]

Surgical Treatment. Patients with mild forms of the anomaly are managed medically, and surgery is reserved for those with progressive worsening of symptoms or those who present with severe forms of the anomaly.[15] Factors associated with higher risk include: patients in Class III or Class IV NYHA, severe cardiomegaly, congestive heart failure, a diagnosis made in infancy with early onset of symptoms, and associated cardiac defects including pulmonary stenosis or atresia.[18,19] The goal of surgery is to restore the right ventricle to a more efficient pumping chamber and is based on a repair to obtain a competent, nonstenotic tricuspid valve.[28,29] This is accomplished by valvuloplasty and annuloplasty as described by Danielson, or by reconstruction of the tricuspid valve and right ventricle as described by Carpentier, or by insertion of a prosthesis. Repair is favored over replacement as it avoids the problems of bleeding and thromboembolic phenomena associated with mechanical valves in this position and the need for anticoagulation. The Danielson repair is accomplished with the patient on cardiopulmonary bypass and moderate hypothermia with hypothermic cardioplegic arrest. Electrophysiologic mapping is initially performed and accessory conduction pathways are divided in patients with Wolff-Parkinson-White syndrome. In addition the atrial septal defect is closed with a patch, the atrialized portion of the right ventricle is plicated, and a plastic repair of the tricuspid valve is performed. Included also is resection of the redundant or excessive right atrial wall. If a plastic repair of the tricuspid valve is not possible, then it is replaced.

A new method of reconstruction described by Carpentier distinguishes the anomaly into four separate types based on 2-D echocardiographic findings. Based on these findings the repair is accomplished utilizing mobilization and repositioning of the tricuspid valve and plication of the atrialized chamber in a longitudinal fashion, restoring the right ventricle to an apparently normal shape.[23]

In patients in whom the anatomy is not favorable for tricuspid valve repair because of significant deformities of the anterior leaflet or extensive fusion to the ventricular wall, valve replacement is selected as the procedure of choice. The valve is replaced utilizing the method described by Barnard and Schrire.[31] A low-profile prosthesis is selected, and, after appropriately sizing the annulus, it is sutured in position utilizing mattress pledgetted sutures. In placing the sutures the atrialized portion of the right ventricle may be plicated, totally obliterating this segment. In the vicinity of the coronary sinus the sutures are placed on the atrial side in an effort to avoid injury to the bundle of His and subsequent third degree heart block.[32]

These methods of repair have been accomplished with acceptable morbidity and mortality. The older methods described by Danielson and also valve replacement have yielded excellent long-term results in most patients in NYHA Class I and II.[33] The method of reconstruction by Carpentier appears to be technically more demanding. As it is much more recent, the follow-up time is not as long; however, the results are also excellent over the initial short-term follow-up periods.[23]

Marked improvement in quality and duration of life can be experienced by patients undergoing surgical repair of Ebstein's anomaly in a timely fashion with acceptable morbidity and mortality.

REFERENCES

1. Ebstein W: Uber einen sehr seltenen Fall von Insufficienz der Valvula Tricuspidalis, bedingt durch eine angeborene hochgradige Missbildung derselben. Arch Anat Physiol Eissensch Med 238–254, 1866.
2. Schiebler GL, Grovenstein JS, Von Mierop LHS: Ebstein's anomaly of the tricuspid valve: Translation of original description with comments. Am J Cardiol 22:867–873, 1968.
3. Arnstein A: Eine seltene Missbildung der Trikuspidalklappe ("Besteinsche Krankheit"). Virchows Arch (Pathol Anat) 266:247–254, 1927.
4. Yater WM, Shapiro MJ: Congenital displacement of the tricuspid valve (Ebstein's disease): Review and report of a case with electrocardiographic abnormalities and detailed histologic study of the conduction system. Ann Intern Med 11:1043–1062, 1937.
5. Keith JO, Rowe RD, Vlad P: Heart Disease in Infancy and Childhood. New York, Macmillan, 1958, p 314.
6. Odgers PNB: The development of the atrio-ventricular valves in man. J Anat 73:643–657, 1938–1939.
7. Netter FH, Van Mierop LHS: Embryology. In Yonkman FF (ed): The Ciba Collection of Medical Illustrations, Vol 5. Summit, New Jersey, Ciba Pharmaceutical Company, 1969, p 125.
8. Anderson KR, Lie JT: Pathologic anatomy of Ebstein's anomaly of the heart revisited. Am J Cardiol 41:739–745, 1978.
9. Becker AE, Becker MJ, Edwards JE: Pathologic spectrum of dysplasia of the tricuspid valve. Features in common with Ebstein's malformation. Arch Pathol 91:167–178, 1971.
10. Lev M, Liberthson RR, Joseph RH, et al: The pathologic anatomy of Ebstein's disease. Arch Pathol 90:334–343, 1970.
11. Genton E, Blount SG Jr: The spectrum of Ebstein's anomaly. Am Heart J 73:395–425, 1967.
12. Anderson KR, Zuberbuhler JR, Anderson RH, et al: Morphologic spectrum of Ebstein's anomaly of the heart: A review. Mayo Clin Proc 54:174–180, 1979.
13. Zuberbuhler JR, Allwork SP, Anderson RH: The spectrum of Ebstein's anomaly of the tricuspid valve. J Thorac Cardiovasc Surg 77:202–211, 1979.
14. Anderson KR, Lie JT: The right ventricular myocardium in Ebstein's anomaly. A morphometric histopathologic study. Mayo Clin Proc 54:181–184, 1979.
15. Watson H: Natural history of Ebstein's anomaly of tricuspid valve in childhood and adolescence: An international co-operative study of 505 cases. Br Heart J 36:417–427, 1974.
16. Anderson RH, Arnold R, Wilkinson JL: The conducting system in congenitally corrected transposition. Lancet 1:1286–1288, 1973.
17. Anderson RH, Becker AE, Arnold R, Wilkinson JL: The conducting tissues in congenitally corrected transposition. Circulation 50:911–923, 1974.
18. Giuliani ER, Fuster V, Brandenburg RO, Mair DD: The clinical features and natural history of Ebstein's anomaly of the tricuspid valve. Mayo Clin Proc 54:163–173, 1979.
19. Kumar AE, Fyler DC, Miettinen OS, Nadas AS: Ebstein's anomaly: Clinical profile and natural history. Am J Cardiol 28:84–95, 1971.
20. Schiebler GL, Adams P Jr, Anderson RC, et al: Clinical study of twenty-three cases of Ebstein's anomaly of the tricuspid valve. Circulation 19:165–187, 1959.
21. Amplatz K, Lester RG, Schiebler GL, et al: The roentgenologic features of Ebstein's anomaly of the tricuspid valve. Am J Roentgenol 81:788–794, 1959.
22. Shiina A, Seward JB, Hagler DJ, et al: Ebstein's anomaly: Two dimensional echo-surgical correlation. Echo predictors of tricuspid valve plication vs. replacement. Circulation 64(Suppl IV):4–237, 1981.

23. Carpentier A, Chauvand S, Mace L, et al: A new reconstructive operation for Ebstein's anomaly of the tricuspid valve. J Thorac Cardiovasc Surg 96:92–101, 1988.
24. Sodi-Pallares D, Marsico F: The importance of electrocardiographic patterns in congenital heart disease. Am Heart J 49:202–217, 1955.
25. Van Lingen B, Bauersfeld SR: The electrocardiogram in Ebstein's anomaly of the tricuspid valve. Am Heart J 50:13–23, 1955.
26. Hernandez FA, Rochkind R, Cooper HR: The intracavitary electrocardiogram in the diagnosis of Ebstein's anomaly. Am J Cardiol 1:181–190, 1958.
27. Watson H: Electrode catheters and the diagnosis of Ebstein's anomaly of the tricuspid valve. Br Heart J 28:161–171, 1966.
28. Hardy KL, May IA, Webster CA, Kimball KG: Ebstein's anomaly: A functional concept and successful definitive repair. J Thorac Cardiovasc Surg 48:927–940, 1964.
29. Timmis HH, Hardy JD, Watson DG: The surgical management of Ebstein's anomaly: The combined use of tricuspid valve replacement, atrioventricular plication, and atrioplasty. J Thorac Cardiovasc Surg 53:385–391, 1967.
30. Danielson GK, Maloney JD, Devloo RAE: Surgical repair of Ebstein's anomaly. Mayo Clin Proc 54:185–192, 1979.
31. Barnard CN, Schrire V: Surgical correction of Ebstein's malformation with prosthetic tricuspid valve. Surgery 54:302–308, 1963.
32. Westaby S, Karp RB, Kirklin JW, et al: Surgical treatment in Ebstein's malformation. Ann Thorac Surg 34:388, 1982.
33. Danielson GK, Furster V: Surgical repair of Ebstein's anomaly. Ann Surg 196:499, 1982.

PEDRO J. DEL NIDO, MD
SIDNEY LEVITSKY, MD

TOTAL ANOMALOUS PULMONARY VENOUS DRAINAGE

From the Division of Cardio-Thoracic Surgery
University of Illinois College of Medicine at Chicago
Chicago, Illinois

Reprint requests to:
Pedro J. del Nido, MD
Division of Cardio-Thoracic Surgery
University of Illinois College of Medicine
Box 6998
Chicago, IL 60680

Total anomalous pulmonary venous drainage (TAPVD) is a rare but serious cardiac malformation, constituting approximately 1% of all congenital cardiac lesions.[23] TAPVD is a condition in which all of the pulmonary venous blood joins the systemic venous system and returns to the right atrium. Left atrial and ventricular filling is accomplished through an atrial septal defect. TAPVD occurs more frequently in isolation but can occur in association with other complex congenital cardiac malformations. Brody in 1942 reviewed 37 cases collected from the literature and described the anatomical findings.[4] The first successful surgical correction was achieved by Muller in 1951[19] by anastomosing the common pulmonary vein to the atrium. Since then, surgeons have employed various techniques to correct this lesion, including circulatory arrest with surface cooling,[5] atrial well technique,[16] and currently deep hypothermia with cardiopulmonary bypass with a period of circulatory arrest. Surgical results have been dramatically improved in the last two decades due largely to improved techniques of cardiopulmonary bypass and perioperative management.

EMBRYOLOGY AND ANATOMY

TAPVD occurs when the common pulmonary vein fails to join the left atrium, depending instead on the persistence of splanchnic communications to drain into the systemic venous system. Embryologic anomalies of the pulmonary veins have been classified into four groups:

(a) drainage is into the left common cardinal system via a persistent left superior vena cava or into the coronary sinus; (b) drainage is into the right common cardinal system with the pulmonary plexus draining into the right horn of the sinus venosus; (c) communications persist between the pulmonary venous plexus and the portal venous system through ductus venosus, umbilical-vitelline structures, or portal vein; and (d) a leftward shift of the interatrial septum, leaving the pulmonary veins to drain directly into the right atrium.[20] The most commonly accepted anatomic classification of TAPVD is based on the level of drainage: (a) supracardiac (45% of cases), with two-thirds of the cases draining into a persistent left superior vena cava, and the rest draining into the azygous or right superior vena cava; (b) cardiac (25%), with most cases draining into the coronary sinus and the rest draining into the right atrium directly; (c) infracardiac (20%), with the common pulmonary vein draining inferiorly through the diaphragm into the portal vein, inferior vena cava, or ductus venosus; and (d) mixed type (5–10%), where the drainage is through two or more routes.[8]

An interatrial communication is required for survival because there is no other source of left atrial filling. The size of the interatrial communication is quite variable, ranging from a small patent foramen ovale to a large septal defect. In those cases where the atrial defect is small, restriction of flow into the left atrium can cause a severe low output state. In this group of patients, a balloon atrial septostomy or urgent corrective surgery is required to correct the poor perfusion and acidosis that is often present. Thus, the site of drainage of the common pulmonary vein is an important determinant for the presence of pulmonary venous obstruction. This is most common with infracardiac drainage, since the capillary bed of the liver is frequently interposed via the portal system between the pulmonary veins and the systemic venous system.

The left atrium and ventricle can be smaller than normal in patients with TAPVD. Rarely, however, is the left ventricular size so small as to be unable to support the systemic circulation, but this finding has been identified as a risk factor in operative survival.[7]

NATURAL HISTORY

The clinical course and age of presentation depend greatly on the extent of pulmonary venous obstruction and pulmonary blood flow. The majority of patients have no anatomic restriction to pulmonary artery blood flow but do have some degree of obstruction to pulmonary venous drainage. The venous obstruction is associated with pulmonary arterial hypertension with an increase in pulmonary vascular resistance. In the group of infants with severe pulmonary venous obstruction, pulmonary edema develops early and they present within the first few days of life with severe cyanosis and congestive heart failure and rarely survive beyond the first 1–2 weeks of life. If the pulmonary venous obstruction is not as severe, there is usually increased pulmonary blood flow and pulmonary hypertension. These infants commonly present in the first 1–3 months of life with congestive heart failure and minimal cyanosis. Although the congestive failure may be controlled with medications, these infants are at high risk for development of pulmonary vascular disease. Additionally, recurrent pulmonary infection is common in this group and they rarely survive beyond 1 year of age. Development of pulmonary vascular disease is very common among the survivors and can range from reversible changes with muscularization of the pulmonary arteries to irreversible changes with endothelial proliferation and occasionally plexogenic lesions.[22]

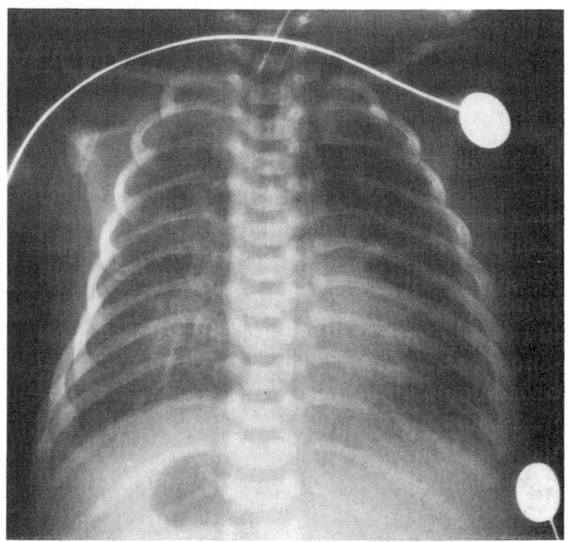

FIGURE 1. Chest x-ray from an infant with infracardiac type TAPVD with obstruction to pulmonary venous drainage. Note the typical venous congestion and ground-glass appearance of the lung fields with a relatively small heart and small right pleural effusion.

There is a small group of patients, however, that do not develop pulmonary arterial hypertension and seem to tolerate their defect well. These children will present at an older age with signs of mild congestive heart failure and some limitation to activity. Most of these cases are of the supracardiac type of anomalous pulmonary venous drainage, and although they may have early findings of pulmonary vascular disease, surgical correction is successful in reversing the process.

CLINICAL FEATURES

The timing of presentation and extent of clinical symptoms present in children with TAPVD depend largely on the severity of pulmonary venous obstruction and pulmonary arterial hypertension. TAPVD in infants can be exceedingly difficult to recognize and differentiate from persistent fetal circulation of the newborn. Respiratory distress can begin as early as a few minutes after birth to several hours. The severity of the respiratory difficulty can also range from moderate distress to profound cyanosis not responding to oxygen. The classic signs of a heaving parasternal cardiac impulse, a loud second pulmonic sound, systolic pulmonary flow murmur, and a diastolic tricuspid flow murmur are seldom present in the newborn but are more frequently seen in older children. The chest x-ray in infants with obstruction usually shows increased vascular markings from venous congestion and a ground-glass appearance with a normal or small cardiac size (Fig. 1). A small pleural effusion can also be present. In older infants the chest x-ray shows increased vascularity from the high pulmonary arterial blood flow, and in children with supracardiac drainage, the mediastinum above the heart is widened due to the large left and right superior vena cava, giving a typical "snowman" appearance to the mediastinum (Fig. 2).

The electrocardiogram usually shows right axis deviation in infants and right ventricular hypertrophy. Reversal of the normal R-wave progression across the precordium is almost always present. Right atrial hypertrophy develops in older infants (usually over 3 months of age).

At present cross-sectional (2-D) echocardiography is the most reliable noninvasive tool for confirming the diagnosis of TAPVD. Visualization of the left

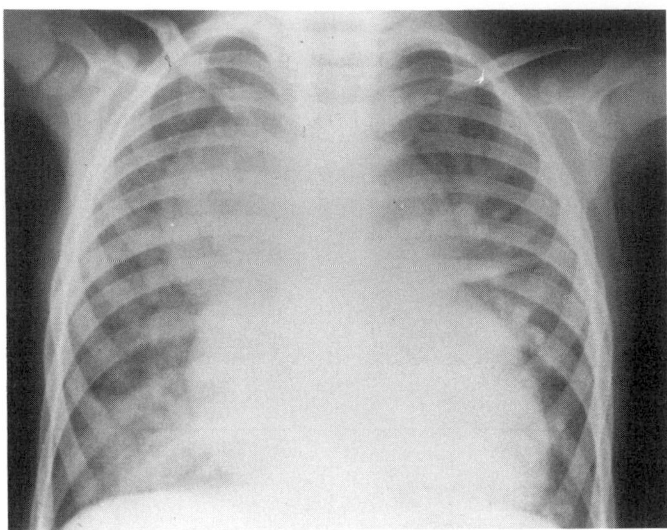

FIGURE 2. Chest x-ray film from an older child with supracardiac type of TAPVD showing a typical "snowman" appearance of the mediastinum. The superior mediastinum is widened by the enlarged persistent left superior vena cava and enlarged right superior vena cava (see Fig. 3A).

atrium and pulmonary veins can be achieved in virtually all patients to exclude TAPVD.[24] The anomalous common trunk behind the heart can also be visualized and the route of drainage frequently seen. In the supracardiac type, the left ascending vein is usually easily visualized, and Doppler examination of that vessel can demonstrate reversal of flow toward the innominate vein and superior vena cava. When the anomalous venous trunk drains into the coronary sinus, a dilated coronary sinus with increased flow velocity by Doppler is easily seen. In the infracardiac type, the venous trunk with caudal blood flow can usually be seen penetrating the diaphragm. Many centers rely solely on clinical and echocardiographic diagnosis of TAPVD prior to performing surgery.[26] This approach avoids the additional stress and time delay due to cardiac catheterization, which is of prime importance in these critically ill newborns.

Cardiac catheterization is usually reserved for those cases where the diagnosis is in doubt, when there are other associated cardiac malformations, or when there is more than one route of pulmonary venous drainage and echocardiography is unable to define the anatomy clearly. Saturation data obtained at cardiac catheterization usually indicate a high right atrial oxygen saturation with similar level of saturation in the left atrium. In fact, all the cardiac chambers usually have the same oxygen saturation. The level of drainage of the pulmonary venous trunk can also be determined frequently by careful measurement of oxygen saturations in the systemic veins before they join the right atrium. In severely cyanotic infants, however, oxygen saturation data can be misleading due to the markedly decreased pulmonary blood flow. The angiographic diagnosis of TAPVD may be made by injecting contrast directly into the main pulmonary artery. In infants with a patent ductus arteriosus and right-to-left shunting, direct branch pulmonary artery injections may be required. The contrast can be observed passing through the lungs into the pulmonary veins and common trunk,

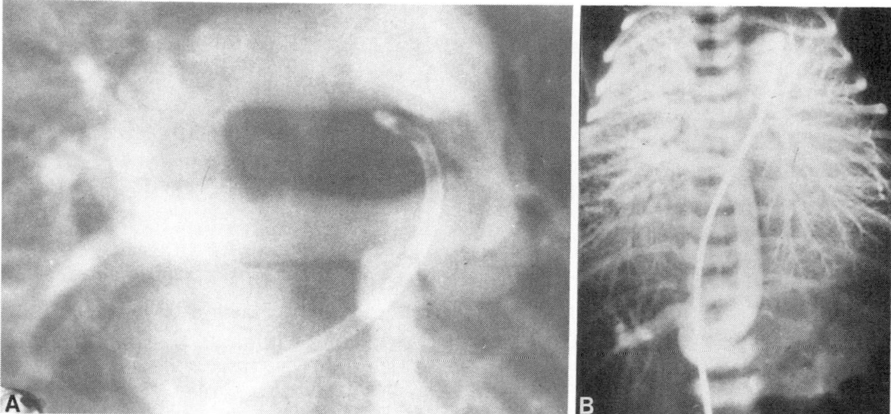

FIGURE 3. Cineangiogram of two children with TAPVD. *A,* Supracardiac type with a persistent left superior cava (Fig. 2). *B,* Infracardiac type with drainage via a descending vertical vein into the portal system.

and the site of drainage can then be determined (Fig. 3). Direct catheterization of the anomalous vein with contrast injection can give sufficient detail to determine if obstruction to drainage is present. This can be more easily done in children with supracardiac and intracardiac types of drainage but is more difficult for the infracardiac type.

PREOPERATIVE MANAGEMENT

Preoperative stabilization is most important in young infants who have some degree of pulmonary venous obstruction or restriction to flow through the interatrial septum. These infants not infrequently present with moderate to severe respiratory distress, profound cyanosis, metabolic acidosis, and renal impairment. Rapid intubation and positive pressure ventilation improve not only the arterial oxygenation but also decrease the work of breathing and therefore oxygen consumption in these critically ill infants. Improved perfusion can usually be achieved by the use of inotropic support, and, in infants with a restrictive interatrial communication, balloon atrial septostomy is recommended to improve left ventricular filling. The atrial septostomy can often be performed in the intensive care unit under 2D-echo guidance, avoiding risky transportation to the catheterization laboratory. The use of prostaglandin E_1 has been advocated to maintain ductal patency and pulmonary artery decompression in young infants.[2] This does, however, carry the risk of worsening the pulmonary congestion by increasing pulmonary blood flow to lungs with venous obstruction.[12]

Most infants managed aggressively early after presentation will improve and tolerate surgical intervention at a later time. If no improvement is seen within a few hours of intensive treatment, surgery should be performed immediately. Any further delay in operative intervention may lead to acute deterioration.

SURGICAL TECHNIQUE

In infants, deep hypothermia with a period of circulatory arrest and removal of the venous cannula afford the best exposure for repair. In older children, bicaval cannulation with moderate hypothermia and low flow cardiopulmonary bypass is most commonly used. Construction of as large an unobstructed anastomosis as possible is most important. The bloodless operative field facilitated by circulatory arrest provides the best condition to perform this anastomosis. The confluence of the pulmonary veins can usually be easily identified posteriorly under the parietal pericardium. This is particularly true when obstruction to venous drainage is present, because the venous confluence is usually filled and tense even on cardiopulmonary bypass. In the supra- and infracardiac types of TAPVD, the draining vertical vein can also be identified and dissected parallel and to the left of the ascending aorta for supracardiac types or as it penetrates the diaphragm in the infracardiac types. There still exists some controversy regarding whether to ligate the vertical vein after repair. Most surgeons ligate the ascending vein in the supracardiac type unless the pulmonary artery pressure is suprasystemic and ventricular function is poor. With the infracardiac types, there has been a report of liver necrosis following ligation of the descending vertical vein. Since obstruction to drainage is more common in the infracardiac types, particularly when drainage is to the portal system, flow through this vein decreases rapidly after surgery and probably ceases after a few days.[27] Even though a large unobstructed anastomosis may have been created, the small size and decreased compliance of the left atrium and ventricle can lead to elevated left atrial pressures early after surgery. The unligated vertical vein may then function as a pressure vent, temporarily decompressing the left atrium.

The technique for repair of TAPVD depends on the anatomical type of venous drainage.

Supracardiac Type

In isolated TAPVD the pulmonary venous confluence is located directly posterior to the left atrium. This finding allows the creation of a direct left atrial to venous confluence anastomosis, regardless of whether the pulmonary venous blood drains via a supracardiac or infracardiac draining vein. Thus the goal of repair of supracardiac TAPVD is to create as large a communication as possible between the common pulmonary vein and the left atrium, close the interatrial septal defect, and ligate the ascending draining vein. The left atrium and common vein are usually approached from the right lateral aspect of the heart, permitting access to the left atrium. A transverse incision in the left atrium is made which can be extended across the interatrial septum and connected to the atrial septal defect (Fig. 4). The pulmonary venous confluence, which is usually located near the superior aspect of the left atrium, is then opened also with a transverse incision parallel to the left atriotomy, and the anastomosis is created using running monofilament absorbable or nonabsorbable suture. The anastomosis can be terminated at the level of the interatrial septum, or if a larger opening is desired, can be extended into the right atrium. The incision in the venous confluence should not be extended into the pulmonary veins themselves, as this can lead to venous obstruction later. Once the anastomosis is completed, the interatrial defect is then closed with a patch of pericardium (Fig. 4) or primarily if the defect is small. The ascending vein is dissected outside the pericardium where it runs parallel and to the left of the aorta, and is then ligated. In cases where the anomalous drainage is into the right superior vena cava directly, the ostium can be closed directly or patched.

An alternative technique for repair is to approach the left atrium and common pulmonary vein between the right superior vena cava and aorta. The

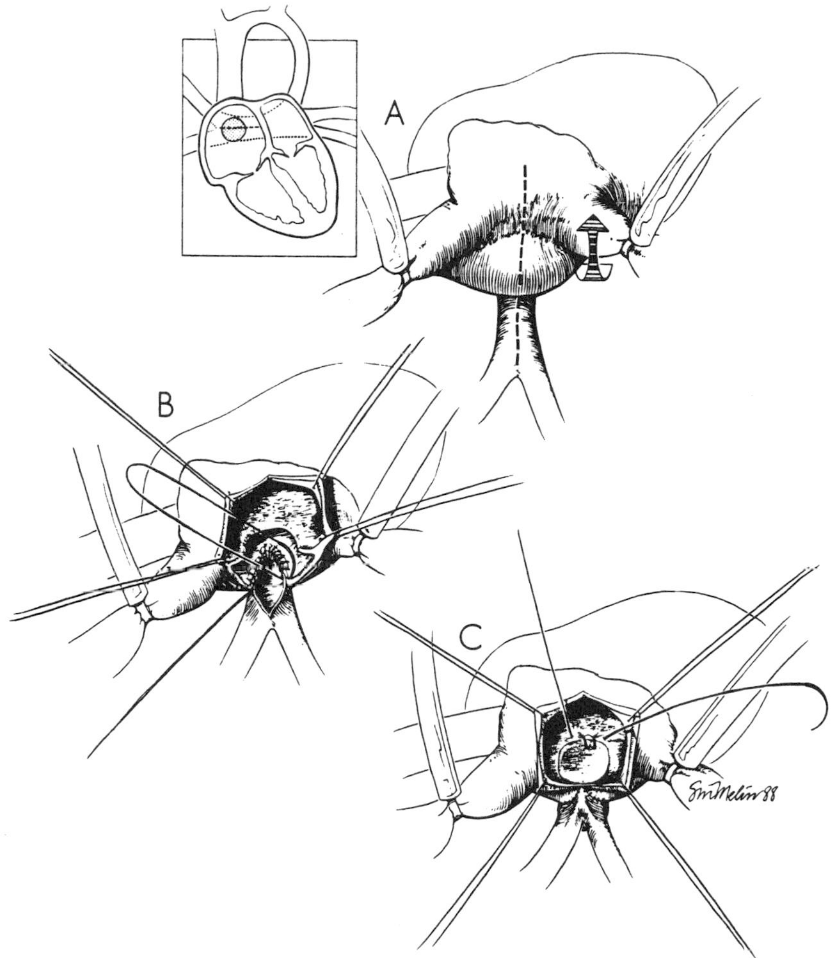

FIGURE 4. Correction of supracardiac type TAPVD with creation of a wide anastomosis from the left atrium into the venous confluence and closure of the atrial septal defect.

left atrium can be opened at the interatrial groove from the right superior cava to the base of the atrial appendage. The anastomosis is then constructed in the same way as described above, and the atrial septal defect is closed through a separate right atriotomy.

Some authors have advocated enlarging the left atrium by extending the anastomosis into the right atrium or using a large patch to close the interatrial defect.[14] However, enlarging the left atrium has not been found to improve survival.[27] Once the repair is completed and the right atriotomy closed, air is evacuated from the heart, the venous cannula reinserted, and the patient rewarmed.

Infracardiac Type

The same approach as for repair of supracardiac TAPVD can be used in the infracardiac type. Exposure to the left atrium and central draining vein can be

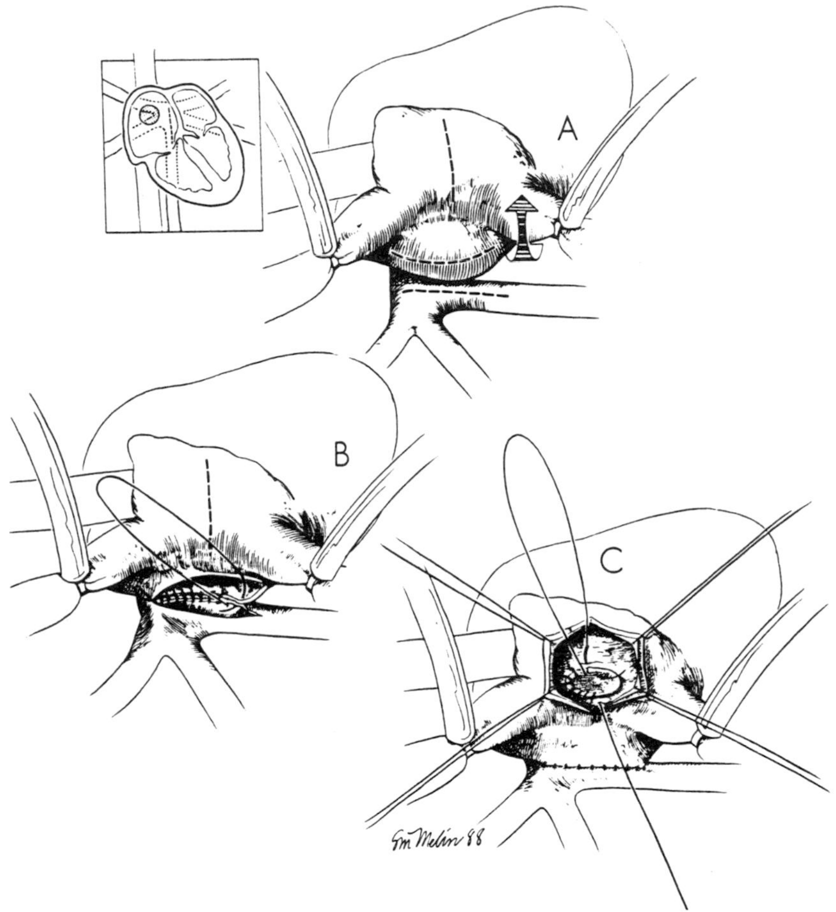

FIGURE 5. Correction of infracardiac TAPVD by creating a large anastomosis between the left atrium and the vertical descending vein followed by closure of the atrial septal defect.

achieved from the right side of the pericardium. The orientation of the draining vein in infracardiac TAPVD often is vertical rather than transverse, and this should determine the left atrial incision (Fig. 5).[15] This difference in orientation of the vertical vein sometimes makes it necessary to extend the venotomy near the orifice of the individual veins in order to achieve an adequate anastomosis. Stellate or curvilinear incisions are sometimes required in order to achieve a sufficiently large anastomosis. Care should be taken, however, not to obstruct or distort the pulmonary veins, particularly in small neonates. Once the venotomy is completed, the left atriotomy is performed in parallel so that there is minimal distortion of the left atrium once the anastomosis is completed. We prefer to approach the veins and left atrium from the right side of the heart, where parallel incisions can be made with the heart minimally retracted (Fig. 5). Once the incisions are made and the anastomosis created, the atrial defect can be closed through a separate right atriotomy. Some surgeons prefer a transverse transseptal incision for this lesion, as this allows enlargement of the left atrium with a patch

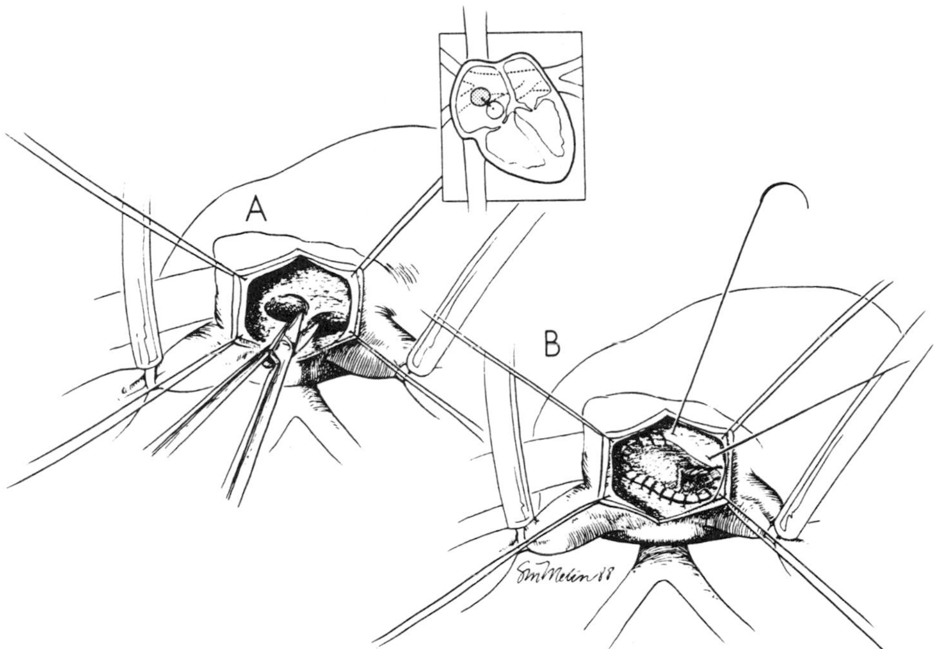

FIGURE 6. Correction of intracardiac TAPVD draining into the coronary sinus. Unroofing of the enlarged coronary sinus into the left atrium is followed by patch closure of the septal defect.

for the septal defect (Fig. 4). Others have proposed that exposure to the left atrium and vertical vein can be achieved by lifting the heart out of the pericardium and retracting it to the right in order to create an adequate anastomosis.[28] However, distortion of the small left atrium and subsequent kinking of the atriovenous anastomosis is a potential hazard with this approach.[11] Once the correction is completed and the patient rewarmed, bypass is discontinued and the vertical vein can then be ligated. A pulmonary artery pressure line is recommended in order to asses the effects of vertical vein ligation on pulmonary vascular resistance. Many surgeons do not ligate this vein because the resistance to flow through it is great enough to prevent significant left to right shunting under normal conditions. Leaving the vein open may serve potentially to decompress the left atrium should the atrial pressures rise acutely. However, division of the vertical vein at the level of the diaphragm is sometimes necessary in order to relieve tension on the anastomosis.

Intracardiac Type

Correction of the intracardiac type of TAPVD is simpler than the other types. When drainage is into the coronary sinus, correction can be done simply by unroofing the coronary sinus into the left atrium and patch closure of the septal defect (Fig. 6). Care must be taken during the closure of the septal defect not to injure the AV node, which lies in close proximity to the edge of the coronary sinus. If the drainage is directly into the right atrium, the interatrial septal defect should be enlarged to accommodate all the pulmonary venous flow, and the flow redirected by means of a pericardial baffle from the venous confluence to the septal defect. If an adequate anastomosis cannot be achieved by this method, an incision should be made between the left atrium and the venous confluence, and the anastomosis enlarged in a similar fashion to the supracardiac type. In rare cases, a left superior vena cava (ascending vein) can also be present with drainage into the coronary sinus. In this situation, the left cava should be ligated and the coronary sinus unroofed if there is no evidence of restriction to pulmonary venous flow into the coronary sinus.[1]

Mixed Type

When the pulmonary venous drainage is via more than one route, a combination of techniques must be used in order to correct this lesion. The type of correction should be individualized based on the appropriate technique for that drainage. In cases where a single lobar vein drains to a different site, this vein can be left without much sequelae. If the left upper lobe vein is separate, the left atrial appendage can be used to complete the correction. This procedure can add significantly to the operative time, however, with little gain.

Some controversy over the suture technique to create the anastomosis has revolved around the use of running versus interrupted sutures. The proposed disadvantage of the continuous technique is that it does not allow for anastomotic growth; however, long-term follow-up studies have not substantiated this claim. We prefer to use a running suture of absorbable monofilament material for this anastomosis.

POSTOPERATIVE CARE

The postoperative management of children with TAPVD is similar to that of other infants undergoing open heart procedures—with two major differences. First, due to the limited size and compliance of the left atrium and ventricle, care must be taken to restrict intravenous volume infusions, since these infants have a great tendency to develop pulmonary edema even after adequate decompression of the pulmonary venous drainage. Second, increased pulmonary vascular reactivity is seen frequently, particularly in infants who had some degree of pulmonary venous obstruction prior to surgery. Monitoring of pulmonary artery pressures in the early postoperative period is strongly recommended for at least the first 24 hours. Pulmonary hypertensive crisis with resultant systemic hypotension has been well described in this group of patients.[10] Mechanical hyperventilation, preferably with a volume cycled ventilator, in the first 24–48 hours after surgery is the simplest method of preventing these pulmonary hypertensive events. Sedation and use of skeletal muscle relaxants and various vasodilators (tolazoline, prostaglandins, phenoxybenzamine, etc.) have also been recommended to control or prevent pulmonary hypertension, but should not be considered substitutes for mechanical hyperventilation.

RESULTS OF SURGERY

Early Results

Operative results have improved mostly in the high-risk infant group as methods of early diagnosis, preoperative stabilization, and timely surgery have improved. Mortality in older infants (> 1 month) has generally been low, ranging from 6–13%.[2,3,13,14] In the younger age group (< 1 month) operative mortality has been higher, primarily due to pulmonary venous obstruction, leading to earlier presentation. Mortality has ranged from 12–42% in this newborn group, depending on the presence and severity of pulmonary venous obstruction.[17,18,21] The site of drainage has also been reported to be an important risk factor, with the infracardiac group having a higher operative risk. In addition, venous obstruction is more common in the infracardiac group, and this may explain the earlier onset of symptoms and higher incidence of postoperative pulmonary hypertension in this group of infants.

The operative technique used for correction has had little influence on early operative mortality. There have been reports of a greater incidence of anastomotic distortion and obstruction when the heart is retracted out of the pericardial sac to create the anastomosis.[6] However, if care is taken to maintain the proper orientation of the left atrium, this problem can be avoided.[27]

Associated cardiac anomalies do have an adverse effect on outcome, particularly in infants with complex cardiac anomalies such as those with the visceral heterotaxy syndromes. In this patient group, the presence of pulmonary venous obstruction can be masked by decreased pulmonary blood flow from pulmonary stenosis or atresia. Early recognition and correction of this problem have led to improved operative results.[9]

Late Results

Late pulmonary venous obstruction is a major complication in the postoperative period, occurring in 3–15% of patients.[27,29,30] Most present within the first 3–6 months after surgery with signs of progressive pulmonary hypertension and occasionally pulmonary edema. The obstruction is most frequently at the anastomotic site but can also be located at the terminal ends of the pulmonary veins. A 2D-echocardiography and Doppler examination can usually detect the presence of late postoperative obstruction and localize the area of stenosis.[25] Surgical intervention is recommended when the obstruction is at the level of the anastomosis, and this approach has yielded satisfactory results.[27] When the obstruction is in the pulmonary veins, the results have not been as encouraging.

The pulmonary vascular changes seen in children undergoing repair have almost always been reversible when the pulmonary venous obstruction has been relieved. Only rarely have cases been reported of irreversible progressive changes continuing after surgical correction.[22] The size of the left heart chambers, although usually small preoperatively, appear to grow to normal size on late follow-up. Similarly, right ventricular size and function return to normal once the pulmonary hypertension resolves postoperatively. Although only a few reports exist with long-term follow-up (10–20 years), most indicate that further complications rarely arise beyond the first year after surgery.[26,29]

REFERENCES

1. Arciprete P, McKay R, Watson GH, et al: Double connections in total anomalous pulmonary venous connection. J Thorac Cardiovasc Surg 92:146, 1986.
2. Barratt-Boyes BG: Techniques and results of treatment in total anomalous pulmonary venous connection. In Parenzan L, Crupi G, Graham G (eds): Congenital Heart Disease in the First Three Months of Life. Bologna, Patron Editore, 1982, p. 461.
3. Berg CA, Jamieson MPG, Pollock JCS: Repair of total anomalous pulmonary venous connection in adults. Thorac Cardiovasc Surg 34:359, 1986.
4. Brody H: Drainage of the pulmonary veins into the right side of the heart. Arch Pathol 33:221, 1942.

5. Cooley DA, Ochsner A: Correction of total anomalous pulmonary venous drainage. Technical considerations. Surgery 42:1014, 1957.
6. Cooley DA, Hallman GL, Leachman RD: Total anomalous pulmonary venous drainage. Correction with the use of cardiopulmonary bypass in 62 cases. J Thorac Cardiovasc Surg 51:83, 1966.
7. Coussement AM, Gooding CA, Carlson E: Left atrial volume, shape, and movement in total anomalous pulmonary venous return. Radiology 107:139, 1973.
8. Darling RC, Rothney WB, Craig JM: Total pulmonary venous drainage into the right side of the heart: Report of 17 autopsied cases not associated with other major cardiovascular anomalies. Lab Invest 6:44, 1957.
9. DeLeon SY, Gidding SS, Ilbawi MN, et al: Surgical management of infants with complex cardiac anomalies associated with reduced pulmonary blood flow and total anomalous pulmonary venous drainage. Ann Thorac Surg 43:207, 1987.
10. del Nido PJ, Williams WG, Villamater J, et al: Changes in pericardial surface pressure during pulmonary hypertensive crisis after cardiac surgery. Circulation 76:III–93, 1987.
11. Fleming WH, Clark EB, Osoley KJ, et al: Late complications following surgical repair of total anomalous pulmonary venous return below the diaphragm. Ann Thorac Surg 27:435, 1979.
12. Freedom RM, Alley PM, Cacesni F, Rowe RD: The prostaglandin challenge: Test to unmask obstructed total anomalous pulmonary venous drainage. Br Heart J 40:90, 1978.
13. Gomes MMR, Feldt RH, McGoon DC, Danielson GK: Total anomalous pulmonary venous connection: Surgical considerations and results of operation. J Thorac Cardiovasc Surg 60:116, 1970.
14. Katz NM, Kirklin JW, Pacifico AD: Concepts and practices in surgery for total anomalous pulmonary venous connection (collective review). Ann Thorac Surg 25:479, 1978.
15. Kawashima Y, Matsuda H, Nakano S, et al: Tree-shaped pulmonary veins in infracardiac total anomalous pulmonary venous drainage. Ann Thorac Surg 23:436, 1977.
16. Lewis FJ, Varco RL, Taufic M, Niazi SA: Total anomalous pulmonary venous return in the infant: Surgical treatment. Presented at the 7th Ruinioni Medico-Chirurgio Internazionelli, Torino, Italy, 1975.
17. Long WA, Lawson EE, Harned HS, Henry GW: Infradiaphragmatic total anomalous pulmonary venous drainage: New diagnostic, physiologic, and surgical considerations. Am J Perinatol 1:227, 1984.
18. Mazzucco A, Rizzoli G, Francasso A, et al: Experience with operation for total anomalous pulmonary venous connection in infancy. J Thorac Cardiovasc Surg 85:686, 1983.
19. Muller WH: The surgical treatment of transposition of the pulmonary veins. Ann Surg 134:683, 1951.
20. Neill CA: Development of the pulmonary veins: With reference to the embryology of anomalies of anomalous venous return. Pediatrics 18:880, 1956.
21. Oelert H, Schafers HJ, Stegman T, et al: Complete correction of total anomalous pulmonary venous drainage: Experience with 53 patients. Ann Thorac Surg 41:392, 1986.
22. Petersen RC, Edwards WD: Pulmonary vascular disease in 57 necropsy cases of total anomalous pulmonary venous connection. Histopathology 7:487, 1983.
23. Rowe RD: Anomalies of venous return. In Keith JD, Rowe RD, Vlad P (eds): Heart Disease in Infancy and Childhood, 3rd ed. New York, Macmillan, 1978, p. 554.
24. Smallhorn JF, Sutherland GR, Tommasini G, et al: Assessment of total anomalous pulmonary venous connection by two-dimensional echocardiography. Br Heart J 46:613, 1981.
25. Stark J, Smallhorn J, Huhta J, et al: Surgery for congenital heart defects with cross-sectional echocardiography. Circulation 68:II–129, 1983.
26. Stark J: Anomalies of pulmonary venous return. World J Surg 9:532, 1985.
27. Williams GR, Richardson WR, Campbell GS: Repair of total anomalous pulmonary venous drainage in infancy. J Thorac Cardiovasc Surg 47:199, 1964.
28. Wright CM, Barratt-Boyes BG, Calder AL, et al: Total anomalous pulmonary venous connection. J Thorac Cardiovasc Surg 75:52, 1978.
29. Yee ES, Turley K, Hsieh WR, Ebert PA: Infant total anomalous pulmonary venous connection: Factors influencing timing of presentation and operative outcome. Circulation 76:III–83, 1987.

L. DOUGLAS COWGILL, MD

ANOMALOUS SYSTEMIC VENOUS RETURN

From the Department of Surgery
Dean Clinic
Madison, Wisconsin

Reprint requests to:
L. Douglas Cowgill, MD
Department of Surgery
Dean Clinic
1313 Fish Hatchery Rd.
Madison, WI 53715

Anomalous systemic venous return is an important, and occasionally confusing, type of congenital heart disease. It includes the unroofed coronary sinus syndrome, and frequently coexists with other anomalies. For purposes of classification four types have been identified: anomalous return to the right atrium, anomalous return to the left atrium, anomalous return to both atria, and combined anomalous systemic and pulmonary venous return.[1]

HISTORY

Persistent left superior vena cava (LSVC) draining to the left atrium was first reported by Winter[2] and Campbell and Deuchar[3] in 1954, and subsequently by Friedlich et al.[4] and Tuchman et al.[5] in 1956. Raghib et al.[6] recognized a pathologic triad of anomalous LSVC draining to the left atrium with absent coronary sinus and atrial septal defect in 1965, and suggested an embryologic cause. The term "unroofed coronary sinus" was first used by Helseth and Peterson in 1974.[7] The same year, an uncommon variant of this syndrome, with large left-to-right shunt through a partially unroofed coronary sinus, was described by Allmendinger et al.[8]

Interruption of the inferior vena cava (IVC) with connection to the superior vena cava (SVC) via the azygous vein (azygous continuation) was reported in 1925 by Miller,[9] and subsequently by many others.[10-12] Anomalous connection of the IVC to the left atrium as an isolated anomaly was reported by Gardner and Cole[13] in 1955 and by Meadows et al.[14] in 1961. Anomalous drainage of both IVC and

SVC to the left atrium was reported by Ring[15] in 1805, and by Taussig[16] in 1960.

The surgical history of anomalous systemic venous return began in 1955 when Hurwitt et al.[17] ligated a persistent LSVC draining to the left atrium, which was also subsequently reported by Davis et al.[18] and Taybi et al.[19] The latter group also performed transfer of the left SVC to the right atrium but no outcome was described. A more complex form of transfer procedure was described by Schumacker et al.[20] in 1967. The so-called tunnel repair was first performed successfully by Rastelli and coworkers[21] in 1965.

Use of a pericardial baffle to isolate systemic from pulmonary venous return was first reported by Miller et al.[22] in 1965 for a patient with total anomalous systemic venous return to the left atrium. This technique was subsequently reported for unroofed coronary sinus syndrome by Helseth and Peterson[7] in 1974. Correction of isolated anomalous IVC drainage to the left atrium was reported by Gallaher and colleagues[23] in 1963. Recently, patients with azygous continuation associated with right-heart obstructive lesions were corrected using a modified Glenn shunt (termed "total cavopulmonary shunt") by Kawashima et al.[24]

INCIDENCE

The most common form of anomalous systemic venous return is persistent left superior vena cava draining to the right atrium via the coronary sinus. Abbott[25] found a 3.6% incidence of persistent LSVC in autopsies of patients with congenital heart disease, whereas Campbell and Deuchar[3] noted a 3% incidence. In the great majority of patients, no connection exists between the LSVC and the right superior vena cava (RSVC). In approximately one-third of patients, associated cardiac defects are present, most commonly atrial septal defect.[2]

Anomalous LSVC to the left atrium is much less common. Winter[2] found only 7 in a study of 170 world literature cases of anomalous LSVC, all of which had associated cardiac defects (usually atrial septal defect). In another 8 cases, the anomalous LSVC drained to the left side of a common atrium.

Incidences of the other systemic venous anomalies are also very low. Interrupted inferior vena cava (azygous continuation) was found in 0.6% of patients with congenital heart defects reviewed by Anderson and associates.[26] In many of these patients positional anomalies of the heart and thoracic and abdominal viscera are present.

EMBRYOLOGY

The normal SVC develops from the transformation of the anterior (precardinal) veins. The paired precardinals drain the segments that will ultimately become the upper extremities, head, and neck, whereas postcardinal veins drain the primitive caudal portions of the embryo (Fig. 1). The pre- and postcardinal veins unite to form the cardinal veins, or ducts of Cuvier, which empty into the sinus venosus. The sinus venosus also receives the common hepatic vein.

The paired precardinals communicate during the eighth week by an oblique cross-channel shunting blood from the left vein to the right. This becomes the innominate vein, and diversion of blood through it normally leads to obliteration of left cardinal vein, with the left duct of Cuvier and left horn of the sinus venosus persisting as the oblique vein of Marshall and coronary sinus respectively. The right anterior cardinal vein and duct of Cuvier become the superior vena cava,

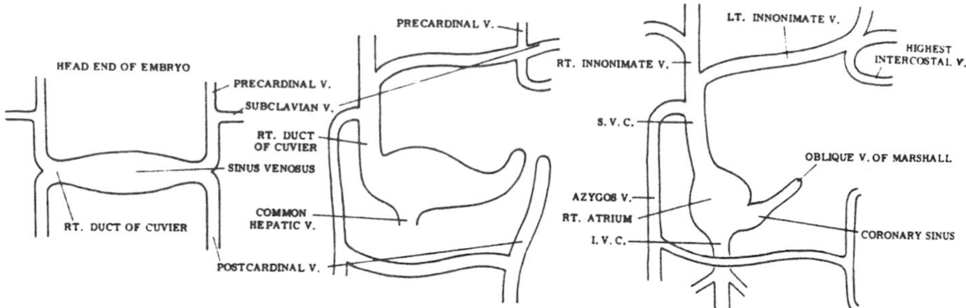

FIGURE 1. Diagrammatic representation of developmental changes of systemic veins. (Modified from Campbell and Deuchar; reprinted with permission from Ann Thorac Surg 165:797–805, 1967.)

the developing IVC and hepatic vein unite, and the right postcardinal vein persists as the azygous. Abnormal development at various stages may lead to persistence of left SVC draining to the coronary sinus (with or without a bridging innominate vein), persistent left SVC draining to the left atrium, obliteration of the right SVC with persistent left SVC, and unroofed coronary sinus.

The embryology of the IVC is more complex, involving contributions from three separate venous systems. It can be divided into four segments: (1) a suprahepatic segment from the right vitelline vein, (2) a hepatic segment from the right subcardinal and right vitelline veins, (3) a renal segment from an anastomosis between the right and left subcardinal veins, and (4) an infrarenal segment from remnants of the lumbar portion of the right subcardinal vein where it joins the iliac (postcardinal) system.[27]

Absence of the IVC occurs when the right subcardinal vein and right vitelline vein fail to connect. The hepatic veins then empty directly into the atrium, while systemic venous blood from below the diaphragm passes directly into the right subcardinal (azygous) vein. This vessel may empty into the right SVC, or less commonly into the left supracardinal (hemiazygous) vein and then into the left superior vena cava. Drainage of the hepatic veins and coronary sinus into the left atrium may also occur in these cases.

ANATOMY

Anomalous Return to the Right Atrium

This group of anomalies causes no functional disturbance, but may be of surgical importance (1) when venous cannulation is necessary for cardiopulmonary bypass, and (2) when a cavopulmonary (Glenn) shunt is to be performed.

The most common type is persistent left superior vena cava draining to the coronary sinus (Fig. 2a). In most cases a right superior vena cava is present as well, but in only 10–25% of individuals is there a bridging left innominate vein. The persistent LSVC descends anterior to the aortic arch and pulmonary artery, enters the pericardium posterior and superior to the left atrial appendage, and merges with the coronary sinus, which is enlarged.

The other important anomaly in this group is interrupted IVC with azygous continuation. As discussed above, when the hepatic and renal segments of the embryonic IVC fail to connect, the IVC connects with either the azygous, or less

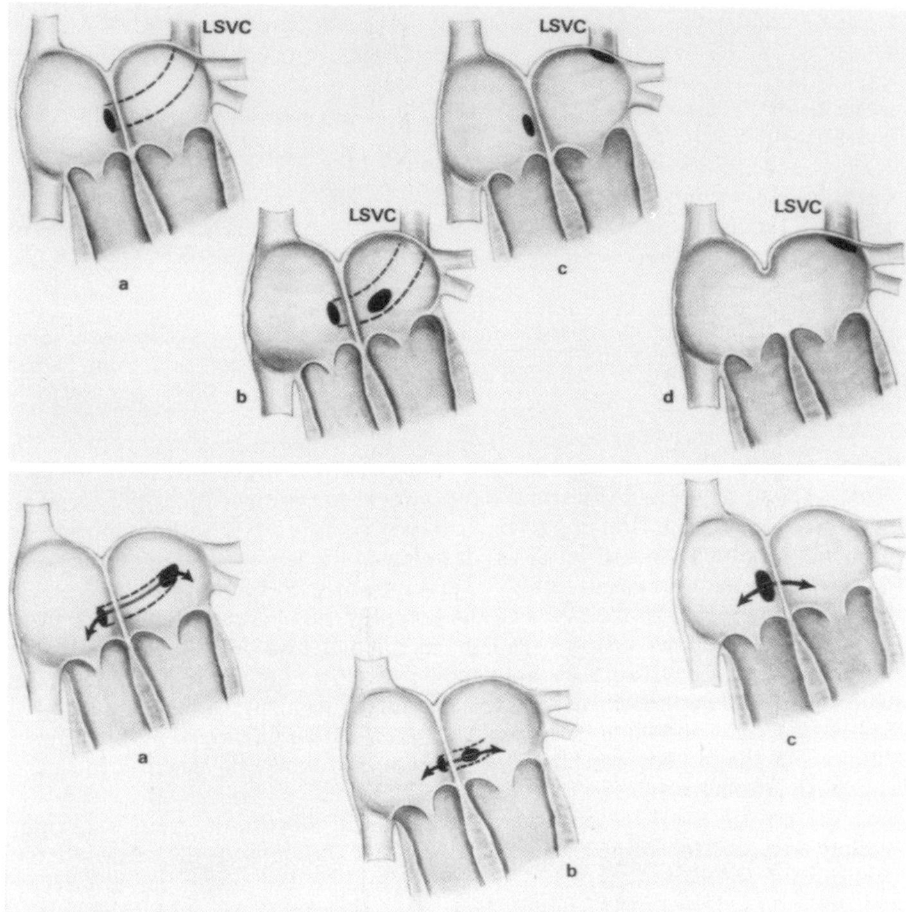

FIGURE 2. (TOP) Anomalous left superior vena cava: (a) draining to the right atrium, (b) draining to the right atrium with unroofed coronary sinus, (c) draining to the left side of a common atrium. (Reprinted with permission from de Leval M: Surgery for Congenital Heart Defects. New York, Grune & Stratton, 1983, pp. 253–260.)

FIGURE 3. (BOTTOM) Various forms of unroofed coronary sinus occurring as isolated anomaly. (Reprinted with permission from de Leval M: Surgery for Congenital Heart Defects. New York, Grune & Stratton, 1983, pp. 253–260.)

commonly, hemiazygous vein, to drain into the RSVC or LSVC respectively, while the hepatic veins drain directly to the right atrium.

Anomalous Return to the Left Atrium

This group, which includes the unroofed coronary sinus syndrome, is functionally significant, most often producing cyanosis from right-to-left shunting, but also capable of left-to-right shunting through associated septal defects. The most common type is persistent LSVC draining to the left atrium, which in unusual cases where the right SVC is absent may drain all of the cerebral and arm venous blood to the left atrium.[33] The vein typically enters the left atrium in the left upper corner, superior to the atrial appendage and anterior to the pulmonary veins (Fig. 2c). In most cases the coronary sinus is absent and an atrial septal defect (ASD) is present, forming a pathologic trial (with the anomalous LSVC) as described by Raghib et al.[6] The ASD is low and posterior on the atrial septum in the usual position of the coronary sinus, but differs from an ostium primum defect in that a rim of septal tissue separates the defect from the atrioventricular valves. A secundum ASD may be present as well, or complete absence of the septum with common atrium may occur (Fig. 2d). The coronary veins drain separately and individually into the atria. When LSVC to the left atrium is present, atrial isomerism and atrioventricular canal defects are common associated anomalies.[1]

If the coronary sinus is present, but a portion of its anterior left atrial wall (left atriovenous fold) is absent, a form of unroofed coronary sinus occurs. The defect may occur anywhere along the course of the coronary sinus. This may be present with or without persistent left SVC. In the former case, both right-to-left (from persistent LSVC) and left-to-right (through unroofed coronary sinus) shunts may occur simultaneously (Fig. 2b). When the defect occurs as an isolated anomaly, a significant and confusing left-to-right shunt may occur as described by Allmendinger et al. (Fig. 3a,b).[8] This type of defect may also occur with tricuspid atresia, and cause failure of Fontan repair by large postoperative right-to-left shunt through the unroofed coronary sinus.[28] Another operative concern with unroofed coronary sinus syndrome may be the position of the atrioventricular node and conduction bundle. Chiu and associates[37] found the best guide to the atrioventricular conduction axis to be the fusion point of the ventricular septum with the atrioventricular junction.

The other rare but important anomaly in this group is drainage of the IVC into the left atrium. This may occur as either direct left atrial entry[38] or as functional left atrial drainage when a prominent eustachian valve shunts IVC blood to the left atrium across a low ASD. Both types of defects were reported by Gallaher et al.[23] Anomalous IVC return to the hemiazygous vein may in turn join an anomalous left SVC and drain to the left atrium. Other rare types include hepatic veins draining to the left atrium and total anomalous systemic venous return to the left atrium with massive right-to-left shunt.[1,16,22,34–36,39]

Occasionally, anomalous venous drainage may occur to both atria, with an azygous continuation of the IVC to the right SVC and left SVC to the left atrium being an example.

Combined Anomalous Systemic and Pulmonary Venous Return

Many anatomical variations are possible in this group, which has been extensively detailed by de Leval et al.[1] The most common subgroup is anomalous SVC and anomalous pulmonary venous connection to the right atrium. Less commonly, there is anomalous SVC to the left atrium and anomalous pulmonary venous connection to the right atrium. Other complex cardiac malformations are common in this group.

CLINICAL COURSE

Anomalous systemic venous drainage to the right atrium is clinically innocuous. For patients with anomalous left SVC to the left atrium, right-to-left shunting causes cyanosis that is usually relatively mild. It should be suspected in patients with right-to-left shunting without evidence of right ventricular hypertrophy. In up to 25% cerebral embolization or cerebral abscess eventually occurs.[29] Cyanosis is severe for those rare patients with anomalous IVC drainage to the left atrium or with total anomalous systemic venous return to the left atrium.

Those patients with unroofed coronary sinus syndrome occurring as an isolated lesion (without anomalous LSVC) may have large left-to-right shunt and congestive failure.[8,30] As noted already, if associated with a right-sided obstructive lesions such as tricuspid atresia it may become apparent only after Fontan repair, in which case substantial right-to-left shunt persists from elevated postoperative right atrial pressure.[28,31,32]

For those patients with multiple anomalies and mixed right-to-left and left-to-right shunts, failure to thrive with congestive failure and cyanosis is usually apparent early in life.

DIAGNOSIS

Until the advent of echocardiography, the diagnosis of anomalous systemic venous return was most often made at cardiac catheterization or cardiac exploration. The demonstration of anomalous venous return can be done by catheter passage (e.g., passage of left arm venous catheter directly into the left atrium) or cineangiogram.

A persistent left superior caval vein is often associated with leftward deviation of the P wave axis and arrhythmias.[33,40–42] Chest x-ray for persistent LSVC may show a crescentic vascular shadow passing from the left border of the aortic arch toward the middle third of the left clavicle,[33] while x-ray for azygous continuation may show a protuberance from an enlarged azygous vein at its junction with the superior vena cava.[26]

Currently, cross-sectional echocardiography is an extremely specific and highly sensitive method of recognizing anomalous systemic venous return,[43] and is also valuable for the detection of abnormal atrial situs.[44] Huhta and colleagues[43] found the sensitivity of cross-sectional echocardiography to be 100% for right SVC, 96% for left SVC, 95% for bilateral SVC, 100% for absence of the suprarenal IVC, and 91% for azygous continuation of the IVC. It is thus the procedure of choice for diagnosis of anomalous systemic venous return.

Another modality, radionuclide angiography, has been used to demonstrate anomalous LSVC to the left atrium, since intravenous injections in the left arm will show much larger right-to-left shunting than injections in the right arm.[45] Finally, two-dimensional (cross-sectional) echocardiography when combined with peripheral intravenous injections of contrast has recently been shown to reliably demonstrate anomalies of systemic venous return.[46] Whether the contrast administration is a necessary supplement could be questioned, however, since the findings of Huhta et al.[43,44] so clearly support two-dimensional echocardiography (without contrast enhancement) for diagnosis of anomalous systemic venous return and abnormalities of atrial situs.

TREATMENT

Anomalous Systemic Venous Return to the Right Atrium

These anomalies cause no physiologic abnormalities by themselves (although they may be associated with more serious cardiac lesions), and consequently require no treatment. They become important, however, during cardiopulmonary bypass and require special attention. For the commonest anomaly, persistent LSVC draining to the coronary sinus, the surgeon has a number of options. If a bridging innominate vein is present, the simplest maneuver is to sling the LSVC as it enters the pericardium, being careful to avoid injury to the left phrenic nerve. When adequate collateral circulation is not present (LSVC pressure rises above 15–20 mm Hg), the choice is between simple aspiration of the noncannulated coronary sinus return with the pump sucker, separate cannulation through the coronary sinus (connected to one of the other caval catheters by a Y connector), direct cannulation where the vein enters the pericardium with a right-angle cannula, and particularly in infants, deep hypothermia with circulatory arrest.

These anomalies may also influence the surgical repair in a number of situations. A cavopulmonary (Glenn) shunt, for example, should not be performed in patients with bilateral superior vena cava because of preferential flow through the persistent LSVC.[20,47] On the other hand, a modified Glenn shunt, termed "total cavopulmonary shunt," has been used successfully for patients with lesions such as univentricular heart associated with azygous continuation by Kawashima et al.[24] In the case of procedures which may leave the coronary sinus on the left side of an atrial patch (e.g., ostium primum repairs or atrial switch operations), a persistent LSVC must be ligated to avoid unacceptable postoperative right-to-left shunt. When ligation causes an unacceptable rise in LSVC pressure, the atrial repair must be altered in these patients so that the coronary sinus drains to the right side, or the anomalous vein reimplanted.

Anomalous Systemic Venous Drainage to the Left Atrium

In most cases these anomalies result in right-to-left shunts with cyanosis and risk of brain abscess and embolization. Occasionally, an unroofed coronary sinus allows significant left-to-right shunt, either directly through an associated ASD or via the coronary sinus. Operation is indicated when shunts are substantial to avoid the above complications.

For the commonest anomaly, persistent LSVC to the left atrium, four approaches have been utilized. Ligation may be performed if LSVC pressure does not rise above 15–20 mm Hg, provided the coronary sinus is not atretic with retrograde coronary venous return through the LSVC.[1,17–19,48] Since an ASD is also usually present, it is closed separately. Another alternative is ASD closure with reimplantation of the LSVC into either the right atrium[19,20] or pulmonary artery.[49] The latter technique may be necessary if intra-atrial repair is not feasible, but presently is an infrequently used technique.

For the majority of patients who will not tolerate LSVC ligation, one of two intra-atrial approaches is preferred. Originally, a tunnel, with or without pericardium, was constructed on the floor of the left atrium to direct the LSVC return to the right atrium, and the ASD closed with a separate pericardial patch which adjoined the tunnel repair (Fig. 4).[21,29] Recently a modification of the tunnel technique has been advocated by Sand and associates,[50] in which the tunnel is constructed along the superior rather than posterior aspect of the left atrium (Fig. 5).

Because of potential obstruction of pulmonary venous return or the mitral valve by the tunnel, or creation of too small a tunnel, in most cases the preferred operation presently is a baffle directing LSVC return to the right atrium and pulmonary venous return to the mitral valve. This was originally performed in a

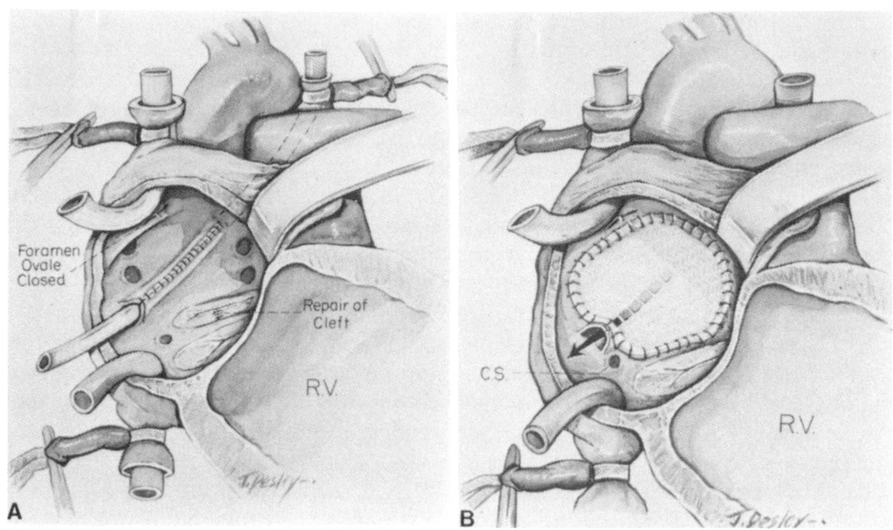

FIGURE 4. *A,* The tunnel technique for anomalous left superior vena cava, here shown with primary repair over a caval cannula. *B,* The atrial septal defect is subsequently closed with pericardium that abuts the tunnel repair. (Reprinted with permission from Mayo Clin Proc 40:528–532, 1965.)

patient with total anomalous systemic venous return by Kirklin's group (Fig. 6)[22] and has been widely employed subsequently by others.[1,7,36,39,51,52] Following institution of total cardiopulmonary bypass, preferably with separate LSVC cannulation, the right atrium is opened and the atrial and caval drainage patterns observed. If necessary for exposure, the ASD is enlarged. A patch (usually pericardium) is inserted from just below the orifice of the LSVC (anterior to the left pulmonary veins), above the mitral valve to divert pulmonary venous return through it, and down to the posterior aspect of the atrial septal defect (Fig. 7). This diverts the LSVC blood anterior to the patch to the tricuspid valve, and completely separates pulmonary from systemic venous return. For patients with a common atrium and absent coronary sinus, the inferior portion of the patch is sutured along the tricuspid valve annulus well to the right before coming posteriorly and superiorly along the floor of the common atrium, leaving the conduction tissue on the left side of the patch.[53]

In patients with partially unroofed coronary sinus, in which a defect in the mid-portion of the coronary sinus allows left-to-right shunt, the defect is repaired either by direct suture or by a patch working through an opening created in the atrial septum.[8] For patients with anomalous IVC return through a defect low in the atrial septum, the repair consists of closure of the ASD with a pericardial or Dacron patch which directs IVC return to the right atrium[1,23,38] This may require resection of the Eustachian valve. As already noted, in patients with total anomalous systemic venous return to the left atrium, a baffle is constructed to an enlarged ASD to separate systemic from pulmonary venous return (Fig. 6).[22,36,39]

Two other types of repair for complex anomalies deserve comment. When anomalous LSVC is associated with partial or complete atrioventricular canal, the inferior portion of the pericardial baffle is sutured to the rim of ventricular

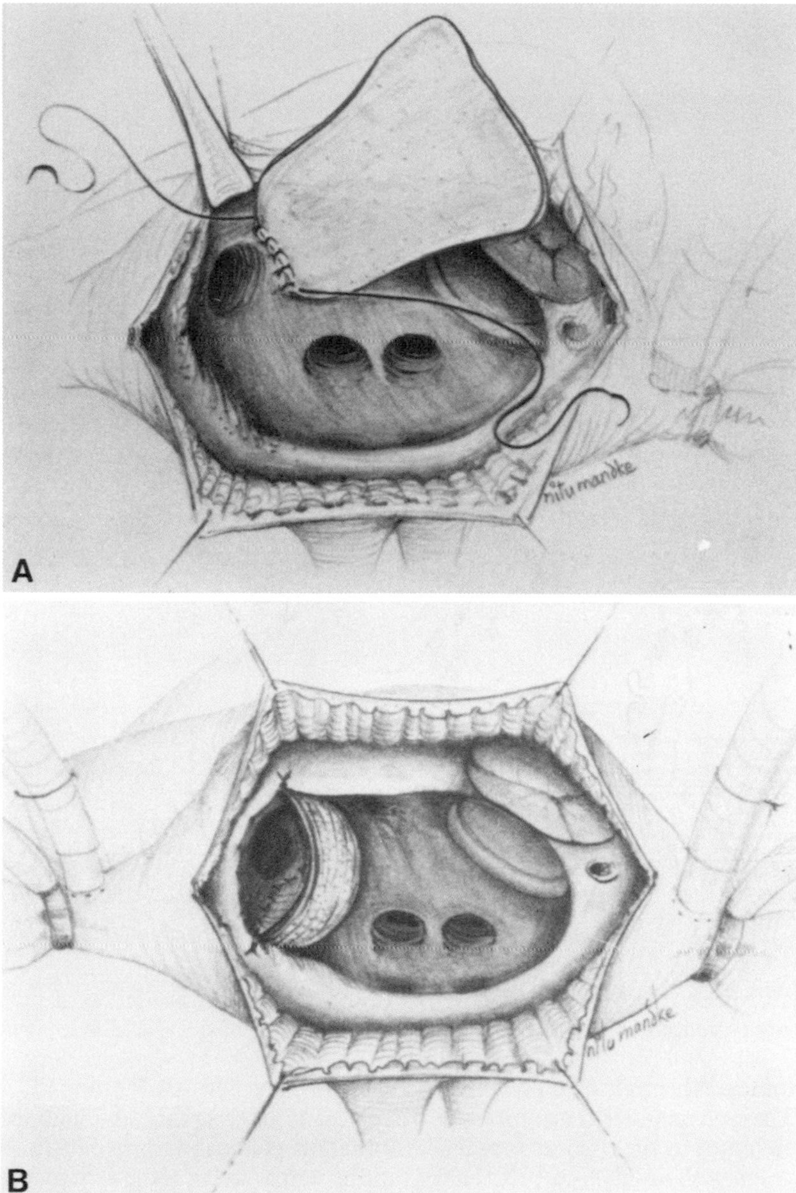

FIGURE 5. Alternative method of tunnel repair along superior rather than posterior aspect of the left atrium using a pericardial patch. (Reprinted with permission from Ann Thorac Surg 42:560–564, 1986.)

septum and atrioventricular valves (for ostium primum defect) or to the top of the Dacron patch used to close the ventricular septal defect (for complete atrioventricular canal). For patients with anomalous systemic venous return associated with transposition of the great arteries undergoing atrial switch repair,

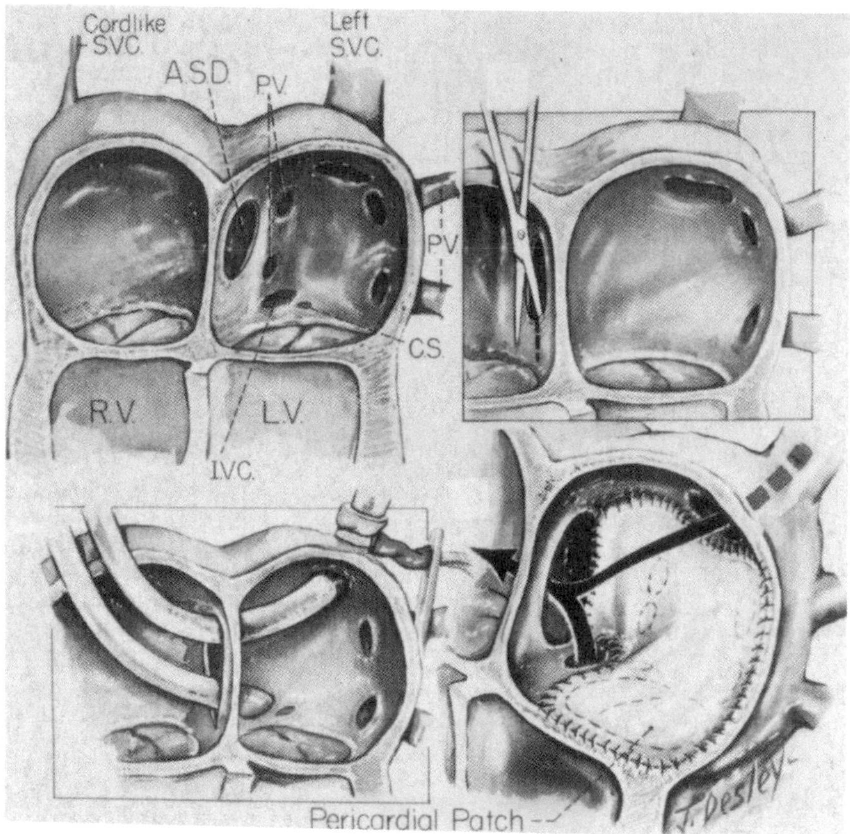

FIGURE 6. Use of a pericardial baffle to correct anomalous left superior vena cava and, in this patient, anomalous inferior vena cava. (Reprinted with permission from Mayo Clin Proc 40:532–538, 1965.)

the baffle is created to direct all systemic venous blood into the left ventricle and pulmonary venous blood into the right ventricle.[1]

Combined Anomalous Systemic and Pulmonary Venous Return

The two major subgroups here are anomalous systemic and pulmonary venous return to the right atrium, and anomalous systemic venous return to the left atrium with anomalous pulmonary venous return to the right atrium.[1] Other complex anomalies are also frequently present.

The principles of repair are direction of all systemic venous return to the pulmonary ventricle and pulmonary venous return to the systemic ventricle with use of a baffle. In addition, any significant extracardiac communication between the systemic and pulmonary veins optimally should be divided, although an isolated pulmonary vein draining to a systemic vein can be left uncorrected with little adverse effect (small left-to-right shunt).[1] The precise identification of intracardiac anatomy is imperative, with special attention to caval and pulmonary venous drainage patterns. In addition to intra-atrial baffle, division and reimplantation of an anomalous systemic vein to which pulmonary veins are joined

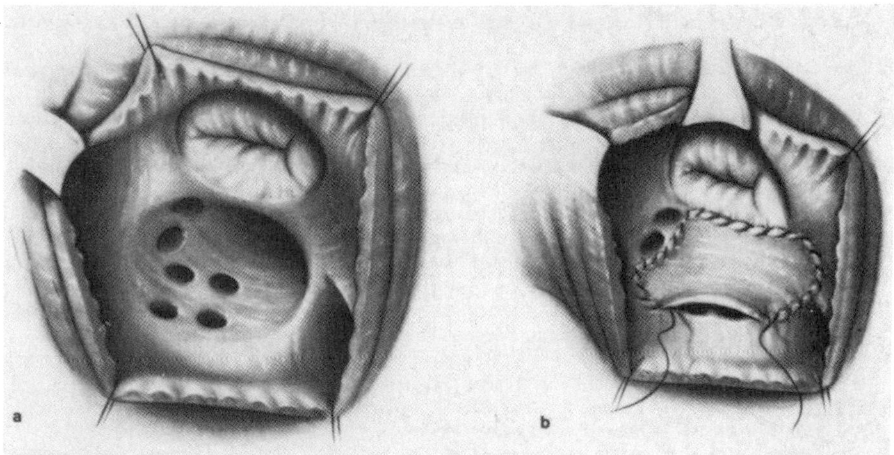

FIGURE 7. Baffle procedure for isolated left superior vena caval drainage to the left atrium and associated atrial septal defect. The anomalous left superior vena cava and left atrial appendage remain anterior to the baffle. (Reprinted with permission from de Leval M: Surgery for Congenital Heart Defects. New York, Grune & Stratton, 1983, pp. 253–260.

may be necessary to completely separate systemic from pulmonary venous drainage.

RESULTS

Results of correction for isolated anomalous LSVC with ASD are excellent,[1,6,29,48] and operative mortality should approach that for ASD alone. When anomalous systemic venous return is present with other complex cardiac anomalies, operative mortality is higher and is related to the associated defects.[1] Because of occasional obstructive complications from tunnel repair, the most common technique currently used is an intra-atrial baffle. The risk of heart block will be higher in patients with common atrium and absent coronary sinus.

REFERENCES

1. de Leval MR, Ritter DG, McGoon DC, Danielson GK: Anomalous systemic venous connection: Surgical considerations. Mayo Clin Proc 50:599, 1975.
2. Winter FS: Persistent left superior vena cava. Angiology 5:90, 1954.
3. Campbell M, Deuchar DC: The left-sided superior vena cava. Br Heart J 16:423, 1954.
4. Friedlich A, Bing RJ, Blount SG Jr: Circulatory dynamics in the anomalies of venous return to the heart including pulmonary arteriovenous fistula. Bull Johns Hopkins Hosp 86:20, 1956.
5. Tuchman H, Brown JF, Huston JH, et al: Superior vena cava draining into left atrium. Am J Med 21:481, 1956.
6. Raghib G, Ruttenberg HD, Anderson RC, et al: Termination of left superior vena cava in left atrium, atrial septal defect, and absence of coronary sinus. Circulation 31:906, 1965.
7. Helseth HK, Peterson CR: Atrial septal defect with termination of left superior vena cava in the left atrium and absence of the coronary sinus. Ann Thorac Surg 17:186, 1974.
8. Allmendinger P, Dear WE, Cooley DA: Atrial septal defect with communication through the coronary sinus. Ann Thorac Surg 17:193, 1974.
9. Miller AJ: Congenital heart disease with partial situs inversus, absence of the inferior vena cava, and other anomalies. Am J Pathol 1:467, 1925.
10. Huseby RA, Boyden EA: Absence of the hepatic portion of the inferior vena cava with bilateral retention of the supracardinal system. Anat Rec 81:537, 1941.

11. Latimer HB, Virden HH: A case of complete absence of the inferior vena cava. J Kansas Med Soc 45:346, 1944.
12. Anderson RC, Heilig W, Novick R, Jarvis C: Anomalous inferior vena cava with azygous drainage: so-called absence of the inferior vena cava. Am Heart J 49:318, 1955.
13. Gardner DL, Cole L: Long survival with inferior vena cava draining into left atrium. Br Heart J 17:93, 1955.
14. Meadows WR, Bergstrand I, Sharp JT: Isolated anomalous connection of a great vein to the left atrium: the syndrome of cyanosis and clubbing, "normal" heart, and left ventricular hypertrophy on electrocardiogram. Circulation 24:669, 1961.
15. Ring: A singular case of malformation of the heart. Med & Physical J 13:120, 1805.
16. Taussig HB: Congenital Malformations of the Heart. Cambridge, MA, Harvard University Press, 1960.
17. Hurwitt ES, Escher DJW, Citrin LI: Surgical correction of cyanosis due to entrance of left superior vena cava into left auricle. Surgery 38:903, 1955.
18. Davis WH, Jordaan FR, Snyman HW: Persistent left superior vena cava draining into the left atrium, as an isolated anomaly. Am Heart J 57:616, 1959.
19. Taybi H, Kurlander GJ, Lurie PR, Campbell JA: Anomalous systemic venous connection to the left atrium or to a pulmonary vein. Am J Roentgenol 94:62, 1965.
20. Schumacker HB Jr, King H, Waldhausen JA: The persistent left superior vena cava: surgical implications, with special reference to caval drainage into the left atrium. Ann Surg 165:797, 1967.
21. Rastelli GC, Ongley PA, Kirklin JW: Surgical correction of common atrium with anomalously connected persistent left superior vena cava: Report of a case. Mayo Clin Proc 40:528, 1965.
22. Miller GAH, Ongley P, Rastelli GC, Kirklin JW: Surgical correction of total anomalous systemic venous connections: Report of a case. Mayo Clin Proc 40:532, 1965.
23. Gallaher ME, Sperling DR, Gwinn JL, et al: Functional drainage of the inferior vena cava into the left atrium—three cases. Am J Cardiol 12:561, 1963.
24. Kawashima Y, Kitamuras, Matsuda H, et al: Total cavopulmonary shunt operation in complex cardiac anomalies. A new operation. J Thorac Cardiovasc Surg 87:74, 1984.
25. Abbott ME: Atlas of Congenital Cardiac Disease. New York, American Heart Association, 1936.
26. Anderson RC, Adams P Jr, Burke B: Anomalous inferior vena cava with azygous continuation (intrahepatic interruption of the inferior vena cava). J Pediatr 59:370, 1961.
27. Langman J: Medical Embryology. Baltimore, Williams & Wilkins, 1963.
28. Rumisek JD, Pigott JD, Weinberg PM, et al: Coronary sinus septal defect associated with tricuspid atresia. J Thorac Cardiovasc Surg 92:142, 1986.
29. Quaegebeur J, Kirklin JW, Pacifico AD, Bargeron LM Jr: Surgical experience with unroofed coronary sinus. Ann Thorac Surg 27:418, 1979.
30. Mantini E, Grondin CM, Lillehei CW, Edwards JE: Congenital anomalies involving the coronary sinus. Circulation 33:317, 1966.
31. Freedom RM, Culham JAG, Rowe RD: Left atrial to coronary sinus fenestration (partially unroofed coronary sinus): Morphological and angiocardiographic observations. Br Heart J 46:63, 1981.
32. Rose AG, Beckman CB, Edwards JE: Communications between coronary sinus and left atrium. Br Heart J 36:182, 1974.
33. Choi JY, Anderson RH, Macartney FJ: Absent right superior caval vein (vena cava) with normal atrial arrangement. Br Heart J 57:474, 1987.
34. Gueron M, Hirsh M, Bowman J: Total anomalous systemic venous drainage into the left atrium. J Thorac Cardiovasc Surg 58:570, 1969.
35. Roberts KD, Edwards JM, Astley R: Surgical correction of total anomalous systemic venous drainage. J Thorac Cardiovasc Surg 64:803, 1972.
36. Pearl WR, Spicer MJ: Total anomalous systemic venous return. South Med J 73:259, 1980.
37. Chiu IS, Hegerty A, Anderson RH, et al: The landmarks to the atrioventricular conduction system in hearts with absence or unroofing of the coronary sinus. J Thorac Cardiovasc Surg 90:297, 1985.
38. Chantepie A, Marchand M, de la Tour R, et al: Inferior caval return to the left atrium with intact atrial septum. Report of two cases operated upon successfully. Arch Mal Coeur 79:684, 1986.
39. Danielson GK, McMullan MH, Kinsley RH, et al: Successful repair of complete atrioventricular canal associated with dextroversion, common atrium, and total anomalous systemic venous return. J Thorac Cardiovasc Surg 66:817, 1973.
40. Lenox CC, Zuberbuhler JR, Park SC, et al: Absent right superior vena cava with persistent left superior vena cava: Implications and management. Am J Cardiol 45:117, 1980.

41. Camm AJ, Dymond D, Spurrell RAJ: Sinus node dysfunction associated with absence of right superior vena cava. Br Heart J 41:504, 1979.
42. Momma K, Linde LM: Abnormal rhythms associated with persistent left superior vena cava. Pediatr Res 3:210, 1969.
43. Huhta JC, Smallhorn JF, Macartney FJ, et al: Cross-sectional echocardiographic diagnosis of systemic venous return. Br Heart J 48:388, 1982.
44. Huhta JC, Smallhorn JF, Macartney FJ: Two dimensional echocardiographic diagnosis of situs. Br Heart J 48:97, 1982.
45. Konstam MA, Levine BW, Strauss HW, McKusick KA: Left superior vena cava to left atrial communication diagnosed with radionuclide angiography and with differential right-to-left shunting. Am J Cardiol 43:149, 1979.
46. Foule R, Bourdillon PD, Somerville J, et al: Anomalous systemic venous return: Recognition by two-dimensional echocardiography. Eur Heart J 4:186, 1983.
47. Mathur M, Glenn WWL: Long-term evaluation of cava-pulmonary artery anastomosis. Surgery 74:899, 1973.
48. Lee ME, Sade RM: Coronary sinus septal defect: Surgical considerations. J Thorac Cardiovasc Surg 78:563, 1979.
49. Foster ED, Baeza OR, Farina MF, et al: Atrial septal defect associated with drainage of left superior vena cava to left atrium and absence of the coronary sinus. J Thorac Cardiovasc Surg 76:718, 1978.
50. Sand ME, McGrath LB, Pacifico AD, et al: Repair of left superior vena cava entering the left atrium. Ann Thorac Surg 42:560, 1986.
51. Sherafat M, Friedman S, Waldhausen JA: Persistent left superior vena cava draining into the left atrium with absent right superior vena cava. Ann Thorac Surg 11:160, 1971.
52. Crenshaw R, Okies JE, Phillips SJ, et al: Partial anomalous systemic venous return. Report of surgical treatment in two cases. J Thorac Cardiovasc Surg 69:433, 1975.
53. Asano K, Sakurai T, Matsuzawa H: Surgical correction of common atrium with anomalously connected persistent left superior vena cava. Jpn Heart J 10:545, 1969.

EDWARD D. VERRIER, MD
FRANK L. HANLEY, MD
KEVIN TURLEY, MD

TRUNCUS ARTERIOSUS

From the Department of Surgery
University of California,
San Francisco

Reprint requests to:
Edward D. Verrier, MD
Department of Surgery
Cardiothoracic Surgery, M 896
University of California,
San Francisco
505 Parnassus Ave.
San Francisco, CA 94143-0118

Persistent truncus arteriosus is a rare anomaly, accounting for less than 1% of all congenital heart defects. In this condition, the systemic, pulmonary, and coronary circulations all arise from a single great vessel, which is connected to the base of the heart by a single, semilunar valve. A ventricular septal defect is an integral part of the defect. Mild cyanosis may be present in infancy because of admixture of saturated and unsaturated blood at the ventricular and great vessel level. The predominant symptoms, however, result from congestive heart failure, which develops as pulmonary blood flow increases in response to the normal drop in pulmonary vascular resistance after birth. Later, if the lesion remains untreated, cyanosis may progress and congestive heart failure abate, as pulmonary hypertension develops due to the excessive pulmonary blood flow. A thorough understanding of the embryology, pathophysiology, and natural history of this congenital heart lesion has led to significant improvements in prognosis following surgical repair over the past decade.

EMBRYOLOGIC AND ANATOMIC FEATURES

Knowledge of embryology is important to understand both the various anatomic configurations of persistent truncus arteriosus and the surgical alternatives available to correct them. The basic defect in persistent truncus arteriosus is absence of the truncal septum. In the developing heart, the truncus arteriosus makes up the distal third of the bulbus cordis and is attached proximally to the conus cordis and distally to the aortic sac. With normal septal development, the truncus arteriosus forms the proximal aorta and pulmonary artery including the valves, the conus cordis forms the left and right ventricular outflow tracts, and the aortic sac forms the origins of the aortic arch and the distal main pulmonary artery trunk. The fourth aortic arches arise from the aortic sac and form aspects of the true aortic arch and great vessels, and the sixth aortic arches also arise from the aortic sac and form the left and right pulmonary arteries. Beginning at 27 days of gestation and extending over the next 10 days, two opposing spiraling ridges of endocardial tissue appear within the truncus arteriosus and approach each other to form the spiral septum, which divides the truncus into aorta and pulmonary artery. At the same time, the conal septum is forming to divide the conus cordis. The truncal and conal septa merge, thus creating right ventricular to pulmonary artery continuity. The aortic and pulmonary valves form at the level of fusion of these two septa. At the other end of the truncus arteriosus, the aortic sac is developing in such a way that the paired sixth aortic arches are migrating to the left and the paired fourth aortic arches are migrating to the right. The enlargement of the aortic sac results in invagination of its roof between these two pairs of arches, resulting in the aorto-pulmonary septum. This septum merges with the truncal septum, thereby completing the separation of aorta and pulmonary artery. The truncus arteriosus defect then can be seen as resulting primarily from a failure of the truncal septum to form; however, abnormalities of the conal septum and of aortic sac invagination also contribute to the defect. The absence of the truncal septum results in a single great vessel and single outflow valve; however, the degree of deficiency of the conal septum will determine the size and position of the ventricular septal defect. This has considerable clinical significance at the time of surgical repair. Likewise, the degree of development of aortic sac septation will determine the configuration of the origin of the pulmonary arteries from the persistent truncus. This configuration also has clinical implications for surgical repair. The variations in configuration of the pulmonary artery origin from the truncus have been formally classified. The earliest accepted classification system for truncus arteriosus was described by Collette and Edwards. In type 1 truncus, a short main pulmonary artery arises from a single orifice, usually on the undersurface of the truncal artery. In type 2, the left and right pulmonary arteries arise from separate orifices, but in close approximation to each other. In type 3, the individual orifices of the left and right pulmonary arteries are widely separated. Types 1 and 2 represent almost 90% of all clinical cases. Originally, a type 4 truncus was described. This is now recognized to be pulmonary atresia with absent central pulmonary arteries, hypertrophied bronchials arising from the descending aorta, and a ventricular septal defect. Hemi-truncus is an unusual variant in which, usually, the right pulmonary artery arises from the ascending aorta and the left pulmonary artery arises from the right ventricle.

The ventricular septal defect in truncus arteriosus is usually high, anterior, large, and located beneath the truncal valve between the two superior limbs of the trabecula septomarginalis (septal bands). The posterior border in such patients is muscle, but depending on the extent of development of the ventriculo-infundibular fold, the defect may extend to the membranous portion of the septum in 30% of the cases. In this situation, the posterior border is adjacent to the tricuspid annulus, and the conduction system lies close to the rim of the defect. Since truncus represents a defect in midline development, other congenital cardiac and systemic anomalies occur commonly with truncus arteriosus, including interrupted aortic arch (13%), atrial septal defect (20%), right aortic arch (20%) and coronary artery anomalies (15%), thymic atresia, and DeGeorge syndrome.

NATURAL HISTORY

Most children die of severe congestive heart failure in infancy. If associated anomalies are present, such as interrupted aortic arch or severe truncal valve insufficiency, death usually occurs in the perinatal period. The rare survivor to adulthood usually dies of cyanosis as pulmonary vascular disease (PVD) progresses, leading to Eisenmenger's syndrome. As in other lesions with increased pulmonary blood flow, failure to thrive and emaciation are common, predisposing to recurrent pulmonary bacterial infections. If untreated, approximately 16% of patients born with truncus arteriosus survive infancy and early childhood to age 5 years without the development of severe pulmonary vascular disease, and are reasonable candidates for corrective surgery at that time. The remainder of the 84% of patients either die in the first year of life (75%) or develop severe pulmonary vascular disease and become inoperable (9%). Of the 16% who arc surgical candidates, some will die at the time of corrective surgery (5%) or will develop pulmonary vascular disease after corrective surgery (3%), leaving 8% of the total as long-term survivors.

Historically, the initial therapeutic approach in these critically ill infants was pulmonary artery banding in an attempt to lower the early mortality. This was accomplished by decreasing pulmonary blood flow, but there was minimal impact on long-term survival. This procedure doubled the first year survival to 50% because it controlled congestive heart failure, but only 20% survived a second corrective operation and were without pulmonary vascular disease at 5 years of age. Of the other 30%, 5% died before corrective surgery, 10% developed severe PVD, precluding correction, and the remaining 15% either died at the time or corrective surgery or developed pulmonary vascular disease after surgery (Table 1). It is difficult to achieve a good clinical result with pulmonary artery banding in truncus arteriosus, because adequate control of the left-to-right intracardiac shunt, without obtaining clinically obvious oxygen desaturation, may not be possible. Even with a clinically effective pulmonary artery band, pulmonary vascular disease will develop in one or both of the pulmonary arteries in greater than 50% of the cases. In addition, pulmonary artery distortion occurs commonly. These unsatisfactory results have stimulated other approaches. Total repair as an initial procedure in the first 6 months of life has lowered the 1-year mortality to 15%. The pulmonary and systemic circulations are separated and progression of pulmonary vascular disease is averted. The major operative risk factors that have been identified are the presence of pulmonary hypertension or truncal valve

TABLE 1. Patients Alive and Well (%)

Treatment	Birth	1 year	5 years
None	100%	25%	8%
Early PA band	100%	50%	20%
Total correction	100%	89%	87%

insufficiency. All children with truncus arteriosus who undergo complete repair in infancy, however, do face further operative procedures and require life-long monitoring.

CLINICAL PRESENTATION

The clinical presentation of truncus arteriosus is determined by the degree of pulmonary blood flow and the presence or absence of associated anomalies. In the neonatal period, pulmonary vascular resistance often remains elevated, and the child will be minimally symptomatic unless the truncal valve is insufficient or an interrupted arch is present. Rarely, pulmonary vascular resistance remains persistently elevated and the child develops symptoms gradually. These children have good weight gain and growth in the early months of life, but usually become cyanotic as pulmonary vascular disease gradually develops. These patients are not operable. This group should be differentiated from an equally rare group of patients who are born with stenosis at the take-off of the pulmonary arteries from the main trunk. These patients have restricted pulmonary blood flow secondary to the stenosis; however, pulmonary vascular resistance is low. They also present with cyanosis, good weight gain, and growth in the early months of life; however, they are excellent candidates for primary repair. Most often, as pulmonary vascular resistance decreases after birth, pulmonary blood flow increases and congestive heart failure ensues. These children present with tachypnea, tachycardia, irritability, poor feeding, lack of weight gain, and recurrent pulmonary infections. Truncal valve insufficiency will compound these symptoms. Respiratory distress may be worsened by bronchial compression, causing atelectasis. Mild cyanosis may be present due to admixture of saturated and unsaturated blood at the ventricular and great vessel level, but cyanosis is not a major clinical issue until pulmonary vascular disease develops.

Physical examination usually reveals an emaciated, pale, excessively sweaty infant with moderate respiratory distress. The heart is large and often overactive, with a systolic thrill along the left sternal border. Auscultation reveals a pansystolic murmur from the ventricular septal defect and a loud ejection click from opening of the large truncal valve. An apical, high-pitched diastolic murmur along the left sternal border usually represents truncal valve insufficiency. An apical gallop may be present but is rare.

The characteristic chest x-ray shows cardiomegaly, increased pulmonary vascular markings, and an absent main pulmonary artery segment. A right-sided aortic arch is present in approximately 20% of patients. The electrocardiogram usually demonstrates biventricular hypertrophy with predominant left ventricular forces when excessive pulmonary blood flow is present or predominant right-sided forces when pulmonary blood flow is diminished (pulmonic stenosis or pulmonary vascular disease). Two-dimensional echocardiography is diagnostic of truncus arteriosus in most cases and can usually delineate the origin of the pulmonary arteries and the degree of truncal valve insufficiency. Echocardiography does not, however, directly evaluate the degree of pulmonary vascular disease.

Cardiac catheterization with angiocardiography is necessary if further clarification is required to determine (1) the pulmonary artery anatomy, (2) the pulmonary vascular resistance, (3) the competency of the truncal valve, and/or (4) aortic arch anatomy (Fig. 1).

Typical hemodynamic findings in infants include a left-to-right shunt at the ventricular level with equal left and right ventricular pressures, and pulmonary

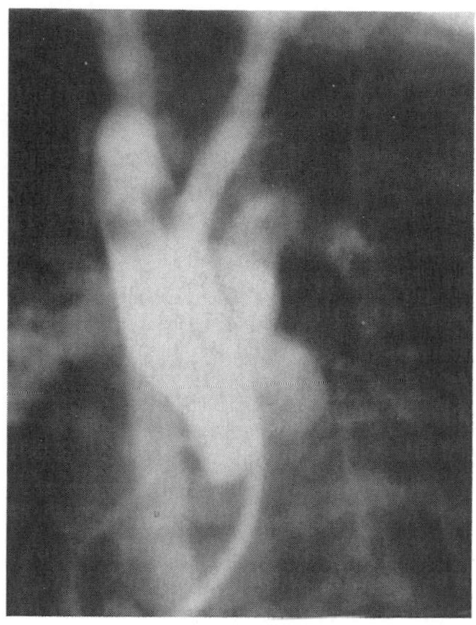

FIGURE 1. Contrast injection in root of truncus, showing competent truncal valve, main pulmonary artery arising from trunk, and aortic arch vessels. Coronary arteries are seen.

artery pressures close to systemic. The elevated pulmonary flow keeps aortic oxygen saturation greater than 85%. Pulmonary vascular resistance is usually only mildly elevated (2–4 Wood units/m^2). If left ventricular pressure is higher than right ventricular pressure, this usually signifies a restrictive ventricular septal defect with malalignment or truncal valve stenosis, both rare conditions. When arterial oxygen saturations fall below 84%, significant pulmonary vascular disease limiting pulmonary blood flow is usually the cause, and the child may not tolerate operative correction. Cineangiocardiography of both ventricles and the aorta delineates the ventricular septal defect anatomy, the pulmonary artery anatomy, and the truncal valve anatomy and physiology. The truncal root contrast injection helps to rule out patent ductus arteriosus, aortopulmonary window, and interrupted aortic arch.

SURGICAL MANAGEMENT

The general philosophy is early corrective surgery in infants with truncus arteriosus. The initial medical management is accomplished with the use of digitalis and diuretics, nutrition, and often ventilatory support. This may temporarily relieve the symptoms of congestive heart failure, allowing the infant to stabilize and grow, but cannot be used for prolonged therapy. Pulmonary vascular disease will develop early, often by 4–6 months of age if repair is delayed.

Pulmonary artery banding is rarely used for palliation and only in unusual circumstances; for example, when another major congenital defect is present, or when there is concomitant serious medical illness, such as bacterial pneumonia. In such a circumstance, the complicated and difficult procedure of bilateral pulmonary artery banding is necessary.

Repair is not recommended in children with fixed pulmonary vascular disease with resistances greater than 8 Wood units/m^2. Another indicator of inoperability is a peripheral arterial saturation of less than approximately 83% in patients without stenosis of the pulmonary arteries. Operative mortality approaches 50% in these situations and pulmonary vascular disease frequently progresses despite closure of the ventricular septal defect and construction of a right ventricle to pulmonary artery conduit. In children with reactive pulmonary vascular disease that responds to oxygen therapy or a pulmonary vasodilator such as priscoline by dropping pulmonary vascular resistance to less than 8 units/m^2, correction is still recommended, although at a higher perioperative risk. If such children survive the difficult operative period, the elevated pulmonary vascular resistance will tend to stabilize or decrease, as the pulmonary arteriolar resistance may be reversible (hypertrophy) rather than fixed (obstructive). Other anatomic considerations that increase operative and perioperative risk are truncal valve insufficiency, truncal valve stenosis with a dysmorphic valve, severe override of the trunk which carries the risk of subaortic stenosis, a ventricular septal defect with perimembranous extension, and a small left ventricular cavity.

The physiologic presentation determines the timing of surgery. A small group of patients develop CHF from birth and require surgery in the neonatal period. The majority of patients can be treated medically, and be operated on between 6 and 12 weeks of age. Another small group of patients has persistently elevated pulmonary vascular resistance and they are never surgical candidates. Surgical correction is based on the pioneering experimental work of Rastelli, who in 1967 demonstrated the technical feasibility of connecting the pulmonary arteries to the right ventricle by use of an ascending aortic homograft. Based on this experimental work, the first successful clinical correction was done later in 1967 by McGoon et al. In spite of these advances, perioperative mortality generally remained in the range of 50%, probably because many infants were corrected after six months of age when pulmonary vascular disease had developed. Further advances were made by Ebert et al., who showed markedly improved survival of 88% after complete repair in a series of 106 infants when surgery was performed before 6 months of age. These results seemed paradoxical at first evaluation, since at this age CHF is most severe and infants appear quite ill. The severe CHF, however, reflects a lower pulmonary resistance and thus a healthy pulmonary vasculature, allowing a smoother postoperative recovery. At a later age, CHF has often abated to some degree and the infants are well-nourished and growing and appear much more robust. The clinical trap is that they appear to be much better surgical candidates at this time; in reality, the reason for the clinical improvement is decreased pulmonary blood flow secondary to development of pulmonary vascular disease. This results in severe postoperative problems and higher mortality. In all series, presently, the pulmonary artery(ies) are detached from the undersurface of the trunk, the ventricular septal defect is closed through a right ventriculotomy, and a valved conduit is used to establish right ventricular to pulmonary artery continuity.

Operative Technique

Most children are anesthetized with an inhalation agent and minimal sedation. Peripheral indwelling arterial and venous catheters are placed percutaneously or by cut-down. The heart is approached through a median sternotomy and the lower half of the thymus is removed to allow space for the new right ventricular to pulmonary artery conduit. Pursestring sutures are placed in the atrial appendage and high on the ascending aorta at the base of the innominate artery, in order to allow room for the aortic cross-clamp. The main pulmonary artery, if possible, or the branch pulmonary arteries are encircled with snares. In infants, the ascending aorta is cannulated with a No. 10 Bardex straight arterial

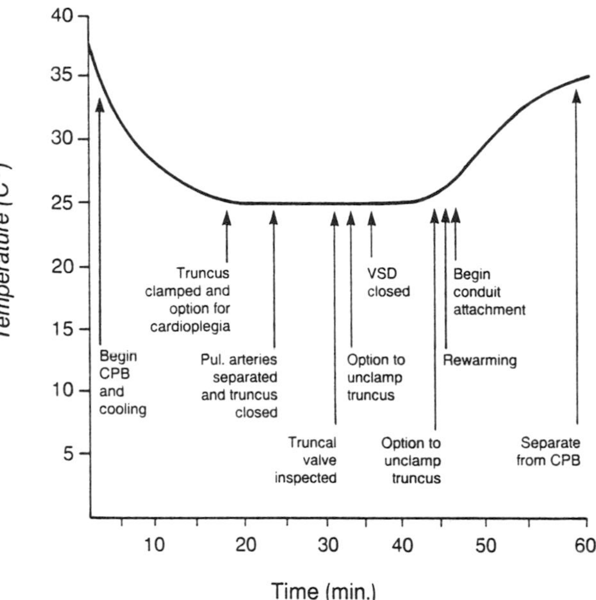

FIGURE 2. Typical sequence of an operation for truncus arteriosus. The truncus cross-clamp can be removed after completing the closure of the truncus defect created after separation of the pulmonary arteries, in which case no cardioplegia is needed. Alternatively, the cross-clamp can remain in place for evaluation and closure of the ventricular septal defect, in which case cardioplegia is used.

cannula and the right atrium with a No. 18 or 20 multi-holed single venous cannula. The left ventricle is occasionally vented through the right superior pulmonary vein, as in older children with significant truncal valve insufficiency. Cardiopulmonary bypass is initiated with the precooled oxygenated blood prime and the patient is systematically cooled to 20–25°C. Deep hypothermia and circulatory arrest are not routinely used.

The pulmonary artery snare(s) is tightened at the onset of bypass to minimize pulmonary blood flow. When myocardial contractility decreases and

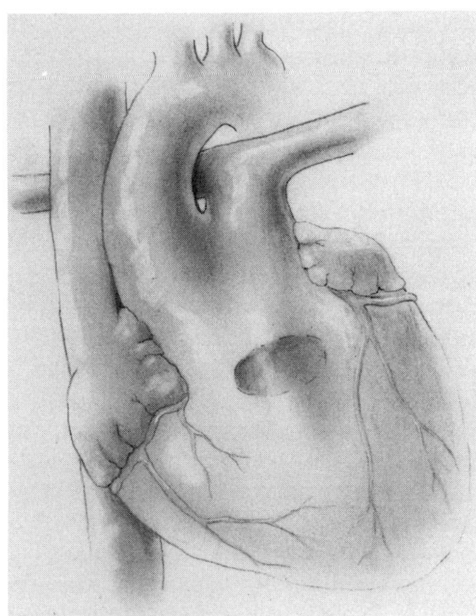

FIGURE 3. Configuration of type 1 truncus arteriosus with persistent trunk, main pulmonary artery segment, and high arterial VSD.

the heart rate slows, the ascending aorta is cross-clamped. Instillation of cardioplegia (4° C) into the proximal aortic route may provide for additional myocardial protection (Figs. 2–4).

The pulmonary arteries are then excised from the truncus. In types I and II truncus, the pulmonary artery orifice is excised, taking care to remove an adequate cuff of aorta to avoid pulmonary artery distortion. The aorta is then closed transversely with care not to injure the truncal valve or coronary arteries, using a continuous simple suture of 5–0 polypropylene. The undersurface of the aorta is the most common site of postoperative hemorrhage and can be somewhat difficult to suture once the right ventricular to pulmonary artery conduit is in place. In type III truncus, a wider cuff of aorta, including the bridge of aorta between the two pulmonary artery orifices, is excised, thereby maintaining continuity between the two pulmonary arteries. Occasionally, an entire ring of truncal tissue must be excised which incorporates both pulmonary artery orifices. The anterior aspect of the ring between the two pulmonary arteries is then excised before reconstructing the right ventricular outflow tract. The truncal artery is then reapproximated with a continuous suture in an end-to-end fashion.

A longitudinal right ventriculotomy is made, starting at the base of the truncus and extending onto the right ventricular free wall. The endocardium tends to evert, so the muscle is undercut to assure an adequate match for the right ventricular proximal conduit anastomosis. Care is used not to injure a major coronary artery. The incidence of the left anterior descending coronary arising from the right coronary artery is much lower than in tetralogy of Fallot; however, large right coronary branches often cross the right ventricle to supply the ventricular septum. Attempts to save these branches of the right coronary artery are made whenever possible. The aortic cross-clamp is then removed, and truncal valve competency is directly evaluated by visualization through the right ventriculotomy. Rarely, the truncal valve is severely incompetent and truncal valve replacement is necessary. Moderate amounts of truncal valve insufficiency are accepted without valve replacement. This situation does increase surgical mortality; however, the mortality is probably less than if valve replacement is added to an already complex operation. Significant truncal valve insufficiency adds considerable complexity to intraoperative management on cardiopulmonary bypass and special attention is required to assure adequate myocardial protection and avoid ventricular distention.

The ventricular septal defect (VSD) is evaluated through the right ventriculotomy and closed with an appropriate-sized prosthetic patch using either a running or interrupted suture technique. If necessary, the aortic cross-clamp may be replaced to visualize the ventricular septal defect. Most of the VSDs associated with truncus arteriosus have a rim of muscle between the defect and the tricuspid annulus, so that complete heart block is a smaller risk than in perimembranous ventricular septal defects. When the VSD does extend to the membranous septum (30%), care must be taken to avoid conduction tissue. The patch is approximated to the rim of the defect and extended superiorly to the cephalic end of the ventriculotomy. This reconstruction incorporates the truncal valve into the left ventricular outflow tract (Fig. 5). If the truncal valve markedly overrides the right ventricle or the VSD is small, the VSD may need to be enlarged inferiorly in order to avoid obstruction of the left ventricular outflow tract at the level of the VSD patch. The aortic cross-clamp, if placed for VSD closure, is removed and rewarming is started. If truncal valve incompetence is

FIGURE 4. Cannulation method for truncus arteriosus. A snare is placed around the pulmonary artery at the start of cardiopulmonary bypass to prevent excessive blood flow to the lungs. The dotted lines indicate the position of the incisions.

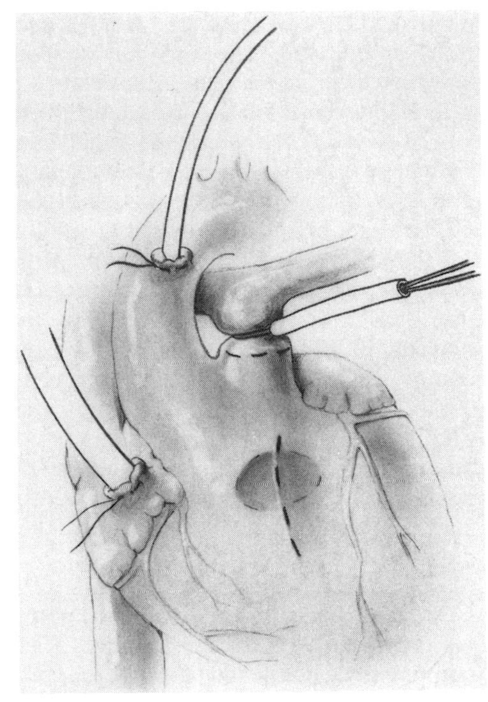

FIGURE 5. The main pulmonary artery has been divided and the proximal aorta oversewn. Patch closure of the VSD is partially completed. Note that the superior aspect of the patch is sewn to the epicardium of the right ventriculotomy incision.

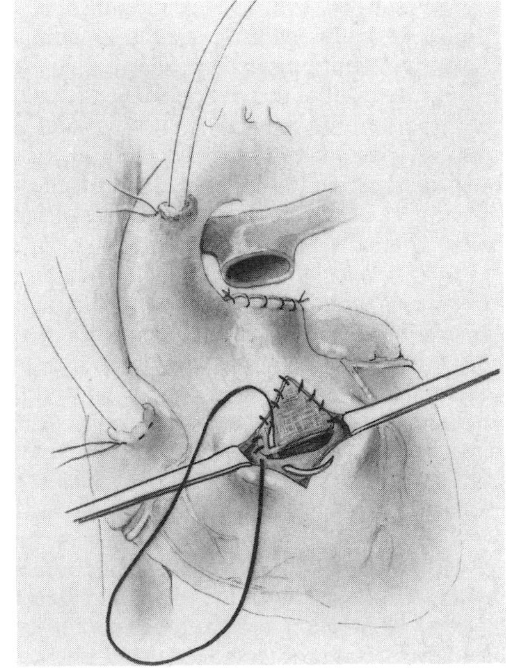

present at all, care must be taken to avoid left ventricular distention when the heart is fibrillating. The heart may require manual compression and early defibrillation even before the right ventricular-to-pulmonary artery conduit is in place.

Right ventricular-to-pulmonary artery continuity is accomplished with a valved conduit. We believe the initial conduit should be valved to minimize early right ventricular failure in the postoperative period, when the large ventriculotomy and wide swings in pulmonary artery resistance predispose to right ventricular difficulties. Our preferred conduit until 1985 was the Dacron tube graft with a porcine heterograft bioprosthesis. More recently, the cryo-preserved aortic allograft (Cryolife) has been used because of its ease of handling and theoretical improved long-term function. When a Dacron conduit with a bioprosthetic heterograft valve is used, it is important not to over-size the graft. The most common size used in infants is 12 mm. Later, in the first year of life, 14-16 mm conduits can be used. The lack of space in the anterior mediastinum may predispose larger conduits to compression once the sternum is closed. The few additional months gained by placing a larger conduit are probably not worth the acute risks related to space problems. Intimal proliferation and valve calcification lead to conduit stenosis in all these Dacron prosthetic conduits, necessitating conduit replacement.

The distal anastomosis between the conduit and pulmonary artery is performed first, using a running 5–0 polypropylene suture. When using a Dacron composite prosthesis, the valve is placed as distally as possible to prevent compression of the metal valve support ring (stent) onto the heart and/or coronary arteries. Occasionally, the distal Dacron graft must be trimmed in an elliptical or T shape in order to accomplish patch angioplasty of the right or left pulmonary artery or both.

The proximal end of the Dacron conduit is then bevelled and anastomosed to the undercut oval right ventriculotomy. This ventriculotomy should be placed high and not be made unnecessarily large, since right ventricular function can be severely compromised. The anastomosis is buttressed with a strip of Teflon felt across the wall of the ventricle when a Dacron composite prosthesis is used. This is important in the small infant to avoid tearing of ventricular muscle from the sutures. The pleura on the left side of the chest is widely opened to allow space for the conduit to move to the left side when the sternum is closed. The close proximity of the conduit to the undersurface of the sternum must be remembered when reentering the mediastinum.

Either fresh antibiotic–preserved or cryopreserved aortic allografts have been used exclusively for the last three years, both for primary and secondary operations (Fig. 6). Surgical considerations are similar to those of the Dacron conduit except suturing and handling are considerably easier with the graft compared with the rigid tube. The anterior leaflet of the mitral valve at the proximal end of the aortic allograft conduit is used to patch the ventriculotomy and no Teflon felt reinforcement is necessary. Occasionally, a pericardial gusset is used to enlarge the mitral valve leaflet if it is too small. The space issue is not as acute using the aortic allograft, since the valve lies partially within the right ventricle and does not project into the anterior mediastinum as much as the Dacron conduit. Most 12–mm Dacron conduits require revision within 5 years after initial placement due to conduit stenosis from pseudointimal hyperplasia or valve degeneration. Similar longevity information concerning small cryopreserved allografts has not been obtained yet; however, there are promising lines of

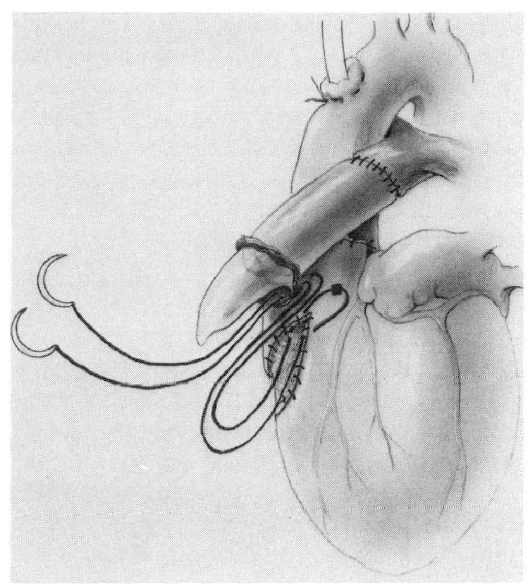

FIGURE 6. The aortic allograft has been sutured to the pulmonary artery. The first suture in the allograft to right ventricle anastomosis has been placed. Note the specific placement of this first suture, which allows the allograft valve to partially sit within the right ventricle, giving the new conduit a very low profile within the anterior mediastinum.

evidence to suggest that they are more durable. None of our initial 12-mm aortic allograft conduits has required replacement with follow-up as long as 3 years (Fig. 7).

Reentering the anterior mediastinum for conduit replacement can be technically challenging because of the dense adherence of the conduit to the undersurface of the sternum. Routinely, minimal dissection of the heart is required in order to cannulate the aorta and right atrium. Additional dissection is required and angioplasties are necessary if the more peripheral pulmonary arteries are stenotic. For conduit replacements, the patient is only moderately

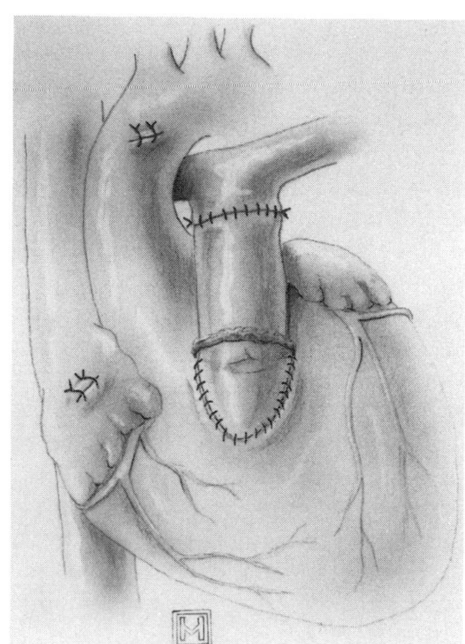

FIGURE 7. The appearance of the heart at the completion of the operation. Note that the anterior leaflet of the allograft mitral valve is used in the anastomosis between the allograft conduit and the right ventricle.

cooled to 28–30° C and fibrillation is induced. The previous Dacron graft is completely excised, with care to preserve the distal native pulmonary artery. A large nonvalved Dacron conduit can be used for this operation if right ventricular function is good and residual pulmonary hypertension or pulmonary artery distortion does not exist. The development of pseudointimal hyperplasia appears to be less in nonvalved conduits, and there is no bioprosthetic valve present to degenerate. It is presently our practice at UCSF, however, to place a fresh or cryopreserved aortic allograft at the time of the conduit replacement.

PERIOPERATIVE MANAGEMENT: CONSIDERATIONS AND COMPLICATIONS

Infants with truncus arteriosus have been difficult to care for despite an operation that is simple in concept. There are specific immediate and long-term surgical and medical management considerations that must be understood to maximize success.

Anesthetic Issues. Preoperative and induction anesthetic issues are similar to those for any child with excessive pulmonary blood flow, which may lower diastolic coronary perfusion pressure, leading to subclinical coronary ischemia. The latter is a potential cause of early postoperative left ventricular dysfunction. Anesthetic issues early after cardiopulmonary bypass concern avoidance of hypoxemia, hypercarbia, and acidosis, which potentiate increases in pulmonary vascular resistance, leading to further hypoxemia and acute right ventricular failure.

Surgical Issues. Major intraoperative surgical considerations include hemorrhage and sternal closure; minor surgical considerations include myocardial protection, coronary artery compression, and conduction injury. Significant hemorrhage is the most common perioperative complication when Dacron grafts are used. Our incidence of reexploration for bleeding approached 40%, probably because the large amount of Dacron consumes clotting factors in these very small babies. Tamponade is a frequent mode of presentation of hemorrhage because mediastinal space is limited due to the relatively large volume of the conduit. If tamponade is suspected because of low cardiac output in the early postoperative period, the lower portion of the incision must be opened. Meticulous surgical technique and the transfusion of clotting factors immediately at the termination of bypass help to minimize this complication. Bleeding has not been a significant issue in the homograft conduits and therefore fresh-frozen plasma, platelets, and cryoprecipitate are usually not required.

If the conduit is too large or is cut too long, compression of the conduit during sternal closure can be significant. The factors leading to compression can be accentuated if myocardial protection is poor or the operation is prolonged, so that the heart and adjoining tissues become edematous. Rarely, the sternum must be left open and covered with skin or Silastic, then reclosed 3–4 days later, when the child has stabilized and the edema has resolved.

Myocardial protection should be a minor issue, because myocardial ischemia is mandatory only during excision of the pulmonary arteries and closure of the aorta. Coronary artery compression has been eliminated with the Dacron conduit by moving the circular metal support stent of the bioprosthesis distally. Finally, injury to the conduction system should be an issue only in those children who have a perimembranous component to the VSD. We have not observed complete heart block in our series.

Medical Issues. Cardiac failure in the postoperative period is usually right ventricular unless truncal valve insufficiency, hypoplasia of the left ventricle, myocardial protection, or coronary artery compression was an intraoperative issue. The right ventricle is vulnerable in the early postoperative period because of closure of the VSD, the large right ventriculotomy, and wide swings in pulmonary artery resistance. Hepatic enlargement and systemic venous distention may be present with subsequent abnormalities of synthetic liver function or coagulation parameters. The noncompliant right ventricle may function better at faster heart rates and smaller ventricular volumes in the early postoperative period; therefore, inotropic agents may be required acutely and digitalis therapy chronically for 2–3 months.

Alterations in pulmonary vascular resistance can be quite striking in the early postoperative period, because the pulmonary vascular bed has been exposed to high pulmonary artery pressures and blood flows prior to repair. In most infants without significant pulmonary hypertension, pulmonary pressures are less than 50% of systemic pressures early after repair. Acidosis, hypercarbia, or hypoxemia, however, will elevate pulmonary artery pressures in this reactive vascular bed and should therefore be avoided. Infants are always mechanically ventilated, initially, with PCO_2s in the range of 30–35 and pHs approaching 7.50. The child is well-sedated, usually with relatively short-acting narcotics such as fentanyl, to avoid the potential risk of a reactive pulmonary vascular crisis. Low-dose isoproterenol is frequently the inotropic drug of choice to maintain pulmonary artery pressure as low as possible.

The majority of these infants are quite malnourished, particularly those in the most favorable hemodynamic subset with low pulmonary vascular resistance and massive pulmonary blood flow. Adequate caloric intake is important, particularly if prolonged ventilation is anticipated. This can usually be accomplished by gavage feedings through a small nasogastric tube; however, total parenteral nutrition may have a role.

Long-term Issues. Long-term complications include the development of pseudointimal hyperplasia of the conduit, bioprosthetic valve degeneration, subacute bacterial endocarditis, truncal valve insufficiency, residual ventricular septal defect, and pulmonary artery growth difficulties. Pseudointimal hyperplasia is the most significant problem with the Dacron grafts. A thick peel develops on the inner surface of the conduit, causing significant stenosis. The etiology of this intimal peel is unclear and no preventive therapy is known. Stenosis is most common at the distal end of the conduit or at the valve level, but the valve leaflets are usually not involved. Dacron conduit replacement is usually required between 36 and 48 months of age. At the present time, the conduit of choice for replacement is an aortic allograft. Pseudointimal hypoplasia does not appear with these grafts, although calcification and valve stenosis may occur.

Two patients developed postoperative subacute bacterial endocarditis with staphylococcal species in the series of 218 cases of truncus arteriosus at UCSF, but both were successfully treated with intravenous antibiotics and did not require excision of the prosthetic material. Small residual ventricular septal defects were not considered a serious complication; however, reoperation of larger defects is critical. Usually, this problem is addressed at the time of conduit revision. Problems with pulmonary artery growth were also minor, as the pulmonary arteries appeared to grow appropriately with the child. Rarely, patch angioplasties or percutaneous transluminal balloon angioplasties are required on the proximal right or left pulmonary artery, particularly in type 2 or 3 truncus.

Truncal valve insufficiency is associated with increased mortality, both early and late, after repair. Truncal valve insufficiency may present problems intraoperatively, as noted previously. In addition, once the ventricular septal defect is closed, the regurgitant volume must be effectively handled by the left ventricle, rather than being shared by both ventricles. This can contribute to poor left ventricular function, both acutely and chronically. If the child has significant truncal valve insufficiency, truncal valve replacement is probably indicated. Such an aggressive approach might have improved our survival statistics.

RESULTS

A total of 218 infants have undergone physiologic repair of persistent truncus arteriosus at the University of California, San Francisco with an operative mortality of 15%. The major determinants of mortality are truncal valve insufficiency and pulmonary hypertension. The minor determinants of mortality include age and weight at the time of surgery. Infants under 3.0 kg or under 1 months of age have a slightly higher mortality, and children who undergo primary correction after the age of 6 months have a significantly increased mortality. This appears to be closely related to the presence of secondary pulmonary vascular disease.

The last 35 children undergoing surgery for truncus arteriosus have received fresh or cryopreserved aortic allografts for their conduits; 20 infants received the allograft at the time of primary correction and 15 at the time of conduit replacement. Perioperative hemorrhage and graft degeneration have been much less as compared with cases in which Dacron conduits were used. Follow-up has been 1 month to 3 years. A larger prosthesis (13–17 mm) frequently can be placed at the first operation when an aortic allograft is used, and pseudointimal proliferation does not appear to be a significant problem.

Long-term follow-up in these 218 children has been rewarding in that complications have been few with a low mortality for conduit replacement and, commonly, regression of pulmonary hypertension after physiologic repair. Pulmonary artery growth has been excellent, although anastomotic distal stenosis can occur. Conduit revision will be required in all children repaired in the first 6 months of life, even when aortic allografts are used. The number of conduit revisions should be less, however, compared with those children who initially received Dacron conduits with porcine bioprostheses. All children must be followed carefully for truncal valve insufficiency. Overall, the outlook for this anomaly, which was uniformly fatal 20 years ago, has dramatically improved.

REFERENCES

1. Appelbaum A, Bargeron LM Jr, Pacifico AD, et al: Surgical treatment of truncus arteriosus, with emphasis on infants and small children. J Thorac Cardiovasc Surg 71:436, 1976.
2. Collett RW, Edwards JE: Persistent truncus arteriosus: A classification according to anatomic types. Surg Clin North Am 29:1245, 1979.
3. Ebert PA, Robinson SJ, Stanger P, Eagle MA: Pulmonary artery conduits in infants under six months of age. J Thorac Cardiovasc Surg 72:351–356, 1976.
4. Ebert PA, Turley K, Stanger P, et al: Surgical treatment of truncus arteriosus in the first 6 months of life. Ann Surg 200:451, 1984.
5. Juaneda E, Hawort SG: Pulmonary vascular disease in children with truncus arteriosus. Am J Cardiol 54:1314, 1984.

6. McFaul RC, Mair DD, Feld RH, et al: Truncus arteriosus and previous pulmonary arterial banding: Clinical and hemodynamic assessment. Am J Cardiol 38:626, 1976.
7. McGoon DC, Wallace RB, Danielson GK: The Rastelli operation: Its indications and results. J Thorac Cardiovasc Surg 65:865, 1973.
8. Mair DD, Ritter DG, Davis GD, et al: Selection of patients with truncus arteriosus for surgical correction. Anatomic and hemodynamic considerations. Circulation 49:144–151, 1974.
9. Marcellati C, McGoon DC, Mair DD: The natural history of truncus arteriosus. Circulation 54:108, 1976.
10. Oldham HN Jr, Kakos GS, Jarmakani MM, et al: Pulmonary artery banding in infants with complex congenital heart defects. Ann Thorac Surg 13:342, 1972.
11. Poirier RA, Berman MA, Stansel HC Jr: Current status of the surgical treatment of truncus arteriosus. J Thorac Cardiovasc Surg 69:169, 1975.
12. Singh AK, DeLeval M, Pincott J, et al: Pulmonary artery banding for truncus arteriosus in the first year of life. Circulation 54(Suppl 3):17, 1976.
13. Van Praagh R, Van Praagh S: The anatomy of common aorticpulmonary trunk (truncus arteriosus communis) and its embryologic implications: A study of 57 necrosy cases. Am J Cardiol 16:406, 1965.

JOHN D. PIGOTT, MD
WILLIAM I. NORWOOD, MD, PhD

HYPOPLASTIC LEFT HEART SYNDROME

Division of Cardiothoracic Surgery
Children's Hospital of Philadelphia
Philadelphia, Pennsylvania

Reprint requests to:
John D. Pigott, MD
Division of Cardiothoracic Surgery
Children's Hospital of Philadelphia
34th Street and Civic Center Blvd.
Philadelphia, PA 19104

Hypoplastic left heart syndrome is a common congenital cardiovascular malformation. In the New England Regional Infant Cardiac Program, hypoplastic left heart syndrome was present in 7% of infants presenting with cardiac disease in the first year of life, ranking it in incidence with patent ductus arteriosus and coarctation of the aorta.[5] Moreover, it is the most common form of the single ventricle complexes.

This malformation is universally lethal without surgical intervention early in life. Recent advances in our understanding of the anatomy and physiology of the disease and developments in surgical management have led to the potential to significantly change the natural history of this disease. The advent of surgical management for patients with hypoplastic left heart syndrome has stimulated interest in a more precise anatomical definition in order to better understand diagnostic, therapeutic, and prognostic implications.[3,8,11,12–14, 16]

ANATOMY

Hypoplastic left heart syndrome encompasses a group of cardiovascular malformations which are characterized by aortic valve atresia, stenosis, or severe hypoplasia accompanied by hypoplasia or absence of the left ventricle. As a consequence, the ascending aorta and aortic arch are characteristically hypoplastic. Mitral atresia and severe hypoplasia usually coexist. Of 100 patients who underwent palliation at the Children's Hospital of Philadelphia, 74% had normally related great arteries with valvar aortic stenosis or atresia and mitral stenosis or atresia. Sixteen percent had a common atrioventricular canal with rightward malalignment of the canal with regard to the muscular ventricular septum and associated aortic valve atresia or stenosis. Ten percent of the patients had double outlet right ventricle with valvar aortic atresia or hypoplasia.[16]

The most likely developmental anomaly in hypoplastic left heart syndrome is a limitation of either left ventricular inflow or left ventricular outflow. Restriction to left ventricular outflow may occur in those patients with isolated aortic valve atresia or double outlet right ventricle with aortic valve atresia. The abnormal blood flow patterns secondary to restriction of flow across the aortic valve will be responsible for the altered development of the remaining cardiac and extracardiac structures. With aortic atresia or severe aortic stenosis and an intact ventricular septum, the left ventricle is characteristically hypoplastic or absent. However, normal left ventricular and mitral valve development may occur in the unusual situation of aortic valve atresia with an associated nonrestrictive ventricular septal defect.

The right atrium, tricuspid valve orifice, and right ventricle are typically enlarged, as are the pulmonary valve orifice and proximal main pulmonary artery.[6,9,19] The pulmonic valve is usually normal, with only 1% of the patients presenting at the Children's Hospital of Philadelphia since 1984 having had valvar pulmonic stenosis. Anomalies of pulmonary venous connection are infrequent but may occur. The interatrial communication is usually a patent foramen ovale or an ostium primum atrial septal defect in the presence of a common atrioventricular canal. Of particular surgical significance is the posterior and leftward displacement of the superior and right lateral attachment of the septum primum vis-à-vis septum secundum. This was noted in the majority of patients with hypoplastic left heart syndrome in an autopsy series.[19]

Coronary arterial anatomy is characterized by a normal origin from the aortic root with a normal distribution pattern. It would appear that ventriculo-coronary connections are rare in patients with aortic atresia, unlike patients with pulmonary atresia with intact ventricular septum.[15] In the presence of aortic valve atresia, the ascending aorta usually measures 1-3 mm in luminal diameter. In patients with aortic valve hypoplasia and stenosis, the ascending aorta is often somewhat larger but usually less than 5 mm in diameter. The proximal main pulmonary artery, ductus arteriosus, and descending aorta form a continuum. The isthmus thus appears as a branch of the thoracic aorta. A posterolateral intimal ridge is present at the junction of the aortic isthmus with the ductus arteriosus and the thoracic aorta in most patients and is not a true coarctation, despite reports to the contrary.[4,6]

PHYSIOLOGY

Fetal circulation is abnormal in patients with hypoplastic left heart syndrome. Systemic circulation depends upon right ventricular output through the ductus arteriosus with retrograde perfusion of the aortic arch. Systemic venous return is usually normal but pulmonary venous blood must return to the right atrium. This characteristically occurs through a foramen ovale or a true atrial septal defect. Thus normal development occurs in utero despite the abnormal fetal circulation.

Postnatal physiology is similar to prenatal physiology except that blood is oxygenated in the lungs. Patency of the ductus arteriosus continues to be necessary for systemic perfusion and an interatrial communication permits oxygenated pulmonary venous blood to mix with systemic venous blood. The joined pulmonary and systemic circulations thus act as separate resistances. Thus the relative pulmonary and systemic flows and hence the degree of hypoxemia are dependent on the relative resistance ratios. The pulmonary vascular resistance is near systemic at birth but decreases naturally over the first few weeks of postnatal life. The degree of patency of the ductus arteriosus and the foramen ovale may significantly alter the physiology in any individual patient. As the ductus arteriosus begins to close naturally, systemic blood flow diminishes and pulmonary blood flow and PaO_2 increase. A restrictive interatrial communication can contribute to a balanced systemic to pulmonary blood flow ratio by elevating pulmonary venous pressure. With large pulmonary blood flow and diminished systemic flow, PaO_2 often exceeds 60 mm Hg and is accompanied by metabolic acidosis. In the absence of lung disease, a PaO_2 of less than 22 mm Hg is associated with very restricted pulmonary blood flow. This can result in metabolic acidosis from profound hypoxemia in the face of satisfactory systemic perfusion. This rare occurrence is seen in the subset of patients with a virtually intact atrial septum with a thick muscular septum primum.

DIAGNOSIS

The diagnosis of hypoplastic left heart syndrome is aided by an understanding of this complex physiology. Cardiovascular examination reveals a dominant right ventricular impulse with a decreased apical impulse. S2 is usually single and increased in intensity. Most patients have a nonspecific soft grade I-III/VI systolic murmur at the left sternal border.[2] The electrocardiogram is notable for revealing right ventricular hypertrophy in most patients. Approximately 50% of patients have a Q-R pattern in VI. In patients with malaligned complete common atrioventricular canal, the Q-R-S axis is leftward and superior. Cardiomegaly is common. Radiographically, pulmonary vascular markings are typically increased. Two-dimensional echocardiography is diagnostic of this congenital cardiac malformation.[7,10,18] The intracardiac anatomy can be examined with subcostal, frontal, suprasternal, left oblique, and right oblique sweeps. A very diminutive ascending aorta is characteristic of this malformation and virtually diagnostic of hypoplastic left heart syndrome.

PALLIATION

Preoperative Therapy

At the time of diagnosis, resuscitation should be initiated by a continuous infusion of prostaglandin E1 intravenously at a dose of 0.05 $\mu g/kg/min$. If metabolic acidosis is present, a single large dose of sodium bicarbonate may be administered. An arterial line should be inserted for monitoring arterial oxygenation and acid base status. The umbilical artery is preferentially used in the newborn in order to preserve the peripheral arteries for future access. The major goal in the preoperative period is to assure adequate systemic perfusion and oxygenation to meet the metabolic demands of the child. The pulmonary vascular resistance may be less than systemic. Lowering of pulmonary resistance by ventilation with high inspired oxygen concentrations should be avoided, as patients with hypoplastic left heart syndrome most often have no abnormality in oxygen transport in the lung, and supplemental oxygen may only serve to decrease pulmonary resistance, and thereby diminish systemic perfusion. Inotropic agents often result in an unfavorable pulmonary to systemic resistance ratio and should be avoided. The most potent metabolic factor to influence the pulmonary vascular resistance has been clinically observed to be pCO_2. In babies with low pulmonary vascular resistance, an effective strategy in most is elective intubation and administration of muscle relaxants. The child can then be hypoventilated to a pCO_2 of 45 to 50 mm Hg, thus elevating pulmonary vascular resistance and increasing peripheral perfusion even in the face of preexisting metabolic acidosis. Mild to moderate interatrial obstruction at the level of a patent foramen ovale is usually beneficial to preoperative hemodynamics by limiting pulmonary venous return. An atrial septotomy should not be performed prior to surgical palliation.

In patients who have had a period of hemodynamic instability or circulatory collapse, stabilization and observation until resolution of renal and hepatic insufficiency are appropriate. In such patients evaluation of the central nervous system may also be appropriate. Due to the occasional association of hypoplastic left heart syndrome with partial chromosomal deletion, a karyotype analysis may be performed. In those rare circumstances in which an intact atrial septum is present, profound hypoxemia may mandate emergent surgical intervention.

Reconstructive Surgery: First Stage

Because the pulmonary vasculature of the newborn is immature, precluding survival from a Fontan procedure, yet systemic circulation is dependent on patency of the ductus arteriosus, palliative surgery is necessary in the newborn (Fig. 1). The goals of palliative surgery are to create unobstructed flow from ventricle to aorta, to regulate pulmonary blood flow and thereby permit pulmonary maturation, and to create an unobstructed interatrial communication. A surgical technique designed to utilize primarily native cardiovascular tissue to palliate this lesion was first described in 1980 and has undergone several modifications.[12] The current technique utilized at Children's Hospital of Philadelphia is initiated by induction of anesthesia with fentanyl and pancuronium.[15] A median sternotomy is performed and the thymus is partially excised. Cannulation for arterial infusion is achieved using the main pulmonary artery just distal to the sinuses of Valsalva. Cardiopulmonary bypass is begun and the infant is cooled to 20° C. Immediately after institution of cardiopulmonary bypass, the right and left pulmonary arteries are occluded with tourniquets to ensure adequate systemic perfusion. The brachiocephalic vessels are exposed and individually occluded, and total circulatory arrest is effected.

All perfusion cannulae are removed, the descending aorta is temporarily occluded, and cardioplegia is infused through the pulmonary artery cannulation site. Septum primum is excised through the atrial cannulation site and the main pulmonary artery is divided at the level of the branch pulmonary arteries. The distal main pulmonary artery is closed with a circular patch of pulmonary artery homograft in order to best maintain continuity between the right and left pulmonary artery branches. The ductus arteriosus is exposed and ligated and transsected at the aortic end. The thoracic aorta is incised distally for 1-1.5 cm. The aortic incision is carried proximally through the isthmus, around the aortic arch onto the ascending aorta to the level of the transsected proximal main pulmonary artery. This aortotomy is gusseted with a tailored patch of pulmonary artery homograft to enlarge the ascending aorta and aortic arch to a normal size and configuration. It is important to augment the junction of the aortic isthmus

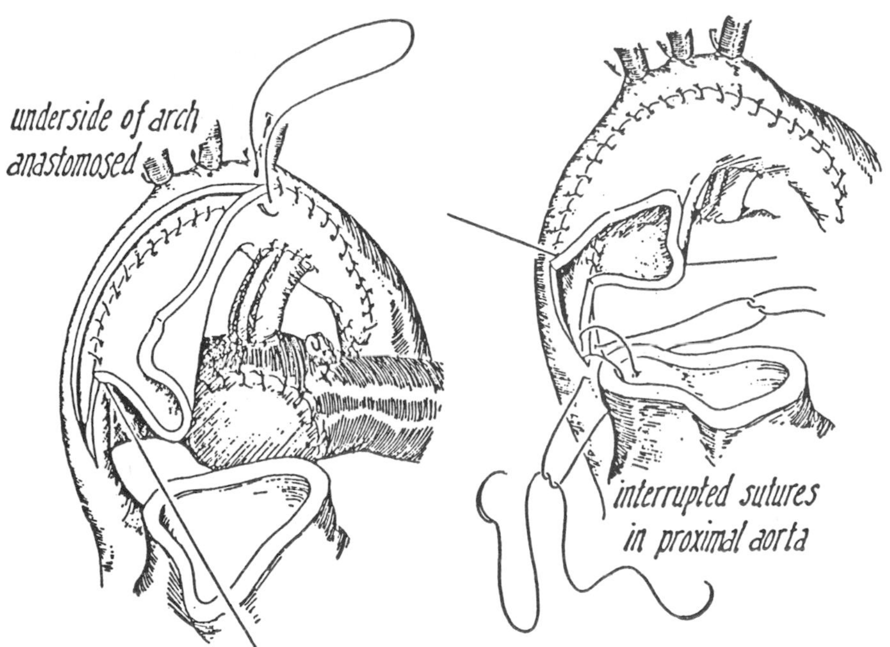

FIGURE 1. Palliation for hypoplastic left heart syndrome includes atrial septectomy and transection of the proximal main pulmonary artery. The aortic arch and ascending aorta are augmented with pulmonary artery allograft, and pulmonary blood flow is provided by a 4-mm central shunt. The right ventricle ejects to the aorta when the proximal main pulmonary artery is associated with the augmented ascending aorta. (From Edmund, Norwood and Low: Atlas of Cardiothoracic Surgery. Philadelphia, Lea & Febiger, 1989, with permission.)

to minimize the development of late distal arch obstruction. A short 4 mm PTFE shunt is interposed between the underside of the augmented aortic arch and the confluence of the branch pulmonary arteries. Pulmonary artery homograft is currently used to gusset the aorta because it is pliable and relatively hemostatic. Reconstruction of the aorta is completed by anastomosis of the proximal main pulmonary artery to the adjacent ascending aorta and pulmonary homograft. Cardiopulmonary bypass is reinstituted and the patient is rewarmed to 37°C. Following discontinuation of cardiopulmonary bypass, a pressure monitoring catheter is placed in the right atrium. Actuarial survival at Children's Hospital of Philadelphia for this phase is currently 78% at 1 month and 61% at 18 months. It is anticipated that with further identification of potential problems and refinement in technique and postoperative care, survival statistics will continue to improve as they have over the last 4 years.

Postoperative Therapy

In the early postoperative period, ventilation is adjusted to achieve a Qp:Qs of approximately 1. The child should be weaned from mechanical ventilation and extubated as soon as tolerated, usually within the first several postoperative days. Oral or nasogastric feeding are begun following surgery. At present digoxin and furosemide are routinely administered to all patients after palliation. After the child is released from the hospital, regular cardiovascular evaluations are important for monitoring anatomical and physiological development. The incidence of aortic arch obstruction is low following augmentation of the distal aortic arch, but, when present, immediate recognition is essential. Palliation necessarily presents the ventricle with a volume load. An additional pressure load often results in rapid deterioration in ventricular function. Physical examination in this circumstance may be misleading. Two-dimensional echocardiography with supersternal imaging of the arch and sequential pulse Doppler interrogation of multiple points along the reconstructed aorta have proved reliable in detecting obstruction. If echocardiography suggests aortic arch abnormalities, cardiac catheterization should be performed to confirm the anatomy and physiology. Surgical relief may be undertaken.

Cardiovascular evaluation should also assess for rapidly progressing cyanosis. This is usually due to limited pulmonary blood flow through the shunt, although cyanosis may rarely occur secondary to a restrictive interatrial communication.[7] Mild tricuspid regurgitation is not unusual and is of limited prognostic import.[1,2] Significant tricuspid regurgitation is poorly tolerated by the already volume-loaded right ventricle. Annuloplasty or valve replacement may be required in patients with moderate to severe tricuspid regurgitation, and has been undertaken in 2% of our patients.

Second Stage: Modified Fontan Procedure

A modified Fontan procedure is performed at approximately 18 months of age. This age was chosen to permit maturation of the pulmonary vascular bed yet to minimize the length of time the right ventricle is subjected to a combined pressure and volume load. Cardiac catheterization is performed prior to this time to evaluate pulmonary vascular resistance, pulmonary arterial anatomy, and ventricular and tricuspid valve function. Preferably pulmonary arterial pressure is measured directly. Pulmonary venous wedge pressures are useful if direct pulmonary artery pressure measurement is unable to be performed. Right ventricular end-diastolic pressure is measured and usually is in the range of 5-8 mm Hg with a pulmonary arterial resistance less than 2.5 Wood's units/m2. Two angiograms are routinely performed: the first is a right ventriculogram, filmed in the anterior-posterior and lateral planes; the second is an aortogram in the mid-portion of the ascending aorta and is filmed anterior-posterior with 30 degrees of cranial angulation. Cranial angulation is optimal for definition of pulmonary arterial anatomy.

The second stage of reconstructive surgery for hypoplastic left heart syndrome is a modified Fontan procedure (Fig. 2). The heart is exposed through a midline sternotomy incision and cardiopulmonary bypass is instituted using ascending aorta and right atrial appendage cannulation sites. The systemic to pulmonary artery shunt is exposed and occluded, and the patient is cooled to 20° C. The pulmonary arteries are exposed and widely incised from the upper lobe branch on the right to the upper lobe branch on the left. An incision is made in the superior aspect of the right atrium at the level of the sulcus terminalis and carried onto the posterior aspect of the right superior vena cava adjacent to the incision in the right pulmonary artery. A suture line is begun at the posterior aspect of the right superior vena cava and right pulmonary artery. The pulmonary arteriotomy and anastomosis between the right atrium and right pulmonary artery are augmented anteriorly with a patch of pulmonary homograft. Through

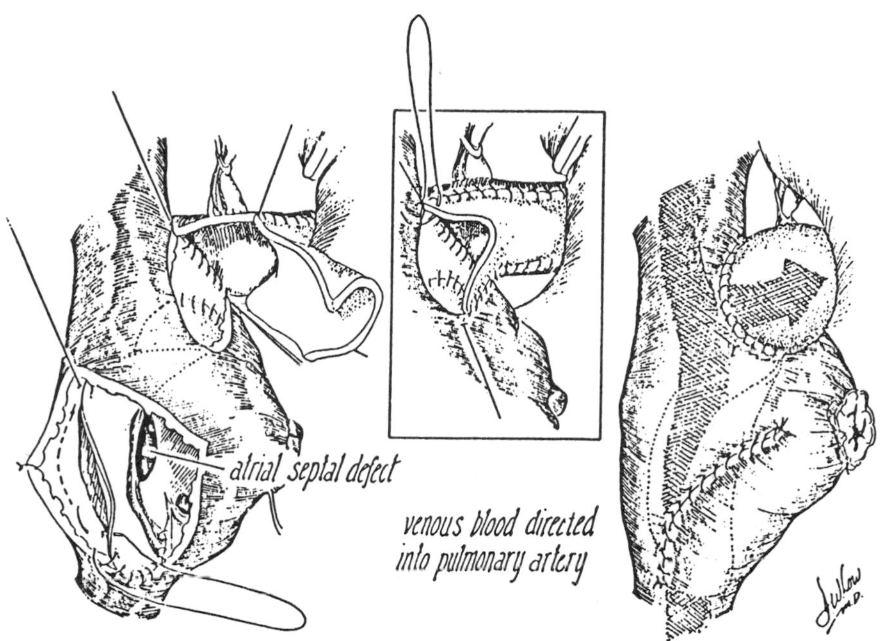

FIGURE 2. A modified Fontan procedure consists of baffling the inferior vena caval return along the right lateral aspect of the right atrium to an augmented anastomosis between the superior right atrium and vena cava and right pulmonary artery. (From Edmund, Norwood and Low: Atlas of Cardiothoracic Surgery. Philadelphia, Lea & Febiger, 1989, with permission.)

a separate lateral right atriotomy, the inferior vena caval blood flow is baffled from the inferior venal caval right atrial inlet to the junction of the superior vena cava using half of a 10-mm diameter PTFE tube graft split longitudinally. This baffling technique minimizes obstruction of pulmonary venous return which can occasionally occur when the pulmonary veins are baffled to the tricuspid valve. Following rewarming and discontinuance of cardiopulmonary bypass, monitoring catheters are placed in the pulmonary artery and right atrial appendage. Management following surgery is similar to that for any patient after a modified Fontan procedure.

CONCLUSION

From October 1984 through October 1988, 62 Fontan procedures have been performed for hypoplastic left heart syndrome on patients managed at Children's Hospital of Philadelphia. Early mortality is 31% with two late deaths. Over the last decade well-defined surgical options have been developed for the treatment of patients with hypoplastic left heart syndrome. The challenge of the future is to better characterize this group of lesions so that the preoperative, operative, and postoperative management may be further improved.

REFERENCES

1. Barber G, et al: What is the fate of the tricuspid valve following palliative surgery for hypoplastic heart syndrome? J Am Coll Cardiol 9:132A, 1987.
2. Barber G, et al: The significance of preoperative tricuspid regurgitation in hypoplastic left heart syndrome. Circulation 74(Suppl II):II–36, 1986.
3. Doty DB, Knott HW: Hypoplastic left heart syndrome—experience with an operation to establish functionally normal circulation. J Thorac Cardiovasc Surg 74:624–630, 1977.
4. Elzenga NJ, Gittenberger de Grott AC: Coarctation and related aortic arch anomalies in hypoplastic left heart syndrome. Int J Cardiol 8:379–393, 1985.
5. Fyler DC: Report of the New England Regional Infant Cardiac Program. Pediatrics 65(Suppl):463, 1980.
6. Hawkins JA, Doty DB: Aortic atresia—morphologic characteristics affecting survival and operative palliation. J Thorac Cardiovasc Surg 88:62--626, 1984.
7. Helton JG, et al: Analysis of potential anatomic or physiologic determinants of outcome of palliative surgery for hypoplastic left heart syndrome. Circulation 74(Suppl I):I-70 to I-76, 1968.
8. Jonas RA, et al: First-stage palliation of hypoplastic left heart syndrome. J Thorac Cardiovasc Surg 92:6–13, 1986.
9. Lehman E: Congenital atresia of the foramen ovale. Am J Dis Child 33:585–589, 1927.
10. Mandorla S, et al: Fetal echocardiography. Prenatal diagnosis of hypoplastic left heart syndrome. G Ital Cardiol 14:517–520, 1984.
11. Moodie DS, et al: The hypoplastic left heart syndrome: Evidence of preoperative myocardial and hepatic infarction in spite of prostaglandin therapy. Ann Thorac Surg 42:307–311, 1986.
12. Norwood WI, Kirklin JK, Sanders SP: Hypoplastic left heart syndrome. Experience with palliative surgery. Am J Cardiol 45:87–91, 1980.
13. Norwood WI, Lang P, Hansen D: Physiologic repair of aortic atresia—hypoplastic left heart syndrome. N Engl J Med 308:23–26, 1983.
14. Norwood WI, Lang P, Castaneda AR, Campbell DN: Experience with operations for hypoplastic left heart syndrome. J Thorac Cardiovasc Surg 82:511–519, 1981.
15. O'Connor WN, et al: Ventriculocoronary connections in hypoplastic left hearts: An autopsy microscopic study. Circulation 66:1078–1085, 1982.
16. Pigott JD, Murphy JD, Barber G, Norwood WI: Palliative reconstructive surgery for hypoplastic left heart syndrome. Ann Thorac Surg 45:122–128, 1987.
17. Roberts WC, et al: Aortic valve atresia: A new classification based on necropsy study of 73 cases. Am J Cardiol 37:753–756, 1976.
18. Sahn DJ, et al: Prenatal ultrasound diagnosis of hypoplastic left heart syndrome in utero associated with hydrops fetalis. Am Heart J 104:1368–1372, 1982.
19. Weinberg PM, et al: Postmortem echocardiography and tomographic anatomy of hypoplastic left heart syndrome after palliative surgery. Am J Cardiol 58:1228–1232, 1986.

DANIEL M. COHEN, MD
ROBERT M. FREEDOM, MD
WILLIAM G. WILLIAMS, MD

CONGENITALLY CORRECTED TRANSPOSITION OF THE GREAT ARTERIES

Daniel M. Cohen, MD
Fellow in Pediatric Cardiovascular Surgery
The Hospital for Sick Children
Toronto, Ontario, Canada

Robert M. Freedom, MD
Professor of Pediatrics, University of Toronto
Chief of Pediatric Cardiology
The Hospital for Sick Children
Toronto, Ontario, Canada

William G. Williams, MD
Associate Professor of Surgery, University of Toronto
Chief of Pediatric Cardiovascular Surgery
The Hospital for Sick Children
Toronto, Ontario, Canada

Reprint requests to:
William G. Williams, MD
Pediatric Cardiovascular Surgery
The Hospital for Sick Children
555 University Ave.
Toronto, Ontario M5G 1X8
Canada

Congenitally corrected transposition of the great arteries (CCTGA) is a cardiac anomaly characterized by atrioventricular discordance and ventriculoarterial discordance. Systemic venous return passes from the right atrium through the mitral valve (right AV valve) into a morphologic left ventricle and is ejected out the pulmonary artery into the lungs. Similarly pulmonary venous return enters the left atrium and passes through the tricuspid valve (left AV valve) into the morphologic right ventricle from where it is ejected out the aorta to the rest of the body. Consequently, the two ventricles are inverted and the great arteries are transposed, and the circulation may be functionally normal. This condition may be encountered in atrial situs solitus or inversus but cannot be found with atrial isomerism because the AV connection is uncertain and cannot be clearly defined as discordant or concordant. Furthermore, the ventricles may be in any position, i.e., levocardia, mesocardia, or dextrocardia. Congenitally corrected transposition of the great arteries may occur as an isolated anomaly with an intact atrial and ventricular septum. More frequently, there may be one or more associated anomalies.

Von Rokitansky (1875)[1] was probably the first to describe a case of CCTGA. Monckeberg (1913)[2] described the anterior position of the atrioventricular (AV) node and Walmsley (1931)[3] recognized many of the basic differences in cardiac morphology, including the specific coronary artery pattern, altered structure of the central fibrous body, and differences in AV conduction.

Thereafter CCTGA was recognized readily by pathologists but further interest remained dormant until the advent of open heart surgery in the 1950s. Anderson and colleagues (1957) provided good clinical documentation of this cardiac anomaly, and included in their report was the first account of a surgical repair involving CCTGA.[4] This was followed by a very comprehensive clinicopathological review published by Schiebler et al. (1961).[5]

INCIDENCE

Stanger et al.[6] reported an incidence of CCTGA of 1.1% in 3000 consecutive autopsies. A report from The Hospital for Sick Children by Bjarke and Kidd provided comparable figures with an incidence of 0.95% in 10535 children with congenital heart disease seen in a 20-year period.[7] Because a number of patients with isolated or uncomplicated CCTGA remain asymptomatic and are likely to remain undiagnosed, they suggested that their figures were probably an underestimate of the true incidence.

Congenitally corrected transposition occurring in association with situs inversus is relatively rare. In the series from The Hospital for Sick Children, 5% cases of CCTGA were associated with situs inversus.[7] Isolated or uncomplicated CCTGA is unusual, occurring only 1-2% of the time, and is nearly always accompanied by intracardiac and/or great artery abnormalities. Although all kinds of cardiac malformations have been described in association with CCTGA, four are so common that they are considered an integral part of this anomaly: ventricular septal defect (VSD), pulmonic stenosis, left-sided AV valve abnormalities, and aberrations in the conduction system.[8] The birthweights of children with CCTGA are usually within a normal range and there is slight male to female preponderance of 1.6:1.[9]

EMBRYOLOGY

Between the 3rd and 4th weeks of embryologic life, the primitive heart tube is fixed by the developing atrium caudally and the conotruncus cephalad.[10] To accommodate additional longitudinal growth, the heart tube folds in its mid-portion between the primitive ventricle and the bulbus cordis. Normally, the cephalic portion of the tube bends in a ventral, caudal direction and slightly to the right (so-called d-looping). If it should bend to the left (l-looping), the proximal part of the tube, or primitive ventricle, from which the left ventricle develops, is displaced to the right side and dorsally. Conversely, the distal part of the tube, or bulbus cordis, which forms the right ventricle, is displaced leftward and ventrally. As a consequence of these embryologic changes the left ventricle comes to lie adjacent to the right atrium and the right ventricle alongside the left atrium (Fig. 1). The interventricular septum assumes a rather oblique orientation from dorsal to ventral and left to right. The conal septum aligns alongside the left border of the trabecular or muscular septum. Regardless of the direction of looping, the apex is oriented to the left and remains so.

Because of the abnormal looping, the conotruncus is twisted from its normal position, so that the right is oriented leftward and vice versa. With division of the truncus arteriosus the aorta emerges from the anatomic right ventricle and the pulmonary artery from the anatomic left ventricle. The aorta runs parallel, to the left, and slightly anterior to the pulmonary trunk.

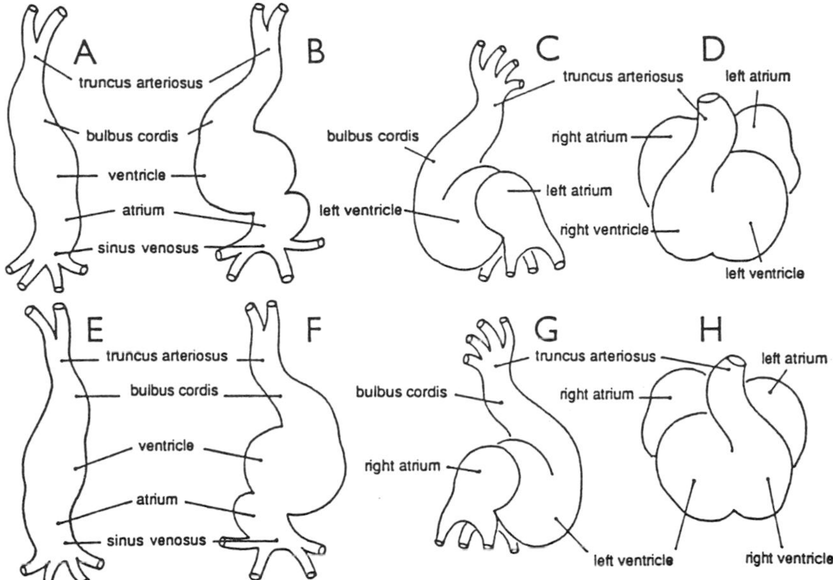

FIGURE 1. Formation of cardiac loop in different stages of development in the normal heart (A,B,C,D) and congenitally corrected transposition (E,F,G,H).

MORPHOLOGY

In atrial situs solitus, the most frequent anatomic arrangement observed in CCTGA is a ventricular l-loop with the aorta arising from an anterior and leftward position relative to the pulmonary trunk (l-transposition). Van Praagh designated this SLL meaning Situs solitus, L-looping, and Levoposition of the aorta.[11] The morphologic left ventricle usually lies to the right and the morphologic right ventricle to the left. In instances in which atrial situs inversus is present, mirror image relations exist, designated IDD or situs Inversus, D-looping, and Dextroposition of the aorta (Fig. 2). While the presence of an anterior, left-sided aorta is suggestive of CCTGA, its presence in this location is not synonymous with the condition.

In atrial situs solitus, the right atrium is connected to a morphologic left ventricle via a morphologic mitral valve with its typically paired papillary muscles.[12] The larger papillary muscle arises from the posterolateral left ventricular free wall and the smaller one arises from the anterolateral free wall, where it may be subject to damage during a left ventriculotomy. The mitral valve is slightly rotated and the commissures are divided into an extensive, anterior, mural leaflet and a shorter, posterior, pulmonary leaflet that is in fibrous continuity with the pulmonary valve. The left ventricle is typically finely trabeculated and the muscular septum usually lies in an anteroposterior orientation.

The left ventricular outflow tract lies beneath the pulmonic valve and is posteriorly positioned. Its right side is formed by the zone of fibrous continuity between the septal leaflet of the mitral valve and the pulmonary valve. The left side is bounded by the membranous septum which separates it from the right ventricle. Anteriorly, there is a prominent recess bounded by the inner curvature of the free ventricular wall. The pulmonary valve lies in a transverse plane to the

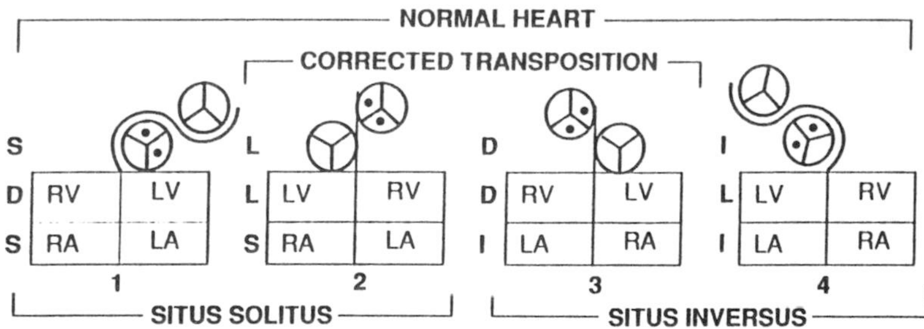

FIGURE 2. Diagrammatic models of four basic hearts. Models 1 and 2 represent situs solitus and 3 and 4 represent situs inversus. Models 1 and 4 correspond with normal anatomy and 2 and 3 with corrected transposition. (LA, left atrium; LV, left ventricle; RA, right atrium; RV, right ventricle.)

right and posterior to the aortic valve, wedged between the mitral and tricuspid valves. It is usually tricuspid and normal in appearance but may be thickened, fused, and occasionally bicuspid.

The left atrium communicates with the morphologic right ventricle via a morphologic tricuspid valve. It is composed of the usual three leaflets: septal, anterior, and posterior. This valve is almost always structurally abnormal, mainly with leaflet dysplasia and thickened chordal attachments. In a few instances a true Ebstein's anomaly exists. The commissures between the leaflets are supported by a medial, anterior, and inferior papillary muscles.

The morphologic right ventricle has characteristic coarse trabeculations and a well-developed infundibulum separating the tricuspid and aortic valves. The aortic valve is usually trileaflet and lies over the infundibulum.

The coronary arteries arise from the aortic sinuses above the facing leaflets of the aortic valve in the right and left posterior positions. The right-sided coronary artery is a morphologic left coronary artery, giving rise to the anterior descending and circumflex branches after a short, left-main artery. The anterior descending artery serves as a guide to the location of the ventricular septum and the circumflex artery encircles the mitral annulus on its posterior aspect. The morphologic right coronary artery arises from the left posterior aortic sinus and terminates in the posterior descending artery on the posterior aspect of the heart. This arterial pattern is an excellent guide to the presence or absence of CCTGA.

The sinus node lies in its normal location at the caval-atrial junction on the right side in atrial situs solitus. The AV conduction tissue in CCTGA is grossly abnormal.[13] A regular (posterior) AV node is found at the apex of the triangle of Koch in front of the ostium of the coronary sinus. Since there is malalignment of the atrial and ventricular septa at this point, the penetrating bundle fails to reach the underlying ventricular septum except in the presence of situs inversus. A second AV node is located anteriorly in the left wall of the atrial appendage close to the mitral annulus near its point of continuity with the pulmonary valve annulus. It gives rise to an AV bundle which penetrates the fibrous trigone and comes to lie beneath the pulmonary valve before descending onto the anterior aspect of the muscular septum where it branches normally (Fig. 3). When there is situs inversus the penetrating bundle almost always crosses the fibrous trigone from the posterior node. The anterior node is also present but does not connect to the bundle of His.

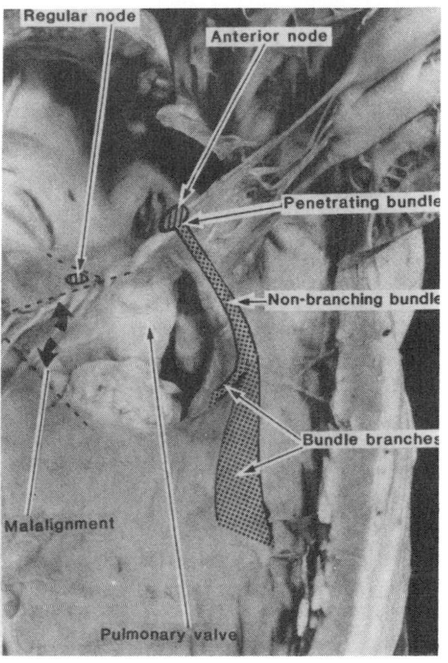

FIGURE 3. Corrected transposition. View of pulmonary outflow tract illustrating the path taken by the nonbranching AV bundle from the anomalously situated anterior node. Note the malalignment between the atrial septum and the inlet ventricular septum. The AV bundle passes anterior and inferior to the pulmonary outflow tract. (Courtesy of Dr. R. H. Anderson, reproduced by permission.)

ASSOCIATED ANOMALIES

Ventricular Septal Defect. This is the most common associated malformation in CCTGA, being present in 88% of cases in combined recent clinical studies (Table 1). Because of the malalignment between the atrial and ventricular septa, the perimembranous septum is large. The VSDs are usually found in the perimembranous septum, but large confluent defects involving the subpulmonic portion of the septum are not uncommon.[14] The pulmonary valve may override to arise in part from the right ventricle. Less commonly, a VSD may be subaortic or in a doubly committed, subarterial position. Rarely, muscular VSDs are encountered. The position of the VSD relative to the great arteries is important in planning appropriate surgical intervention. The VSD may be wholly or partially obstructed by fibrous tissue derived from the tricuspid valve or by an aneurysm of the membranous septum. An isolated VSD is unusual. In about 50% of cases pulmonic stenosis is present as well, and in about 50%, left AV valve abnormalities may be observed.[14] Since the conduction tissue passes inferior to the pulmonary valve on the morphologic left ventricular side, sutures should be placed on the right ventricular aspect of the defect to avoid AV block during surgical repair.

Pulmonic Stenosis. Pulmonic outflow tract obstruction has been observed in 62% of cases of CCTGA with situs solitus (Table 1). It occurs as an isolated anomaly in less than 20% of patients with CCTGA and is seen usually in association with a VSD or left AV valve abnormality.[9] Pulmonary stenosis appears to be clinically significant in 25% of patients. Stenosis may be of valvar origin, in which case the leaflets are thickened and fused, and the valve may be tricuspid or bicuspid. Subvalvar stenosis may be of several different types. A dynamic stenosis may occur as a consequence of LV hypertrophy. Subvalvar membrane may be present or an aneurysm of the membranous septum may

TABLE 1. Summary of Recent Literature and Review of Toronto Experience with AV Discordant Hearts

	No. of pts.	Preop. CHB	Postop. CHB	VSD	PS	TI	% Op. Mort.	% Late Mort.
Boston 1982 (38)	23	5	6	20	19	5	9	14
Iowa 1983 (34)	10	1	1	7	6	4	0	10
N.Y. 1982 (39)	18	0	2	17	14	6	11	12
Rochester 1979 (33)	53	7	24	53	39	10	26	NA
London 1979 (32)	13	0	2	13	9	2	15	18
Birmingham 1983 (40)	74	15	36	52	34	15	7	17
Toronto 1988	75	10	12	66	43	16	9	15
No. pts.	266	38	83	228	164	58		
% pts.		14%	31%	88%	62%	22%	11%	15%

CHB = congenital heart block; VSD = ventricular septal defect; PS = pulmonary stenosis; TI = tricuspid insufficiency.

obstruct the outflow tract.[15,16] Fibrous tissue tags arising from the pulmonary or mitral valves or projecting through a VSD from the tricuspid valve could cause subvalvar pulmonary stenosis.

Left AV Valve (Tricuspid) Abnormalities. Left AV valve abnormalities are encountered in 22% of patients with CCTGA, of which 80% have insufficiency as the principal hemodynamic problem. The frequency of left AV valve abnormalities increases with age. Structural abnormalities are seen in nearly 90% of autopsy reports,[12] and include abnormalities of the valve cusps, abnormal chordae, absence of valve tissue, or Ebstein-like anomalies.[17,18] The latter constitute the less severe end of the spectrum of Ebstein's malformation with dysplasia and downward displacement of the valve leaflets and attachment to the ventricular wall, especially the posterior and septal cusps. True Ebstein's malformation with thinning of the inlet portion of the ventricle has been recorded but is quite rare. Approximately 75% of the left AV valve abnormalities are seen in conjunction with VSD.[9]

Conduction and Rhythm Abnormalities. Atrioventricular conduction abnormalities occur in 14% of patients with CCTGA. The incidence is progressive with age and its presence may alter from moment to moment, either spontaneously or under the influence of different stress conditions such as exercise, infection, or pregnancy. AV block may exist as an isolated phenomenon or in combination with one or more of the other intracardiac anomalies.[19] First-degree AV block is seen in 20-30% of patients.[20] Second-degree AV block is encountered much less frequently; however, its presence is suggestive of CCTGA, because it is rarely detected in other forms of congenital heart disease. Complete AV block is found in 15-25% of cases, often developing in the first decade of life. The incidence of WPW syndrome in patients with CCTGA is higher than in the general population. Both types A and B have been reported with equal frequency.[19]

Other Associated Anomalies. Other associated anomalies seen in patients with CCTGA include atrial septal defects, patent ductus arteriosus, obstructive anomalies of the aortic arch, supravalvar left atrial ring producing tricuspid stenosis, overriding or straddling AV valves, and anomalies of both pulmonary and systemic venous return. Hearts with superior and inferior ventricles and crossed AV connections may also have AV and VA discordance.

CLINICAL PRESENTATION

The clinical presentation of CCTGA is not specific and is influenced entirely by the presence of associated anomalies. Indeed, isolated CCTGA may pass unrecognized for many years, presenting de novo with a conduction disturbance or the onset of a previously undetected murmur because of worsening left AV valve regurgitation. Occasionally, the diagnosis is suspected because the position of the heart is abnormal. More than 50% of patients with dextrocardia and situs solitus have CCTGA.[21] Because the associated anomalies are so frequent and potentially severe, more than 70% of children are symptomatic in the first year of life.[22]

Most children are referred for evaluation of a heart murmur. Even in patients with isolated CCTGA, an ejection murmur may be audible because of the abnormal architecture of the pulmonary outflow tract. Three distinct clinical groups are recognized based upon whether pulmonary blood flow is increased, decreased, or normal. The first group includes patients with VSD and no significant pulmonary stenosis. They have a substantial left-to-right shunt and have signs and symptoms compatible with congestive heart failure or failure to thrive. Patients with significant pulmonary outflow tract obstruction have decreased pulmonary blood flow and right-to-left shunting. They present with cyanosis and clubbing. Patients with normal pulmonary blood flow may have isolated CCTGA, tricuspid insufficiency, or combination of VSD and mild pulmonary stenosis. Patients with isolated left AV valve insufficiency present with a clinical picture not dissimilar from mitral insufficiency in a heart with normal segmental relationships.

The first sound is normal because the AV valves are normally oriented. Because the pulmonary valve is positioned more medially and posteriorly, the pulmonary component of the second heart sound may be soft or inaudible. Conversely, the position of the aortic valve leftward and anteriorly produces a louder second sound in the second intercostal space to the left of the sternum, giving the erroneous impression of pulmonary hypertension. The recognition of a murmur suggestive of mitral insufficiency in children should alert the physician to the possibility of CCTGA; congenital mitral insufficiency is rare except in CCTGA, and a rheumatic origin is unlikely, especially if the murmur has been present from an early age.

DIAGNOSTIC MODALITIES

Electrocardiogram. The ECG is not pathognomonic for CCTGA, but several unusual characteristics may be observed. As a result of the high incidence of AV conduction disturbances, AV block of all degrees is seen. Furthermore, different degrees of AV block may be present at different times in the same patient. Reversal of the normal precordial Q wave pattern is encountered because of inversion of the ventricular surfaces and the bundle branches: Q waves are seen in the right precordial leads and are absent in the left precordial leads.[23] The ECG pattern observed in CCTGA may be influenced greatly by the hemodynamic alterations that occur with associated cardiac malformations. His bundle recordings may be of value in determining the location of the abnormal pathways in AV conduction disturbances and the WPW syndrome.

Chest Radiography. The atrial situs usually can be determined from the location of the liver and stomach or from the bronchial anatomy. The position of the heart in the chest is important, since dextrocardia in situs solitus or

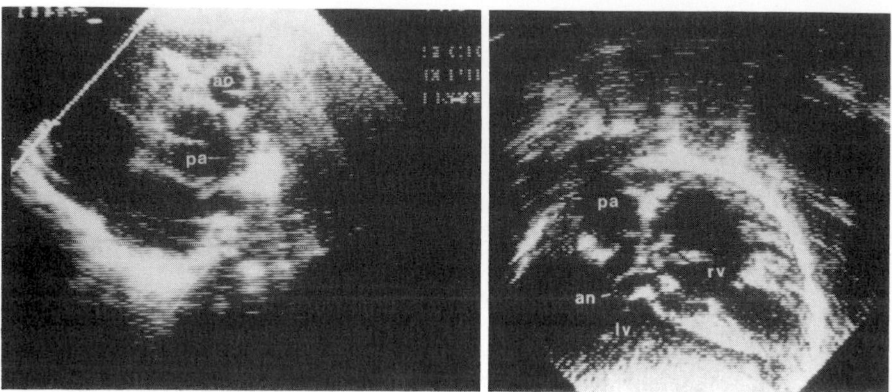

FIGURE 4. Corrected transposition. *Left,* Precordial short axis view showing the aorta (Ao) anterior and to the left of the pulmonary artery (PA). *Right,* Subcostal long axis view showing an aneurysm (An) of the membranous septum protruding into the subpulmonary region.

levocardia in situs inversus strongly suggests the presence of CCTGA. The ventriculoarterial connection cannot be elicited from the plain x-ray directly, but the configuration of the vascular pedicle in CCTGA results in an unusual appearance of the superior mediastinum, i.e., narrow superior mediastinal shadow. The hemodynamic status of the patient may be expressed in terms of changes in the cardiac contour, size, and pulmonary vascular markings. A routine chest x-ray will not provide information regarding the atrioventricular connections.

Echocardiography. The diagnosis of CCTGA may be established by two-dimensional echocardiography. Initially, it is important to establish atrial situs by showing the systemic veins draining into the right atrium and the pulmonary veins draining into the left atrium. Once this has been accomplished, it is necessary to show that each atrium is connected to a separate ventricle and that this connection is inappropriate. The demonstration of a right AV valve in fibrous continuity with the posterior great artery is almost diagnostic of AV discordance.[24] Ventriculoarterial discordance can be established by demonstrating the aortic valve arising from a morphologic right ventricle and the pulmonary valve from a morphologic left ventricle (Fig. 4). Echocardiography is extremely useful in delineating the associated lesions, straddling AV valves, and ventricular size and contractility (Fig. 5).

Cardiac Catheterization and Angiography. Cardiac catheterization will elicit the abnormal architecture of CCTGA and document associated lesions. Furthermore, it is of great importance in determining the patient's hemodynamic status. As on echocardiography, the various cardiac segments and their discordant connections must be identified angiographically in order to establish the diagnosis of CCTGA. The identification of the atria is derived mainly from the morphology of the atrial appendages. The discordant atrioventricular connection is suggested by the course of right heart catheter as it passes through the right AV valve, making a sharp bend upward and medially to enter the pulmonary outflow tract. This is confirmed by ventricular angiography of the typical triangular shape of the finely trabeculated LV and continuity between the

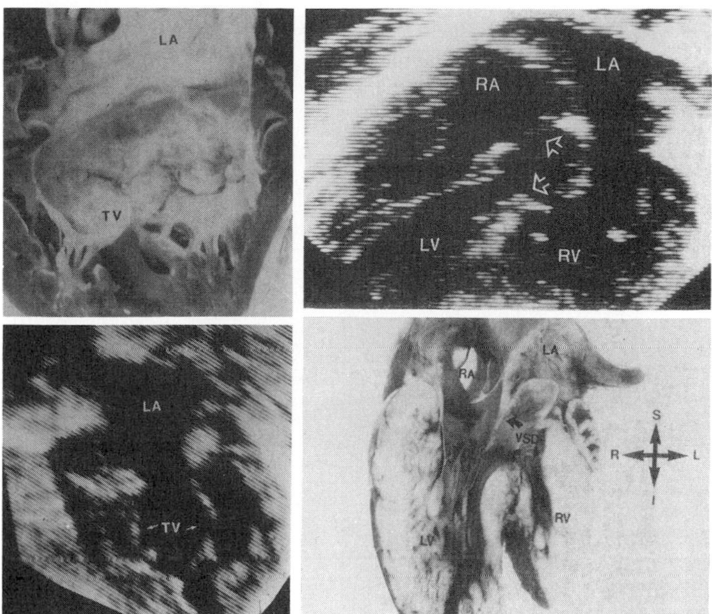

FIGURE 5. *Left side,* Apical four-chamber view showing an Ebstein's malformation of the tricuspid valve (TV). Note the shortened chordae and endocardial sclerosis of the left atrium (LA). Echocardiographic findings correlate with the anatomic specimen. *Right side,* Apical four-chamber view showing the AV valves at the same level and the large perimembranous inlet VSD demarcated by the arrows. Note the discordant AV connections. Echocardiographic findings correlate with anatomic specimen.

pulmonary and mitral valves. Because the axis of the ventricular septum is rotated, the entire length of the ventricular septum is usually seen in the anteroposterior projection.[25] The morphologic right ventricle is a triangular structure with a rounded and heavily trabeculated apex. The aortic valve arises superiorly and is separated from the left AV valve by the crista supraventricularis (Fig. 6).

The distribution pattern of the coronary arteries so typical of CCTGA is readily identified angiographically. In situs solitus, the morphologic left coronary artery arises from the right facing coronary sinus and divides into circumflex and anterior descending branches. The circumflex artery encircles the mitral orifice and the anterior descending artery delineates the ventricular septum. The morphologic right coronary artery arises from the left facing coronary sinus and gives off conal and marginal branches before terminating on the posterior aspect of the heart as the posterior descending artery. In situs inversus the situation is reversed and the distribution of the coronary arteries resembles the normal coronary arterial pattern in a patient with situs solitus.

NATURAL HISTORY

The natural history of CCTGA depends on the presence or absence of associated lesions. Since 99% of patients diagnosed with CCTGA have associated lesions, it is unusual to encounter a situation in which the hemodynamics are normal. Even patients born with isolated CCTGA seem to acquire structural changes

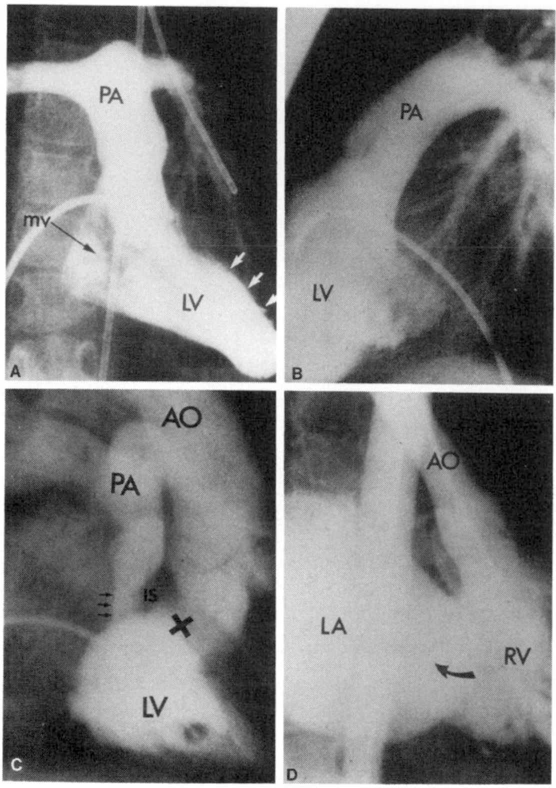

FIGURE 6. Corrected transposition. *A,* Left ventriculogram in AP view with situs solitus. The left ventricle occupies an inferior and right-sided position. The chamber is triangular in shape and the mitral valve is located superiorly and towards the right. The ventricular septum is located to the left and superiorly (arrows). The pulmonary outflow tract is connected to the morphologic LV and in fibrous continuity with the MV. *B,* Left ventriculogram in lateral view with situs solitus. The left ventricle is connected to the PA and the PV is in fibrous continuity with the MV. *C,* Left ventriculogram in RAO view with large VSD demarcated (X) and subpulmonary stenosis bound by the infundibular septum (IS) and the mitral valve. *D,* Right ventriculogram in RAO view with situs solitus demonstrating the connection between the right ventricle (RV) and the aorta (Ao). Marked left AV valve regurgitation is demonstrated (arrow).

during life, mainly involving the left AV valve and conduction tissue. Of the adults studied with an isolated lesion, 33% develop significant hemodynamic changes secondary to mitral insufficiency and about 40% develop complete AV block.[19]

The morphologic right ventricle in CCTGA functions as the systemic pumping chamber. Although it is difficult to prove that the abnormal workload to which this ventricle is subjected is detrimental to overall cardiac performance or life expectancy, studies have suggested that a functional deterioration does take place with time.[26] Benson et al., however, subjected a small group of patients with isolated CCTGA to exercise stress testing and radionuclide assessment of ejection fraction. In this study the responses observed were similar to those observed in the general population.[27,28] Examples of asymptomatic individuals surviving to 73 years have been documented.[29]

The natural history of patients with CCTGA and large VSD is poor, with congestive heart failure occurring early in life and accounting for the high mortality in the first year. Pulmonary stenosis in the presence of a VSD may protect the pulmonary vascular bed at the expense of producing cyanosis early in life and these patients have a natural history similar to that of tetralogy of Fallot.

The natural history of patients with left AV valve abnormalities is not clear. It seems that this valve nearly always shows structural changes but remains competent in the first few years of life. Functional changes increase during the second and subsequent decades of life, perhaps secondary to the structural abnormalities or due to the onset of ventricular dysfunction.

About 5-10% of infants with CCTGA have complete AV block at birth, which increases at a rate of 2% a year. At least 45% of patients have first-or second-degree AV block at birth. With time, prolongation of the PR interval develops, even in some patients with normal intervals originally, and may result in intermittent or permanent complete AV block.[19,20] Only about 40% of patients retain a normal conduction pattern throughout their lives.

TREATMENT

Isolated CCTGA is associated with normal circulation and is compatible with prolonged survival. No treatment should be necessary, barring the onset of complications. Therapeutic intervention is usually necessary for most of the associated anomalies, and management differs little from that for similar lesions and normal AV and VA connections.

Most of the associated anomalies can be repaired surgically with a relatively low risk; however, surgical intervention may not be necessary immediately and the initial institution of medical management may be more appropriate (for example, infants with excessive pulmonary blood flow because of a VSD may be managed medically prior to subjecting them to surgical repair).[30] Also for some infants in whom an intraventricular repair is contemplated, an initial palliative procedure may be preferable, allowing the child to grow to a size at which corrective surgery may be performed more precisely with a lower risk.

Palliation

Pulmonary artery banding now is rarely required to control congestive heart failure, as primary repair is usually considered the procedure of choice. Palliative shunts may be necessary in neonates with severe cyanosis and we prefer a modified Blalock-Taussig shunt on the side of the superior vena cava.

A permanent cardiac pacing system is implanted in all patients with symptomatic complete AV block at the time of palliation or repair, even in the absence of symptoms. An atrial sensing and ventricular inhibited (VDD) pacing system is used if the SA node is normal. In the presence of sinus node dysfunction, an atrial demand and ventricular inhibited (DDD) pacemaker may be used, although a ventricular demand pacemaker with activity mode sensing is a reasonable option and is preferred in the presence of atrial fibrillation.

Other associated anomalies such as coarctation or PDA are treated in the conventional way, and the presence of AV discordance should not influence the timing or conduct of these operations.

Repair of Associated Lesions

VSD Repair. VSD is best approached in most cases via the right atrium. Other approaches such as via the anterior surface of the morphologic LV, pulmonary valve, aortic root, or morphologic RV may be required.[31-33] In approximately two-thirds of cases, the VSD can be repaired through the intact mitral valve. If exposure is suboptimal, the base of the anterior leaflet of the mitral valve can be opened. In patients with situs inversus, the VSD is most easily and safely approached through the aortic valve. A major hazard with VSD repair is the abnormal location of the conduction tissue; interference with it can be avoided by keeping the sutures on the morphologic RV side of the septum. With situs inversus the risk of AV block is much lower. The repair is accomplished using a Dacron patch with a continuous or interrupted suture technique.

Pulmonary Stenosis. Relief of pulmonary stenosis presents a special problem in CCTGA because of the posterior position of the pulmonary outflow tract, wedged between the two AV valves and crossed anteriorly by the conduction tissue. When the pulmonary valve is stenotic, it is approached best via a pulmonary arteriotomy, and pulmonary valvotomy is performed in the usual manner. Also, fibrous subvalvar tags, subvalvar fibrous membrane, or aneurysms of the membranous septum can be excised via the same route. Most commonly, however, the obstruction is subvalvar. Relief of significant stenosis due to a small pulmonary annulus or obstructing subpulmonary tissue is best relieved using a valved conduit between the morphologic LV and pulmonary artery. Doty et al. have proposed a posterior spiral incision across the pulmonary annulus, extending into the subvalvar myocardium with or without an orthotopically placed valve in order to avoid a valved conduit.[34]

When a left ventriculotomy is performed, the incision should be guided via transatrial exposure of the anterior wall of the ventricle and should be carried from the mid-portion of the ventricle toward the apex, avoiding the coronary branches. On the opening of the ventricle, care should be taken to avoid the anterior papillary muscle.

Left AV Valve Repair. Exposure of the left AV valve may be awkward because of its more anterior location, but it is approached usually from the right side via the left atrium below Waterston's groove. Although attempts at repair by annuloplasty are rarely successful, they should be attempted in favorable situations.[35] The presence of Ebstein's anomaly has been thought to be a contraindication to valve replacement, mainly because of the volume of the systemic ventricle.

The presence of left AV insufficiency and systemic ventricular dysfunction is a difficult problem. A combination of tunneling the VSD to the aorta, a Mustard procedure, and an RV to PA conduit is an attractive approach and has been used in two children by Ilbawi.[36]

Other Anomalies. Significant straddling of one AV valve or the presence of a hypoplastic ventricle is a contraindication to a biventricular repair; a modified Fontan procedure is preferred.[37]

RESULTS

An updated review of our own experience and a review of the recent literature is summarized in Table 1. The operative mortality for intracardiac repair in patients with AV discordance is higher than that for repair of an identical lesion with AV concordance. The combined operative mortality of the seven series listed was 11% for initial repair. However, the ability to maintain long-term stable results appears to be compromised. In our series there was a 27% frequency of reoperation associated with a 23% operative mortality (Fig. 7). The indications for reoperation were varied but the vast majority were due to left AV valve insufficiency (41%), conduit stenosis, and residual VSDs. The issue of whether the right ventricle can function as a systemic pumping chamber long term has not been a problem for us. The occurrence of complete AV block prior to surgery and after repair is a problem. Fourteen percent of patients had AV block before operation and 31% developed it following initial repair in the complete list of patients tabulated. An additional 10% of our patients developed AV block following reoperation. The basic anatomic malformation precludes

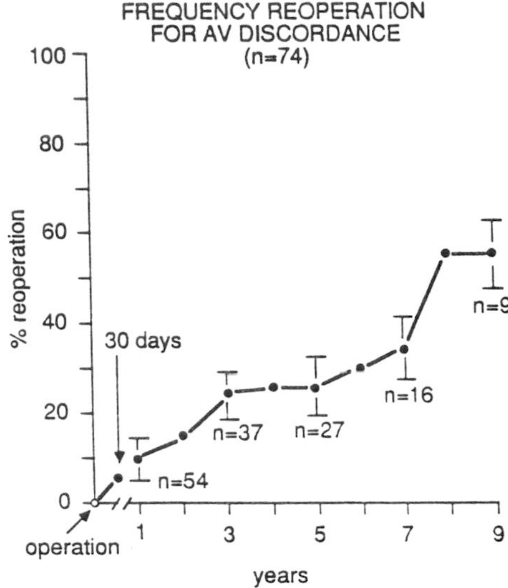

FIGURE 7. Frequency of reoperation after repair of intracardiac lesions in association with AV discordance. After 5 years 28% required reoperation.

avoiding AV block completely, but a knowledge of the anomalous course of the conduction bundle in CCTGA along with the judicious placement of sutures and ventriculotomy aid in reducing this problem. Fortunately the ability to pace these patients in the early postoperative period as well as the availability of improved pacing technology long term have provided a more stable rhythm and better overall patient survival. The overall 5-year survival in our group of patients with AV discordance was 80% (Fig. 8).

OTHER VENTRICULOARTERIAL CONNECTIONS WITH AV DISCORDANCE

With Double Outlet Right Ventricle. Both great arteries arise from the morphologic right ventricle and the only egress of blood from the morphologic left ventricle is through the VSD. Since the right ventricle is the systemic ventricle and is connected to the left atrium, which receives pulmonary venous blood, cyanosis is not a necessary result but is usually produced by the associated pulmonary stenosis. The aorta is usually anterior and leftward, and the pulmonary artery is no longer wedged posteriorly between the AV valves, and overrides the VSD such that more than 50% overlies the left-sided right ventricle. Usually both posterior and anterior nodes persist and a sling of conduction tissue is present encircling the VSD. From a clinical standpoint, this anomaly resembles CCTGA in most respects (Fig. 9).

With Double Outlet Left Ventricle. Both great arteries arise from the morphologic left ventricle. Since the left ventricle is the pulmonary ventricle and is connected to the right atrium, which receives systemic venous blood, cyanosis is an obligatory finding. The VSD is doubly committed with more than 50% of the aorta arising from the left ventricle (Fig. 9).

With Single Outlet of the Heart. This encompasses three separate entities: truncus arteriosus, single pulmonary trunk, and aortic atresia or single aortic trunk and pulmonary atresia. The first two are rare. AV discordance with pulmonary atresia is associated with a VSD. Cyanosis and tachypnea develop shortly after birth.

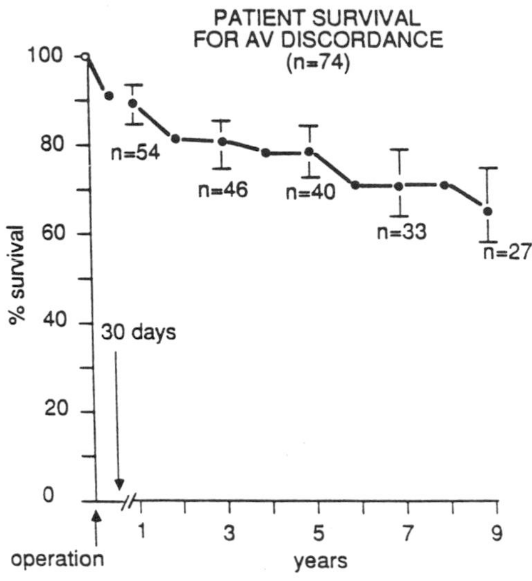

FIGURE 8. Actuarial survival of 74 patients with AV discordance after intracardiac repair of associated lesions. Survival at 5 years is 80% ± 5% with 40 patients at risk.

With Ventriculoarterial Concordant Connections. Ventriculoarterial concordant connections in patients with AV discordance is very rare and is of two types: isolated ventricular inversion and isolated atrial inversion. The systemic and pulmonary circulations are in parallel and the physiology is similar to complete TGA. In isolated ventricular inversion, the aorta lies to the right and posterior to the pulmonary artery and arises from a right-sided morphologic left ventricle. Usually there is a large VSD and pulmonary stenosis is absent. When the ventricular septum is intact, severe cyanosis is present soon after birth. The presence of a large VSD produces moderate cyanosis and is accompanied by congestive heart failure. (Fig. 9). In isolated atrial inversion, there is atrial situs inversus with visceroatrial discordance.

ANATOMICALLY CORRECTED MALPOSITION OF THE GREAT ARTERIES

This is a rare defect characterized by an abnormal spatial relationship between the great arteries, which still arise from their morphologically appropriate ventricles.[41] Most frequently it is found in situs solitus with the aorta arising from

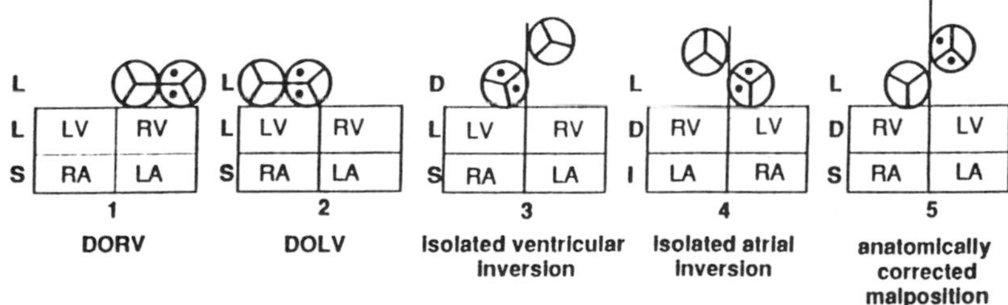

FIGURE 9. Diagrammatic models representing other ventriculoarterial connections with AV discordance and concordance (DORV = double outlet right ventricle; DOLV = double outlet left ventricle).

the normally positioned posterior morphologic left ventricle. However, the aorta is more anterior than normal and lies to the left of the pulmonary artery (Fig. 9). Surgical repair is necessary to correct associated defects only. Its importance lies in the fact that it can be mistaken for congenitally corrected transposition, since both have the L-position of the aorta. The presence of a right aortic arch should alert one to its presence, as it is found in more than 30% of cases; it is rare in CCTGA. VSD is present in virtually all cases and pulmonary outflow tract obstruction is common. Mitral and aortic discontinuity is the rule, with a subaortic conus separating the two valves. The coronary artery anatomy is unusual in that there is a high incidence of abnormal coronary artery distribution and single coronary artery. The conduction tissue is located in its usual posterior position, and left juxtaposition of the atrial appendages is seen in 30% cases.

REFERENCES

1. Von Rokitansky K: Die Defecte der Scheidewande des Herzens. Wilhelm Braumuller, Vienna, 1875.
2. Monckeberg JG: Zur Entwicklungsgeschichte des Afrioventrikular-systems. Verhandlung der Deutschen Pathologischen Gesellschaft 16:228–249, 1913.
3. Walmsley T: Transposition of the ventricles and the arterial stems. J Anat 65:528–540, 1931.
4. Anderson RC, Lillehei CW, Lester RG: Corrected transposition of the great vessel of the heart. Pediatrics 20:626–646, 1957.
5. Schiebler GL, Edwards JE, Burchell HB, et al: Congenital corrected transposition of the great vessels: A study of 33 cases. Pediatrics 27:849–888, 1961.
6. Stanger P, Rudolph AM, Edwards JE: Cardiac malpositions. An overview based on a study of five necropsy specimens. Circulation 56:159–172, 1977.
7. Bjarke BB, Kidd BSL: Congenitally corrected transposition of the great arteries. A clinical study of 101 cases. Acta Pediatr Scand 65:153–160, 1976.
8. Van Praagh R: What is congenitally corrected transposition? N Engl J Med 282:1097–1098, 1970.
9. Friedberg DZ, Nadas AS: Clinical profile of patients with congenital transposition of the great vessels. A study of 60 cases. N Engl J Med 282:1053–1059, 1970.
10. Langman J: Medical Embryology, 3rd ed. Baltimore, Williams and Wilkins Co., 1975, pp 206–209.
11. Van Praagh R, Layton WM, Van Praagh S: The morphogenesis of normal and abnormal relationships between the great arteries and ventricles. Pathologic and experimental data. In Van Praagh R, Takao A (eds): Etiology and Morphogenesis of Congenital Heart Disease. Mt Kisko, NY, Futura, 1980.
12. Allwork SP, Bentall HH, Becker AE, et al: Congenitally corrected transposition of the great arteries: Morphologic study of 32 cases. Am J Cardiol 38:910–923, 1976.
13. Anderson RH, Arnold R, Wilkinson JL: The conduction tissue in congenitally corrected transposition. Lancet 1:1286, 1973.
14. LoseKoot TG, Anderson RH, Becker AE, et al: Congenitally corrected transposition. In Ventricular Septal Defect. Edinburgh, Churchill Livingstone 1983, ch 15.
15. Krongrad E, Ellis K, Steeg C, et al: Subpulmonary obstruction in congenitally corrected transposition of the great arteries due to ventricular membranous septal aneurysms. Circulation 54:679–683, 1976.
16. Levy MJ, Lillehei CW, Elliot LP, et al: Accessory valvular tissue causing subpulmonary stenosis in corrected transposition of great vessels. Circulation 27:494–502, 1963.
17. Van Mierop LMS, Alley RD, Kausel HW: Ebstein's malformation of the left atrioventricular valve in corrected transposition with subpulmonary stenosis and ventricular septal defect. Am J Cardiol 8:270–274, 1961.
18. Becker AE, Becker MJ, Edwards JE: Pathologic spectrum of dysplasia of the tricuspid valve. Features in common with Ebstein's malformation. Arch Pathol 91:167–178, 1971.
19. LoseKoot TG, Anderson RH, Becker AE, et al: Congenitally corrected transposition. In Rhythm and Conduction Disturbances. Edinburgh, Churchill Livingstone, 1983, ch 18.
20. Kirklin JW, Barratt-Boyes BG: Cardiac surgery. In Congenitally Corrected Transposition of the Great Arteries. New York, John Wiley & Sons, 1986, ch 42.
21. Squarcia U, Ritter DG, Kincaid OW: Dextrocardia: Angiographic study and classification. Am J Cardiol 32:965–977, 1973.

22. Kidd BSL: Congenitally corrected transposition of the great arteries. In Keith JD, Rowe RD, Vlad P (eds): Heart Disease in Infancy and Childhood, 3rd ed. New York, MacMillan, 1978.
23. Ruttenberg MD, Elliot LP, Anderson RC, et al: Congenital corrected transposition of the great vessels. Correlation of electrocardiograms and vector cardiograms with associated cardiac malformations and hemodynamic states. Am J Cardiol 17:339–354, 1966.
24. Anderson RH, Beardshaw JA, Gibson DG: Echocardiography of primitive ventricle and corrected transposition. In Lundstrom NR (ed): Echocardiography in Congenital Heart Disease. North Holland, Elsevier, 1978.
25. Freedom RM, Culham JAG, Moes CAF: The Angiography of Congenital Heart Disease. New York, MacMillan, 1984.
26. Graham TP Jr, Parrish MD, Boucek RJ Jr, et al: Assessment of ventricular size and function in congenitally corrected transposition of the great arteries. Am J Cardiol 51:245, 1983.
27. Benson LN, Bonet J, McLaughlin P, et al: Assessment of right ventricular function during supine bicycle exercise after Mustard's operation. Circulation 65:1052–1059, 1982.
28. Benson LN, Burns R, Schelbert HR, et al: Radionuclide angiographic evaluation of ventricular function in isolated CCTGA. Presented at Second World Congress of Pediatric Cardiology, New York, June 1985.
29. Lieberson AD, Schumacher RR, Childress RM, et al: Corrected transposition of the great vessels in a 73 year old man. Circulation 39:96–100, 1976.
30. Bonfils EA, Guller B, McGoon DC, et al: Corrected transposition: Surgical treatment of associated anomalies. Ann Thorac Surg 17:200–209, 1974.
31. Olinger GN, Maloney JV: Trans-pulmonary artery repair of ventricular septal defect with congenitally corrected transposition of the great arteries. J Thorac Cardiovasc Surg 78:515–759, 1980.
32. DeLeval MR, Bastos P, Stark J, et al: Surgical technique to reduce risks of heart block following closure of ventricular septal defect in atrioventricular discordance. J Thorac Cardiovasc Surg 78:515–526, 1979.
33. Marcelletti C, Maloney JD, Ritter DG, et al: Corrected transposition and ventricular septal defect. Ann Surg 191:751–759.
34. Doty DB, Trusedell SC, Marvin WJ: Techniques to avoid injury of the conduction tissue during surgical treatment of corrected transposition. Circulation 68(Suppl II):63–69, 1983.
35. Williams WG: Congenitally corrected transposition of the great arteries. In Arciniegas E (ed): Pediatric Cardiac Surgery. Chicago, Year Book, 1985, pp 285–295.
36. Ilbawi M: Personal communication, 1988.
37. Gale AW, Danielson GK, McGoon DC, et al: Modified Fontan operation for univentricular heart and complicated congenital lesions. J Thorac Cardiovasc Surg 78:831–838, 1978.
38. Westerman GR, Lang P, Castaneda AR, et al: Corrected transposition and repair of associated intracardiac defects. Circulation 66(Suppl I):197–202, 1982.
39. Hwang T, Bowman F, Malm J, et al: Surgical repair of congenitally corrected transposition of the great arteries. Results and follow-up. Am J Cardiol 50:781–785, 1982.
40. Fox LS, Kirklin JW, Pacifico AD, et al: Intracardiac repair of cardiac malformations with atrioventricular discordance. Circulation 54:1223–1227, 1976.
41. Rittenhouse EA, Tenckhoff L, Kawabori I, et al: Surgical repair of anatomically corrected malposition of the great arteries. Ann Thorac Surg 42:220–228, 1986.

DAVID N. CAMPBELL, MD
DAVID R. CLARKE, MD

TRANSPOSITION OF THE GREAT ARTERIES

The Atrial Switch (Baffle) Procedure*

From the Department of Surgery
Section of Cardiovascular Surgery
University of Colorado Health Services Center
Denver, Colorado

Reprint requests to:
David N. Campbell, MD
Section of Cardiovascular Surgery
University of Colorado Health Sciences Center
4200 E. Ninth Ave.
Denver, CO 80262

Since the successful introduction of the arterial switch technique by Jatene from Brazil in 1975,[1] the use of this procedure has increased dramatically over the last few years, leaving many congenital cardiac surgeons to wonder why the atrial switch procedure has not taken its rightful place in the dusty archives of past but no longer useful cardiac procedures. Nothing could be further from reality. The atrial switch techniques of Senning and Mustard still provide a very useful addition to the armamentarium in the surgical management of congenital heart disease even in 1989.

HISTORICAL PERSPECTIVE

The first surgical attempt to palliate transposition of the great arteries (TGA) came in 1950 when Blalock and Hanlon in Baltimore[2] described a technique for closed resection of the atrial septum to allow for better mixing between pulmonary venous and systemic venous blood. Though suggested by Albert[3] in the *Surgical Forum* in 1954, the complete physiologic correction of this lesion was not completed until 1958, when Ake Senning in Stockholm[4] used the posterior portion of the atrial septum as a flap to create the "arterial atrium" and the wall of the right atrium to form the "venous atrium" in a 9-year-old boy with transposition with intact ventricular septum (TGA-IVS). On May 16, 1963, Mustard in Toronto accomplished a successful repair in a 2-year-old girl using a

** Note: A companion article on the Arterial Switch Procedure by Dr. Magdi Yacoub will appear in the June 1989 issue of this series. Because of time constraints, it was unable to be included in this issue.*

pericardial baffle to recreate the "venous atrium." A small VSD was also closed. After this report was published in 1964,[5] the Senning procedure fell out of favor, and the Mustard procedure became the standard method for repair of TGA. Undoubtedly, this had to do with the fact that the initial results with the Senning procedure, particularly in the major American centers, were disappointing at best.

In 1966, Rashkind in Philadelphia[6] changed the initial management of infants when he and Miller introduced balloon atrial septostomy (BAS). Prior to this, only surgical manipulation and resection of the atrial septum to allow mixing at the atrial level via the methods of Blalock and Hanlon (1950)[7] and Edwards and Bayerson (1965)[8] were available to improve the oxygen saturation and to resolve the metabolic acidosis in newborns who were symptomatic from poor cross-circulation.

The Rashkind procedure allowed most newborns to be managed medically until 6 months to 1 year of age when they could safely undergo an atrial switch procedure. This time frame seemed optimal because the risk of operating on these infants under 6 months of age was still significant, and the complication rate involving pulmonary venous obstruction was higher in younger repairs; waiting longer than 6 months after newborn BAS subjected the infants to risk of late death. Vlad and Lambert (1973)[9] indicated that over half of these children had systemic arterial saturations less than 60% 6 months or later following BAS.

Through the early 1970s arrhythmia complications and baffle obstruction remained significant problems with the Mustard procedure. Despite the revision described by the Toronto group,[10] in which the sinoatrial node artery was preserved by leaving a rim of septum superiorly between the tricuspid valve and the superior vena cava surface, other centers continued to report these complications.

In 1977, Quaegebeur and Brom in Leiden[11] authored a paper in *Thorax* entitled "Revival of the Senning Operation in the Treatment of Transposition of the Great Arteries." Their results suggested that baffle obstruction was "exceedingly rare" on the pulmonary venous side and "nearly impossible" on the systemic venous side when the Senning procedure was utilized. Also, the incidence of arrhythmias was "slightly less" than with the Mustard procedure. This sparked renewed interest in the Senning procedure in the early 1980s. Each center and each surgeon has a "favorite," but as further technical refinements have been implemented there is essentially no difference between the two procedures.

ANATOMY OF COMPLETE TRANSPOSITION OF THE GREAT ARTERIES

Quite simply, simple or complete TGA describes a condition in which the pulmonary artery arises from the left ventricle and the aorta arises from the right ventricle. In 1967, Van Praagh[12] pointed out that true transposition entailed three basic features: (1) lack of continuity between the aortic and mitral valves, (2) presence of a subaortic conus, and (3) absence of the subpulmonary conus. Anderson defines it as atrioventricular concordance and ventriculoarterial discordance. The atrial chambers are connected appropriately but the appendages may be juxtaposed. A probe patent foramen ovale is usually present, the leaflets of the mitral and tricuspid valves "face" each other along a broader area of septum, and the overall septum is much straighter than normal.[13] Of clinical significance is the course of the sinoatrial (SA) nodal artery. It usually arises from the right coronary artery close to the mouth of the orifice, travels into the anterior limbus of the fossa ovalis toward the cavoatrial junction, and then passes either anteriorly or posteriorly to join the SA node. Concerning the infundibular morphology, not all transposed hearts have a subaortic conus, while a few (less than 10%) have a subpulmonary conus, usually leading to stenosis. This commonly occurs when a VSD is present. As pointed out by Van Praagh, great artery anomalies such as double outlet, single ventricle and corrected transposition are better classified as malposition of the great arteries because they do not meet the simple criteria stated at the beginning of the section: that the two great arteries are separated by the ventricular septum and they arise from the wrong ventricle.

CLASSIFICATION OF TRANSPOSITION OF THE GREAT ARTERIES

Associated Anomalies

When trying to classify complete TGA, several methods are available to define categories. Anatomically, the presence or absence of associated anomalies comprises four major groups: (1) intact ventricular septum, (2) intact ventricular septum and pulmonary stenosis usually on a dynamic basis, (3) ventricular septal defect, and (4) ventricular septal defect and pulmonary stenosis. Fifty percent of these hearts fall into the first category, in which the ventricular septum is intact and there is no structural pulmonary stenosis, i.e., simple TGA. Ten percent of the overall group of TGA demonstrate left ventricular outflow tract obstruction (LVOTO), 30% have associated VSD, and the other 10% have both VSD and LVOTO.[14]

These associated anomalies are of significance, especially when evaluating the procedure of choice and planning the optimal time for operative intervention. One of the primary reasons for subgrouping the associated anomalies in infants is the variable development of early pulmonary vascular disease (PVD). There is clearly an accelerated progression of PVD in TGA.[15-17] Recent studies suggest that even infants with intact ventricular septum may develop early PVD.[18,19] As age increases, the incidence of PVD rises with all the different subgroups of transposition; however, transposition with VSD has the highest incidence of early PVD. Obviously, these children (TGA-VSD) require early intervention (about 3 months of age) to prevent the progression of this fatal complication. Again, infants with intact ventricular septum should undergo operation between 6 months and 1 year of age. Unfortunately, the presence of a patent ductus arteriosus (PDA) can influence this, and if the ductus is large, the infant should undergo complete repair early (between 3 and 6 months). Complete repair rather than ductus ligation alone is necessary, for ligation of the ductus leaves the child severely hypoxemic, and acidosis commonly follows. Finally, the presence of LVOTO does not ensure protection against PVD.

Clinical Presentation

A second method of classification is based on the amount of mixing between the two parallel circuits. Rowe[20] suggested, as early as 1968, that there are essentially three hemodynamic groups: (1) those with poor mixing, i.e., intact ventricular septum; (2) those with adequate communication, i.e., VSD or large PDA; and (3) those with LVOTO. The clinical presentation of each of these three groups is dependent upon the physiology of the lesion, and the signs and symptoms of each group are distinctly different.

Group 1. In general, TGA is the most likely diagnosis when a newborn presents in the first week of life with cyanosis, and it is the most common type of fetal cyanotic heart disease in the first year of life. Severe cyanosis in a newborn with TGA almost assures the diagnosis of intact ventricular septum without adequate mixing between the two separate circulations (restrictive patent foramen ovale). Tachypnea, tachycardia, and acidosis follow shortly, but there is little evidence of congestive heart failure. Supplemental oxygen does not help the tachypnea and tachycardia, and, in fact, the failure of 100% oxygen to increase the initial oxygen saturation of an infant (a flat shunt study) confirms the presence of cyanotic heart disease rather than pulmonary disease. Except for cyanosis, these newborns appear quite normal: birth weight is average, pulses are full and normal, and cardiac sounds are nonspecific. Unless adequate communication is ensured by BAS, surgical septectomy, or complete repair, a downward spiral continues in which congestive heart failure may or may not become apparent and death occurs.

Group 2. Infants with moderate-sized VSD or large PDA usually do not present in the first few weeks of life, and the cyanosis is barely noticeable. When symptoms develop, they are secondary to congestive heart failure. Respiratory distress, tachypnea, tachycardia, and hepatomegaly are often present. As with infants with intact ventricular septum, these infants are well nourished, their pulses are full and strong, and again the cardiac sounds are nondiagnostic, but there is usually a loud harsh holosystolic murmur. If a large PDA is present, a machinery-type murmur may be heard. Mild to moderate cyanosis is present, but when these babies cry, the cyanosis becomes extreme.

Group 3. This is the group with obstruction of the left ventricular outflow tract which becomes pulmonary stenosis because of the transposed arteries. Usually these infants present later, cyanosis is variable, and heart failure is rare because blood flow to the lungs is moderately decreased. Various types of obstruction occur and include valvar stenosis, subvalvar stenosis, and rarely supravalvar pulmonary artery stenosis. Subvalvar stenosis is the more common type and occurs most often in conjunction with ventricular septal defect.[13] It is usually the result of the posterior malalignment of the outlet septum into the left ventricular outflow tract. This "balance" flow pattern, physiologically similar to tetralogy of Fallot, is the reason these children present later and do not have heart failure.

DIAGNOSTIC TECHNIQUES

Chest X-ray. The classic findings on the roentgenogram of a baby with TGA are increased vascular markings in the lung fields, enlarged heart, and a silhouette referred to as an "egg-on-its-side." Most often, however, the chest film in nondiagnostic. The egg-on-its-side appearance is secondary to the often-present anterior-posterior relationship of the aorta and pulmonary artery, which causes a narrow great vessel silhouette.

Electrocardiography. Again, the electrocardiogram is nondiagnostic and often normal for a newborn (right ventricular hypertrophy pattern). However, this pattern does not regress as it does in normal babies.

2-D Echocardiography and Echo Doppler. With the increasing accuracy of both echocardiographic equipment and echocardiographers, the diagnosis can be assured noninvasively. However, balloon septostomy is not carried out with 2-D echo alone at the present time. Several centers are currently clinically evaluating this technique (BAS performed in a cath lab but with echo only), and it is only a matter of time before it will become routine.

Cardiac Cineangiography. This remains the gold standard, not so much for confirmation of diagnosis any more, but for the completion of a safe, successful balloon septostomy. In complex transposition, VSD and PDA can also be easily seen, but while left LVOTO can also be diagnosed, 2-D echocardiography with echo Doppler is probably more definitive for this problem today.

SURGICAL TECHNIQUES

General Preparation. The patient is anesthetized in routine fashion with fentanyl, endotracheal intubation, and halothane inhalation. If deep hypothermia and circulatory arrest (DHCA) are to be utilized, then methylprednisolone 30 mg/kg and phenytoin 7 mg/kg are given intravenously, and the head is packed in ice. Deep hypothermia and circulatory arrest are used primarily when the weight of the child is less than 4.5 kg or when unusual anatomy is present, such as a persistent left superior vena cava, making cannulation itself more difficult.

After sternotomy, the pericardium is opened and the patient is systemically heparinized with 3 mg/kg. Activated clotting times (ACT) are checked to confirm adequate heparinization. For DHCA, single aortic and single venous cannulation (usually with a right-angled cannula) are utilized. If cardiopulmonary bypass (CPB) is chosen, then two right-angled cannulae are utilized, one in the superior vena cava proper and one in the inferior vena cava at the diaphragm. Care is taken not to injure the SA node area. When CPB is carried out, the systemic temperature is lowered to 20° C rectal and blood cardioplegia is used. No cardioplegia is used with DHCA. Instead, during DHCA systemic temperature is lowered to 17° C rectal and intermittent topical cooling is used after the pump is shut off and the patient is exsanguinated into the pump oxygenator. Prior to establishment of bypass, the ductus arteriosus is ligated if one is present.

Senning Procedure. Once the aorta is cross-clamped, the right atrial incision is made as shown in Figure 1. The longitudinal portion of the right atrial incision is made in an oblique fashion, with the inferior edge at least two-thirds the diameter of the inferior vena cava in distance from the intra-atrial groove. The left atrium is opened just lateral to the intra-atrial groove from the superior edge of the right superior pulmonary vein to the inferior edge of the right inferior pulmonary vein. Often a piece of wall is excised to provide as large an opening as possible. This is the limiting factor for blood flow from the pulmonary veins

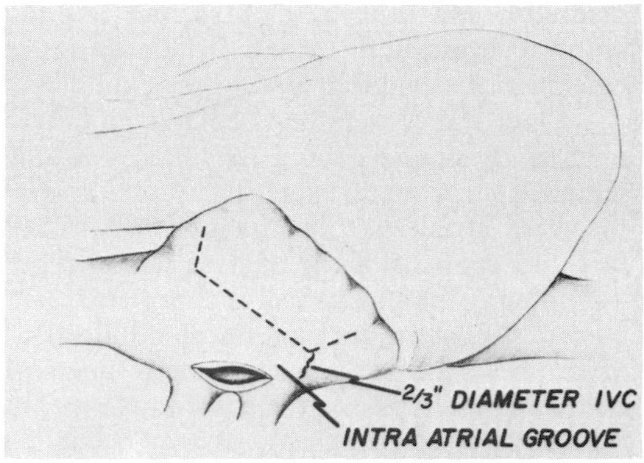

FIGURE 1. The right atrial incision is completed. In fact, once this is accomplished, the rest of the procedure becomes routine. The opening in the left atrium at the right superior and inferior pulmonary vein is made as large as possible.

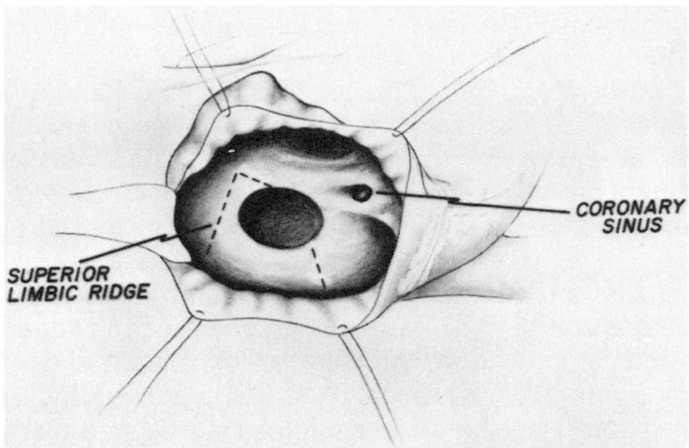

FIGURE 2. The entire remaining atrial septum is excised in the area of the dotted lines. Care is taken not to excise through the atrial wall. If the techniques of Barratt-Boyes or Subramanian are to be used, incisions are made in the area of the dotted line, but the tissue is not excised. Instead, the tissue is used as a flap.

to the tricuspid valve, and the opening must be adequate to carry all the systemic flow.

With the right atrium open, the superior edge of the true septum is excised in total along the limbic ridge (Fig. 2). The coronary sinus is cut back and a piece of Gor-Tex is fashioned in the design of a surfboard to reconstruct the atrial septum. This is anchored into place, leaving the left pulmonary veins below the patch and the mitral valve above the patch. The advantage of the Gor-Tex patch is speed and simplicity; however, the disadvantage is the retention of a foreign body inside the heart. If the surgeon wishes to use only native tissue, several techniques have been described to use tissue already present inside the heart for the septal flap. One technique described by Barratt-Boyes[21] involves incising the septal flap in a very similar fashion to that shown in Figure 2, but leaving the attachment to the true septum (very much like a hinge) at the intra-atrial groove laterally. This flap of tissue is then incised like opening a book upside down, and the piece of tissue is sewn into position similar to the Gor-Tex patch superiorly, medially, and inferiorly. A second technique described by Subramanian[22] involves inversion of the left atrial appendage and using this tissue anchored to the superior septal flap as the neoseptum.

Once the neoseptum is completed (Fig. 3), the systemic venous channel is formed by anastomosing the infero-lateral edge of the right atrium to the remaining true septal ridge. The suture line is started inferiorly (Fig. 4), bringing the right atrial edge in juxtaposition with the eustachian remnant and then traveling cephalad along the true septal ridge to the remaining limbic ridge. The pulmonary venous channel is completed by folding the medial right atrial flap over to the lateral incision in the pulmonary veins (Fig. 5) and completing the anastomosis inferiorly, laterally, and superiorly. One word of caution: care must be taken in completing the anastomosis cephalad along the area of the superior vena cava. Two complications may occur if too much tension is placed on the

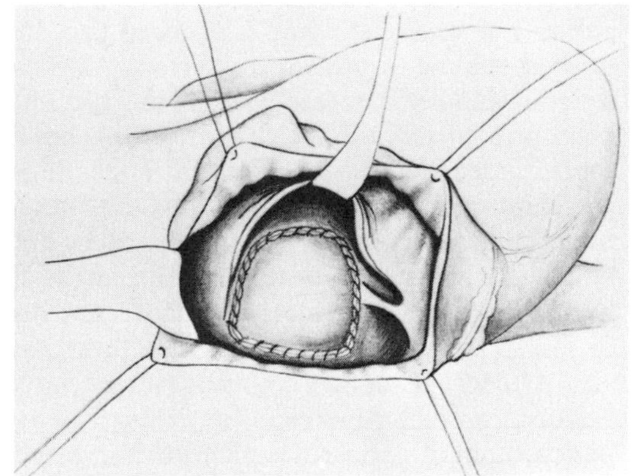

FIGURE 3. The Gor-Tex is sewn into position after the coronary sinus is cut back.

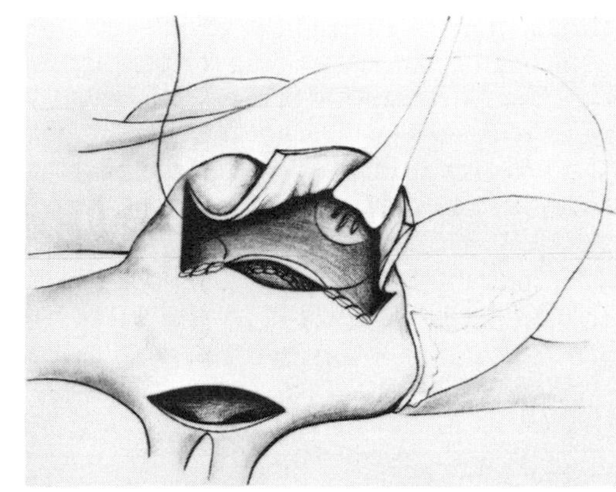

FIGURE 4. Starting at the eustachian remnant, the venous tunnel is completed by sewing the lateral right atrial wall to the remaining true atrial wall medially. Care must be taken to place the suture line in the floor of the cut-back coronary sinus to avoid injury to the AV node.

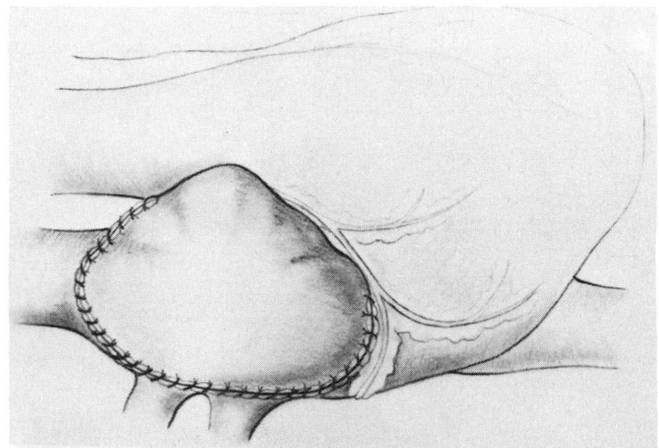

FIGURE 5. The medial right atrial flap is sewn to the right pulmonary veins to complete the procedure.

suture line or the stitches are placed too deep: (1) the sinoatrial node may be injured, leading to sick sinus syndrome, and (2) the superior vena cava–right atrial junction can be narrowed, leading to superior vena cava syndrome. If DHCA has been utilized and all anastomoses have been completed, the venous cannula is repositioned in the true left atrial appendage (now the right atrial appendage), the child is placed back on bypass, and rewarming with the cross-clamp off is undertaken. Pacing wires and chest tubes are placed and bypass is discontinued when appropriate. Occasionally, the suture line can be carried well up onto the pericardium, if the tissue planes have not been violated around either the SVC or IVC. If this is done, care must be taken not to injure the phrenic nerve.

Mustard Procedure. General preparations are similar to those for the Senning procedure except that after opening the sternum and exposing the pericardium, a pericardial patch is harvested (Fig. 6). The patch is shaped in a trouser fashion. One leg (A to B) is tailored to be twice the diameter of the SVC. The other leg (C to D) is tailored to be twice the diameter of the IVC.

After the aorta is cross-clamped, a V-shaped incision as described by Barratt-Boyes is completed in the right atrium, and the wedge is carried well into the juncture of the right superior and inferior pulmonary veins (Fig. 7). This provides a generous opening for the pulmonary venous atrium.

The atrial septum is excised (Fig. 8). The right superior portion of the area of resected atrial wall is not reapproximated as was done in the past, because this is unnecessary unless the atrial wall is perforated during the septal excision. A coronary sinus cutback is performed routinely to enlarge the inferior vena cava pathway and to allow the suture line to be placed safely in the floor of the coronary sinus without injury to the atrioventricular node (Fig. 9). The pericardial patch is sewn into position, starting just above the left superior pulmonary veins

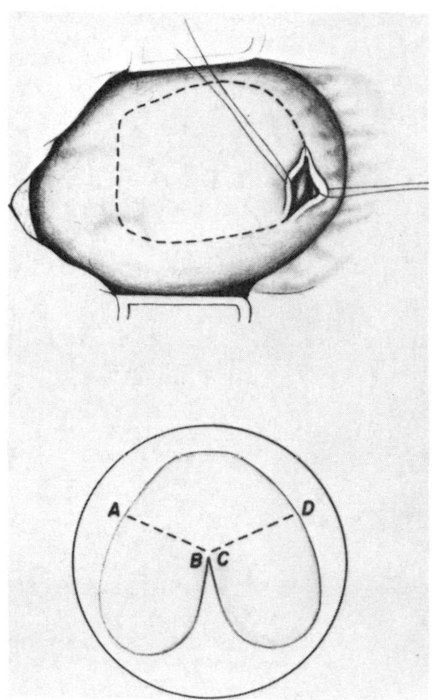

FIGURE 6. The pericardial patch is harvested. A to B and C to D are measured diameters twice the SVC and IVC, respectively.

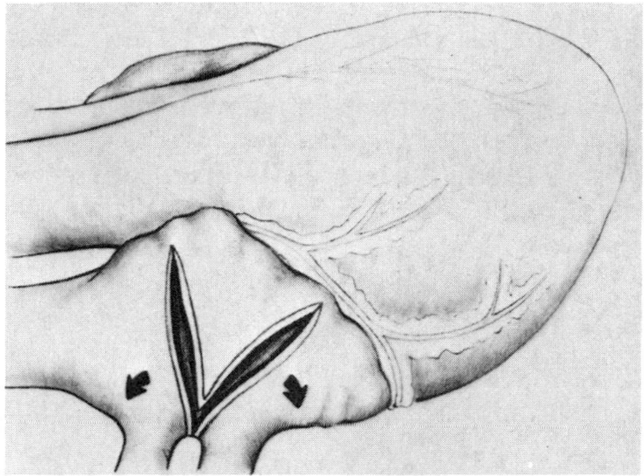

FIGURE 7. The right atrial incision is completed.

FIGURE 8. The atrial septum is excised along the edges as indicated by the dotted lines. Tissue is left in the area of the limbars medially to prevent damage to the SA node artery.

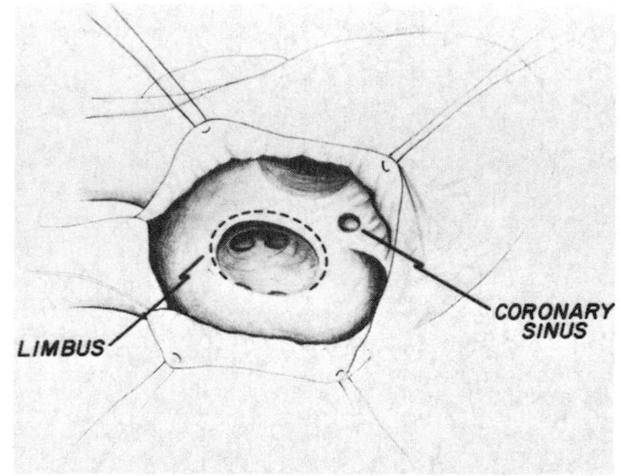

FIGURE 9. The coronary sinus is cut back carefully but well into the left atrium.

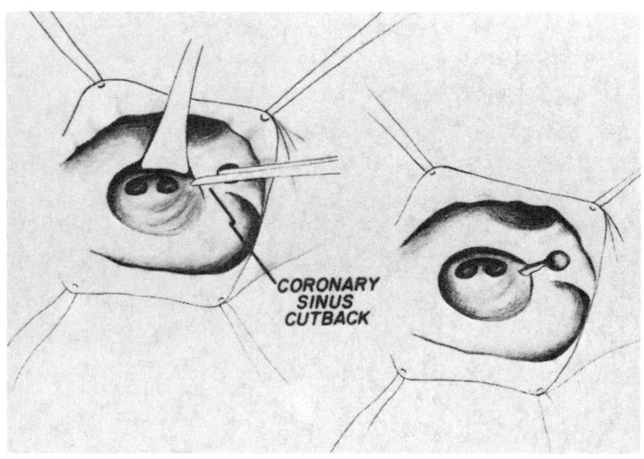

and just below the left atrial appendage (Fig. 10). Care should be taken to avoid narrowing the throat of the superior vena cava by being sure to run the suture line horizontally below the superior ridge of excised septum prior to crossing the intra-atrial ridge to enclose the superior vena cava. Once the baffle is completed (Fig. 11), the right atrial flap is advanced into the apex of the previously opened junction between the right superior and inferior pulmonary veins, much like a V-Y plasty (Fig. 12).

FIGURE 10. The pericardial patch is sewn into position, starting in the left atrium above the left pulmonary veins and below the left atrial appendage.

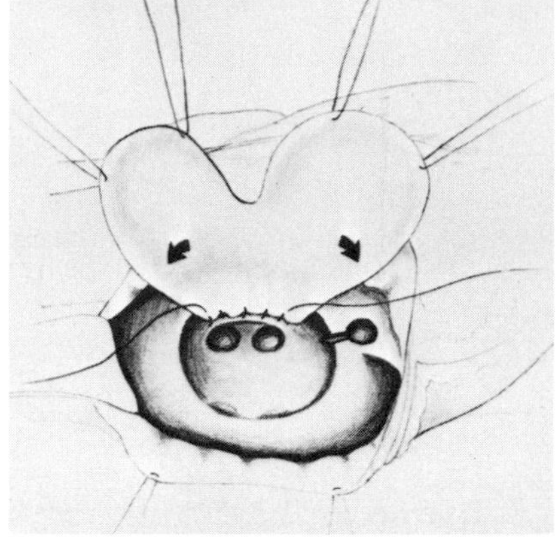

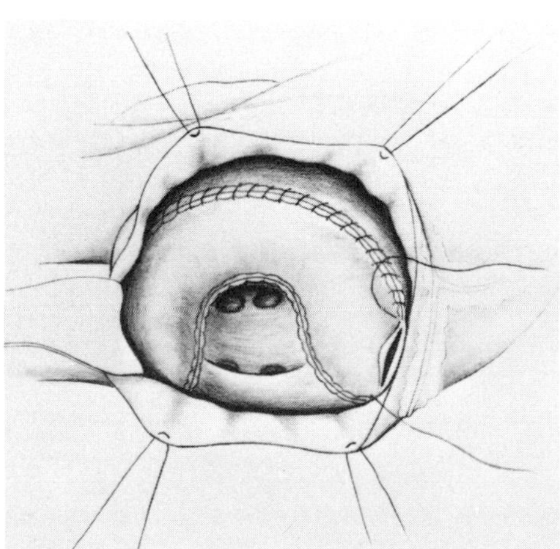

FIGURE 11. The venous tunnel is completed.

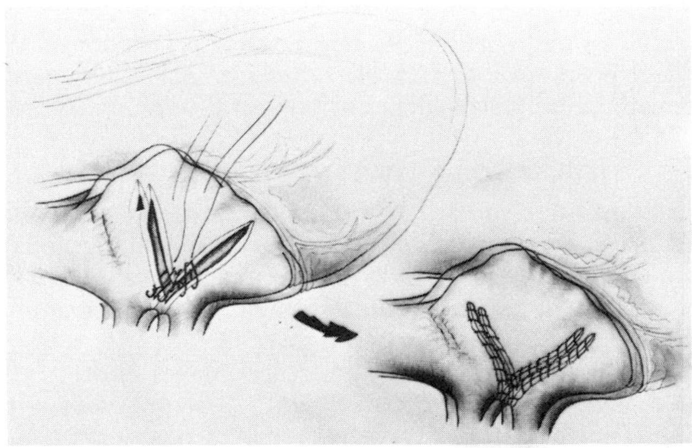

FIGURE 12. The right atrium (neo-left atrium) is reclosed in a V-Y fashion.

RESULTS

The results for complex procedures are not as good as they are for simple TGA-IVS. Therefore, one must keep in mind that the following discussion is directed toward simple transposition repair.

Operative Mortality. Through the years, the operative mortality for both the Mustard and the Senning procedures when performed for uncomplicated TGA in the first year of life has been similar (Tables 1 and 2). An early survival rate of greater than 90% should be expected in any major center experienced in these procedures.[10,23–32]

A recent study from the Congenital Heart Surgeons Society[33] encompassing 20 institutions analyzed the early mortality in simple TGA during an 18-month period from 1985 to June 1986 and found no deaths in 21 infants who underwent Mustard repair and 4 deaths in 35 infants who underwent a Senning repair (11% operative mortality). Granted this does not take into account the few children

TABLE 1. Early Mortality for Mustard Procedure in Simple TGA

Center	Patients	Mortality
LA Childrens (1975)	81	4.9%
Detroit Childrens (1979)	82	4.8%
Hospital for Sick Children, Toronto (1988)	100	1.0%
Boston Childrens (1977)	61	11.0%
Great Ormond Street, London (1980)	307	9.0%

TABLE 2. Early Mortality for Senning Procedure in Simple TGA

Center	Patients	Mortality
Great Ormond Street, London (1982)	44	0
Leiden (1980)	37	2.7%
Boston (1978)	57	5.0%
UCSF (1981)	16	0
Bergamo (1978)	23	0

who die either very early in life around the time of BAS or later while waiting for elective atrial switch repair. However, in the first instance they likely would not survive any procedure, and in the latter instance closer observation and earlier repair can reduce this incidence of preoperative mortality.

COMPLICATIONS FOLLOWING OPERATION

Complications following atrial switch procedures are common to both the Mustard and the Senning procedures and include systemic venous obstruction, pulmonary venous obstruction, dysrhythmias, tricuspid valve insufficiency, right ventricular dysfunction, and late death. Though individual institutional reports may suggest better results with one procedure or the other for each complication, the reality is that the occurrences are about the same for both.

Systemic Venous Pathway Obstruction. Systemic venous pathway obstruction is the most common form of vascular obstruction, and the most common systemic venous pathway obstruction is superior vena cava obstruction. Often this is asymptomatic secondary to decompression by the azygos vein. However, increased head circumference, bluish discoloration of upper body and head, and/or right chylothorax may be noted. The actual incidence following the Mustard procedure is probably 10–15%, although the range varies from 6% to nearly 50% (Table 3).[29,32,35] Age and size of the child at repair have been suggested as independent variables for caval obstruction by Barratt-Boyes et al.,[35] Stark et al.,[36] and Kron et al.[37] However, others have not found the incidence of caval obstruction to be any higher in infant repairs.[32] Baffle obstruction in the Mustard procedure is more likely due to type of material used (Dacron having a higher incidence of obstruction than pericardium), shape of the baffle, and technique of baffle placement along the cut superior septal edge (limbus). Reoperation for symptomatic caval obstruction (often involving both SVC and IVC) is necessary in only about 10–20% of patients with significant caval obstruction. The incidence of isolated inferior caval obstruction is quite low, being in the range of 1–3%.

This high incidence of superior vena cava obstruction caused several centers to switch to the Senning procedure in the late 1970s, and although the incidence of caval obstruction has been somewhat less, it is still significant (Table 3). In the Boston experience, it was 13%, and of these patients 40% required reoperation. Most likely improper surgical technique is the major factor responsible for baffle obstruction when it occurs, although the anatomy of the Mustard repair—particularly when the recently described Toronto technique is used, leaving a

TABLE 3. Systemic Venous Obstruction

Center	Procedure	Initial Operative Survivors	Percent Occurrence	Reoperation	Reop. Death
Toronto	Mustard	98	9	0	0
UCSF	Senning and Mustard	52	25	2/28	0
Boston	Mustard	59	54	11/59 (17%)	1/11
Boston	Senning	54	13	3/54 (5%)	2/3
Bergamo	Senning	45	0	0	0
Zurich	Senning	220	4	8/8 (100%)	0

superior septal ridge to protect the SA node artery—lends itself to a higher incidence of SVC obstruction.

Pulmonary Venous Obstruction. Although systemic venous obstruction can uncommonly be a very serious complication, pulmonary venous obstruction is often lethal. Fortunately, it is relatively uncommon (Table 4). In the Toronto experience, between 1976 and 1985, 3 of 115 children developed pulmonary venous obstruction following Mustard repair and two required reoperation. In the Detroit experience, 4 of 61 (6.5%) developed pulmonary venous obstruction following initial Mustard repair; two died following reoperation and one died without reoperation. In the Boston experience with the Senning procedure, 6 of 54 (11%) had pulmonary venous obstruction and 4 of 6 required reoperation, and one child died before a reoperation could be done. The Boston experience with the Mustard procedure was similar in that 6% developed pulmonary vascular obstruction and all required reoperation. The Bergamo group and the Leiden group reported no pulmonary venous obstruction in their early experience with the Senning procedure, but the Zurich group did report pulmonary venous obstruction in 4 of 220 patients following Senning repair, all of whom required reoperation. When pulmonary venous obstruction occurs, it is usually within the first postoperative year and is almost always symptomatic. Generally, it occurs secondary to shrinkage of prosthetic material used to enlarge the pulmonary venous atrium, and, therefore, this technique should be avoided if possible.

Early Postoperative Arrhythmias. Various types of dysrhythmias have been reported following the atrial switch procedure, including junctional rhythm, atrioventricular conduction abnormalities (including complete heart block), sick sinus syndrome, and ectopic tachyarrhythmias. The incidence of early postoperative rhythm disturbances has decreased through the years as technical modifications have accompanied better understanding of the electrical circuits within the heart and the vascular supply to SA and AV nodes. The Los Angeles Childrens Group[23] reduced their incidence of postoperative dysrhythmias following Mustard procedure from 65% to 43% in the mid-1970s by: (1) direct cannulation of the superior vena cava, avoiding pressure and torque on the SA node and its arterial blood supply, (2) sparing the leftward portion of the atrial septum during excision of the true atrial septum so that the integrity of the anterior internodal pathway could be preserved, and (3) excising the coronary sinus well into the left atrium and placing the baffle around the rim of the

TABLE 4. Pulmonary Venous Obstruction

Center	Procedure	Initial Operative Survivors	Percent Occurrence	Reoperation	Reop. Death
Toronto	Mustard	98	3	3/3 (100%)	1/3
Detroit	Mustard	61	6.5	2 (50%)	0
Boston	Mustard	59	6	4/4 (100%)	1/4
Boston	Senning	54	11*	4/6 (66%)	0/4
Bergamo	Senning	45	0	0	0
Leiden	Senning	25	0	0	0
Zurich	Senning	220	2	4/4 (100%)	0

* One child died before reoperation could be carried out.

coronary sinus portion to avoid the AV node (early 1970s). The Toronto group described their modification to protect the SA nodal artery and internodal pathway by leaving a rim of septum superiorly between the superior vena cava and the tricuspid valve, and, by the late 1970s, their incidence of early dysrhythmias had dropped from 35% to 11%.

The data on early dysrhythmias following Senning repair are similar. Deanfield et al. from Great Ormond Street, London[38] analyzed the cardiac rhythm in 46 survivors of the Mustard procedure and 54 survivors of the Senning procedure. Early dysrhythmias occurred equally in both groups. Eighty-four percent of the patients were in normal sinus rhythm at time of discharge. When postoperative patients were studied using Holter monitoring, the incidence of arrhythmias was found to be low, with ventricular premature contractions occurring in 20% of the simple Senning patients and 7% of the simple Mustard patients. Atrial premature contractions occurred in 7% of the Mustards and 4% of the Sennings. Supraventricular tachycardias occurred in less than 3% of the patients.

Late Postoperative Arrhythmias. In the same study,[38] at 5 to 8 years following operation, only 56% of children in the Senning group and only 66% of children in the Mustard group were in sinus rhythm. The majority of those not in sinus rhythm were in junctional rhythm. However, the incidence of active arrhythmias on Holter remained low. The Great Ormond Street group concluded that: (1) progressive loss of sinus rhythm occurs after intra-atrial repair of transposition by both the Mustard and Senning operations, despite modifications to surgical technique over the years. (However, they could not demonstrate the loss was associated with increase in either tachyarrhythmia morbidity or late mortality.) (2) Therefore, at present, the progressive loss of sinus rhythm should not be viewed as a powerful reason for abandoning intra-atrial repair.

Right Ventricular Dysfunction. Anatomically and physiologically, the right ventricle was designed to function in a low pressure system, and, when required to handle the job of the systemic ventricle for a lifetime, as it is with the atrial baffle procedure for TGA, eventual failure of the ventricle seems only reasonable. Nevertheless, with long-term follow-up the incidence of significant right ventricular dysfunction late after repair is relatively low, being about 10% in several series and similar with both the Mustard and Senning procedures.[27,39] Tricuspid valve incompetence is also low and more often is related to injury of the tricuspid valve at the time of operation, usually for closure of a VSD rather than inability to function long term in the systemic circulation.

Late Death (Sudden Death). Although the incidence is quite low, the majority of late deaths have occurred suddenly and, despite the suggestion to the contrary by the Great Ormond Street group, they are probably secondary to acute arrhythmias. The rest of the deaths are related to chronic congestive heart failure. The incidence of late death is about 1% per year. The long-term survival following the Mustard repair in Toronto[27] at 1 year, 10 years, and 20 years is 90%, 83%, and 80%, respectively, while the long-term survival for the Senning procedure is exactly the same for the Zurich group,[39] being 89% at 10 years and 82% at 20 years. Of those who survive long term, over 90% are in New York Heart Association (NYHA) functional class I, despite the type of procedure performed. Therefore, the general outlook for these children following repair is quite good. Long-term results like this are unknown for the arterial switch procedure.

CONCLUSIONS

To paraphrase Mark Twain, the reports of the death of the atrial baffle are greatly exaggerated. As can be seen from the excellent results in simple TGA repair, both the Mustard and the Senning procedures can be performed routinely by the majority of surgeons with an early operative mortality approaching less than 5%, low morbidity, and long-term survival at 20 years of approximately 80%. Although up to 10% of these children will develop systemic ventricular (right ventricular) dysfunction, the rest remain in NYHA class I and are asymptomatic. It is questionable whether this justifies the change away from a procedure that has such commendable results to a procedure that has high early operative mortality and for which long-term (20-year) follow-up is just not available. For those centers that still consider the atrial baffle as the procedure of choice, it will be difficult to convince them to change and, in fact, it would likely be unethical to force them to change to a procedure at this time that has a significant early learning curve mortality. The choice between Mustard or Senning is purely the surgeon's choice, and, despite the fact that technical consideration can be argued ad infinitum, results are similar, giving neither procedure the edge.

Finally, the use of the atrial switch procedure in infants with TGA and VSD is much more controversial. It is on this level that the results for the atrial baffle techniques and the arterial switch procedure more clearly approximate each other. In fact, it was this group of children with significant VSD in whom the interest in the arterial switch first began in the United States because the operative mortality was two or three times that for simple TGA and long-term results were much less encouraging. Time may give the advantage to the arterial switch for these less fortunate patients.

REFERENCES

1. Jatene AD, Fontes VF, Paulista PP, et al: Anatomic correction of transposition of the great vessels. J Thorac Cardiovasc Surg 72:360, 1976.
2. Blalock A, Hanlon CR: The surgical treatment of complete transposition of the aorta and the pulmonary artery. Surg Gynecol Obstet 90:1, 1950.
3. Albert HM: Surgical correction of transposition of the great vessels. Surg Forum 5:74, 1954.
4. Senning A: Surgical correction of transposition of the great vessels. Surgery 45:966, 1959.
5. Mustard WT: Successful two stage correction of transposition of the great vessels. Surgery 55:469, 1964.
6. Rashkind WJ, Miller WM: Creation of an atrial septal defect without thoracotomy: A palliative approach to complete transposition of the great arteries. JAMA 196:992, 1966.
7. Blalock H, Hanlon CR: The surgical treatment of complete transposition of the aorta and pulmonary artery. Surg Gynecol Obstet 90:1, 1950.
8. Edwards WS, Bargeron LM Jr: More effective palliation of transposition of the great vessels. J Thorac Cardiovasc Surg 49:790, 1965.
9. Vlad P, Lambert EC: Late results of Rashkind's balloon atrial septostomy in transposition. In Kirklin JW (ed): Advances in Cardiovascular Surgery. New York, Grune and Stratton, 1973, pp 29–36.
10. Trusler GA, Williams WG, Izukawa T, Olley PM: Current results with the Mustard operation in isolated transposition of the great arteries. J Thorac Cardiovasc Surg 80:381, 1980.
11. Quaegebeur JM, Rohmer J, Brom AG: Revival of the Senning operation in the treatment of transposition of the great arteries. Thorax 32:517, 1977.
12. Van Praagh R, Vlad P, Keith JD: Complete transposition of the great arteries. In Keith JD, Rowe RD, Vlad P (eds): Heart Disease in Infancy and Childhood, 2nd ed. New York, Macmillan, 1967, p 682.
13. Anderson RH, Becker AE, Tucchese FE, et al: Morphology of Congenital Heart Disease. New York, Annuity Park Press, 1983, Ch. 6.
14. Fyler DC: Report of the New England regional infants cardiac program. Pediatrics 65:375, 1980.

15. Norfeld EA, Paul MM, Mustin AJ, Idriss FS: Pulmonary vascular disease in complete transposition of the great arteries: A study of 200 patients. Am J Cardiol 34:75, 1974.
16. Forey C, Greco JM, Libi-Sylvia M: Variability of pulmonary vascular disease in certain malformations of the heart. In Kidd BSL, Keith JD (eds): The Natural History and Progressive Treatment of Congenital Heart Defects. Springfield, IL, Charles C Thomas, 1971, p 300.
17. Clarkson PM, Nantze JM, Warchill JC, Barratt-Boyes BG: The pulmonary vascular bed in patients with complete transposition of the great arteries. Circulation 53:539, 1976.
18. Planth WH Jr, Naclas AS, Bernhard WF, Fyler DC: Changing hemodynamics in patients with transposition of the great arteries. Circulation 42:131, 1970.
19. Dakier JB, Stanger P, Heymann MA, et al: Early onset of pulmonary vascular obstruction in patients with cardiopulmonary transposition and intact ventricular septum. Circulation 51:875, 1975.
20. Kidd BSL: Complete transposition of the great arteries. In Heart Disease in Infancy and Childhood. New York, MacMillan, 1978, p 590.
21. Kirklin JW, Barratt-Boyes BG: Transposition of the great arteries. In Kirklin JW, Barratt-Boyes BG (eds): Cardiac Surgery. New York, John Wiley and Sons, 1986, Ch. 39.
22. Levinsky L, Srinwasan V, Alvarez-Diaz F, Subramanian S: Reconstruction of the new atrial septum in the Senning operation: New technique. J Thorac Cardiovasc Surg 81:131, 1981.
23. Lewis AG, Lindesmith GF, Takahashi M, et al: Cardiac rhythm following the Mustard procedure for transposition of the great vessel. J Thorac Cardiovasc Surg 73:919, 1977.
24. Takahashi M, Lindesmith FG, Lewis AB, et al: Long term results of the Mustard procedure. Circulation 56(II):85, 1977.
25. Arciniegas E, Farooki ZQ, Hakimi M, et al: Results of the Mustard operation for dextro-transposition of the great arteries. J Thorac Cardiovasc Surg 81:580, 1981.
26. Trusler GA, Williams WG, Izukawa T, Olley PM: Current results with the Mustard operation in isolated transposition of the great arteries. J Thorac Cardiovasc Surg 80:381, 1980.
27. Williams WG, Trusler GA, Kirklin JW, et al: Early and late results of a protocol for simple transposition leading to an atrial switch (Mustard) repair. J Thorac Cardiovasc Surg 95:717, 1988.
28. Egloff LP, Freed MD, Dick M, et al: Early and late results with the Mustard operation in infancy. Ann Thorac Surg 26:474, 1978.
29. Marx GR, Hougen TS, Norwood WI, et al: Transposition of the great arteries with intact ventricular septum: Results of Mustard and Senning operations in 123 consecutive patients. J Am Coll Cardiol 1:476, 1983.
30. Stark J: Concordant transposition-Mustard operation. In Surgery for Congenital Heart Defects. London, Grune & Stratton, Ltd., 1983, p 331.
31. Pacifico AD: Concordant transposition-Senning operation. In Surgery for Congenital Heart Defects. London, Grune & Stratton, Ltd., 1983, p 345.
32. Mahony L, Turley K, Ebert P, Heymann MA: Long term results after atrial repair of transposition of the great arteries in early infancy. Circulation 66:253, 1982.
33. Parenzan L, Locatelli G, Altieri G, et al: The Senning operation for transposition of the great arteries. J Thorac Cardiovasc Surg 76:305, 1978.
34. Castaneda AR, Trusler GA, Paul MH, Blackstone EH, Kirklin JW, and the Congenital Heart Surgeons Society: The early results of treatment of simple transposition in the current era. J Thorac Cardiovasc Surg 95:14, 1988.
35. Clarkson PM, Neutze JM, Barratt-Boyes BG, et al: Late postoperative hemodynamic results and cineangiocardiographic findings after Mustard atrial baffle repair for transposition of the great arteries. Circulation 53:525, 1976.
36. Stark J, Silove ED, Taylor JFN, Graham GR: Obstruction to systemic venous return following the Mustard operation for transposition of the great arteries. J Thorac Cardiovasc Surg 68:742, 1974.
37. Kron IL, Rheuban KS, Joob AW, et al: Baffle obstruction following the Mustard operation: Cause and treatment. Ann Thorac Surg 39:112, 1985.
38. Deanfield J, Camm J, Macartney F, et al: Arrhythmia and late mortality after Mustard and Senning operation for transposition of the great arteries. J Thorac Cardiovasc Surg 96:569, 1988.
39. Turina M, Siebenmann R, Nussbaumer P, Senning A: Long term outlook after atrial correction of transposition of great arteries. J Thorac Cardiovasc Surg 95:828, 1988.

L. DOUGLAS COWGILL, MD

ATRIAL ISOMERISM

From the Department of Surgery
Dean Clinic
Madison, Wisconsin

Reprint requests to:
L. Douglas Cowgill, MD
Department of Surgery
Dean Clinic
1313 Fish Hatchery Rd.
Madison, WI 53715

The usual disposition of the viscera is termed situs solitus, while mirror-imaging of thoracic and abdominal viscera results in situs inversus. When normally asymmetrical organs such as liver and stomach, or paired organs such as lungs and cardiac atria develop symmetrically, Van Mierop and associates[1] introduced the term "situs ambiguus." If the lungs and atria have a right-sided pattern, right isomerism is present, and is associated with asplenia. A left-sided pattern is associated with polysplenia (left isomerism). Because of their common association with major cardiac defects, a brief discussion of their patterns is provided. It is worth noting that exceptions to the correspondences of atrial with thoracic isomerism, as well as exceptions to correspondence of atrial/thoracic with abdominal visceral morphology, may occur.[2,3] Considerable disagreement also has arisen over the proper designation of the atria in the presence of situs ambiguus, ranging from one view that the atria cannot be properly named in this situation,[4] to another that an atrial septum is necessary for precise identification,[3,5] with the most popular view being that the atria may be defined solely on the basis of atrial appendage morphology.[1,2,5,6]

RIGHT ISOMERISM

The lungs typically, but not always, have three lobes bilaterally with relatively short mainstem bronchi that are posterior and superior (eparterial) to the main pulmonary artery.[7,8] Abdominally, the liver is symmetrical and horizontal, the stomach tends to be near the midline, and the spleen is absent.[6]

The right-sidedness is also reflected in the atrial appendages, which are blunt with a broad junction with the smooth-walled atrium. A prominent muscle band protrudes from the appendage into the cavity of the chamber, the crista terminalis.[9] The conduction tissue is abnormal, usually with bilateral sinus nodes.[10] Two AV nodes may also be present, with a sling of conduction tissue between them.

Associated anomalies are multiple and complex. Extracardiac forms, often obstructed, of total anomalous pulmonary venous return occur frequently[9] and affect the natural history and surgical mortality very significantly.[11] Anomalous systemic venous return, including interrupted inferior vena cava and bilateral superior vena cava, occurs occasionally but not as frequently as with left isomerism. Common atrium and AV canal defects occur in about 95% of patients, and about half have a single ventricular chamber.[6,12,13] An intact ventricular septum is very uncommon. Severe pulmonary stenosis or atresia is nearly always present, so that most patients are cyanotic, also contributing importantly to the dire natural history. Ventricular discordance (transposition) or double-outlet right ventricle is also common.

Over one-third of untreated patients with right isomerism die of cardiac causes in the first week of life, and about 80% die by the end of 1 year.[13] In addition to the severe cardiac anomalies, an increased susceptibility to infection from the asplenic state is present.[12]

LEFT ISOMERISM

The lungs are usually bi-lobed with relatively long main-stem bronchi that are anterior and inferior (hyparterial) to the pulmonary artery. The abdominal organs tend less toward symmetry than in asplenia.[6] The stomach is seldom midline, the liver often has a major portion to one side, and considerable abdominal heterotaxia (e.g., malrotation) may be present. Multiple spleens are usually situated adjacent to the stomach, resembling a cluster of grapes or a bi-lobed or tri-lobed spleen.[6,13,14] Biliary atresia occurs with some frequency in cases of polysplenia.[15]

The atrial appendages are long and thin with constrictions along their length.[9] The junction with the smooth portion of atrium is more constricted than in right isomerism, and a crista terminalis is not present. The sinus node is hypoplastic and abnormally located, whereas the atrioventricular bundle arises from either a solitary AV node (with a D-loop ventricular arrangement) or paired AV nodes (with L-loop [ventricular inversion] or univentricular hearts).[10] Complete heart block is common with left isomerism.[16]

Major cardiac anomalies occur in over half of patients, with anomalies of systemic venous return (bilateral superior vena cava, interrupted inferior vena cava with azygos continuation) being especially common.[12,14] Conversely, extracardiac total anomalous pulmonary venous connection is rare. About one-half of patients have common atrium and other types of AV canal defects, and while single ventricle occurs in only 15%, double-outlet right ventricle is common.[12] Although pulmonary stenosis is not nearly as common as with asplenia (thus patients are less frequently cyanotic), obstructive lesions of the morphologic left side of the heart (valvular or subvalvular aortic stenosis, coarctation, mitral stenosis, cor triatriatum) occur in one form or another in over 50%.[14] Ventricular septal defects and absent coronary sinus are also frequent.

Since not all patients with polysplenia have cardiac anomalies, prognosis is better than for asplenia. Nevertheless 50% of patients in one series died by 4 months of age, and 75% before age 5.[14]

DIAGNOSIS

Thoracic isomerism is best identified by posteroantertior (PA) and lateral chest x-rays. The PA projection determines the relative lengths of main-stem bronchi, with L/R ratios of 1.5 or less supporting thoracic isomerism, while ratios of 2 or greater indicate thoracic lateralism. Bilateral short bronchi suggest right isomerism, whereas long bronchi suggest left isomerism. The lateral projection determines the relationship of the main bronchus with the pulmonary artery, an anterior inferior bronchus consistent with left isomerism and a posterior superior bronchus consistent with right isomerism.[1,7,12,17,18]

The most helpful laboratory test is the presence of Howell-Jolly bodies in routine blood smear, indicating asplenia. Atrial situs may be determined indirectly by thoracic and abdominal information from two-dimensional echocardiogram.[19] For example, interrupted inferior vena cava with azygos continuation suggests polysplenia.

MANAGEMENT

Patients with atrial isomerism, especially right-sided, frequently have complex inoperable problems, and until recently surgical endeavors have been infrequent. Some of the issues, particularly related to cyanotic lesions associated with obstructed total anomalous pulmonary venous return, are discussed in the first chapter and will not be repeated here.

Three general reviews are recommended for surgical principles of atrial isomerism.[12,20,21] In addition, specific problems associated with asplenia and polysplenia have been discussed in detail by many others.[11,22-26] According to Marcelletti et al.[20] the following major principles guide management:

1. Appropriate surgical palliation is probably the option of choice as initial treatment of symptomatic patients with cardiac defects associated with isomerism (an important subgroup to exclude are those with obstructed total anomalous pulmonary venous drainage, in whom shunts alone have very poor results,[11,26] as discussed in Chapter 1).
2. Anatomical repair should be offered at an appropriate age to patients with intracardiac anomalies that are correctable using techniques of proven efficacy.
3. Fontan correction should be considered for patients with restricted pulmonary blood flow who have two atria and two AV valves, or two atria and atresia of the right AV valve, whose ventricular anatomy precludes anatomical repair.
4. Patients whose anatomy would require atrial septation or ventricular exclusion using a large complex prosthetic patch along with an atriopulmonary conduit should probably be treated by initial or repeated palliative operations. When complex atrial baffles are used in Fontan repairs, the importance of avoiding obstruction to either systemic or pulmonary venous drainage is paramount.[12,21]

REFERENCES

1. Van Mierop LHS, Eisen S, Schiebler GL: The radiographic appearance of the tracheobronchial tree as an indicator of visceral situs. Am J Cardiol 26:432, 1970.
2. Caruso G, Becker AE: How to determine atrial situs? Considerations initiated by 3 cases of absent spleen with a discordant anatomy between bronchi and atria. Br Heart J 41:559, 1979.
3. Lev M, Liberthson RR, Eckner FAP, Arcille RA: Pathologic anatomy of dextrocardia and its clinical implications. Circulation 37:979, 1968.

4. Van Praagh R: Terminology of congenital heart disease. Circulation 56:139–143, 1977.
5. de Tommasi SM, Daliento L, Ho SY, et al: Analysis of atrioventricular junction, ventricular mass, and ventriculoarterial junction in 43 specimens with atrial isomerism. Br Heart J 45:236, 1981.
6. Stanger P, Rudolph AM, Edwards JE: Cardiac malpositions. Circulation 56:159, 1977.
7. Landing BH, Lawrence TK, Payne VC, Wells TR: Bronchial anatomy in syndromes with abnormal visceral situs, abnormal spleen and congenital heart disease. Am J Cardiol 128:456, 1971.
8. Partridge MC, Scott O, Deverall PD, Macartney FJ: Visualization and measurement of the main bronchi by tomography as an objective indicator of thoracic situs in congenital heart disease. Circulation 51:188, 1975.
9. Macartney FJ, Zuberbuhler JR, Anderson RH: Morphological considerations pertaining to recognition of atrial isomerism: Consequences for sequential chamber localization. Br Heart J 44:657, 1980.
10. Dickinson DF, Wilkinson JL, Anderson KR, et al: The cardiac conduction system in situs ambiguus. Circulation 59:879, 1979.
11. De Donato R, di Carlo D, Squitieri C, et al: Palliation of cardiac malformations associated with right isomerism (asplenia syndrome) in infancy. Ann Thorac Surg 44:35, 1987.
12. Kirklin JW, Barratt-Boyes BG: Atrial isomerism. In Cardiac Surgery. New York, John Wiley & Sons, 1986, pp.1333–1344.
13. Rose V, Izukawa T, Moes CAF: Syndrome of asplenia and polysplenia: A review of cardiac and non-cardiac malformations in 60 cases with special reference to diagnosis and prognosis. Br Heart J 37:840, 1975.
14. Peoples WM, Moller JH, Edwards JE: Polysplenia: A review of 146 cases. Pediatr Cardiol 4:129, 1983.
15. Chandra RS: Biliary atresia and other structural anomalies in the congenital polysplenia syndrome. J Pediatr 85:649, 1974.
16. Garcia OL, Mehta AV, Pickoff AS, Tamer DF, et al: Left isomerism and complete atrioventricular block: A report of 6 cases. Am J Cardiol 48:1103, 1981.
17. Soto B, Pacifico AD, Souza AS Jr, et al: Identification of thoracic isomerism from the plain chest radiograph. Am J Roentgenol 131:995, 1978.
18. Deanfield J, Leanage R, Stroobant J, et al: Use of high kilovoltage filtered beam radiographs for detection of bronchial situs in infants and young children. Br Heart J 44:577, 1980.
19. Huhta JC, Smallhorn JF, Macartney FJ: Two-dimensional echocardiographic diagnosis of situs. Br Heart J 48:97, 1982.
20. Marcelletti C, Di Donato R, Nijveld A, et al: Right and left isomerism: The cardiac surgeon's view. Ann Thorac Surg 35:400, 1983.
21. Pacifico AD, Fox LS, Kirklin JW, Bargeron LM: Surgical treatment of atrial isomerism. In Anderson RH, et al (eds): Paediatric Cardiology, 5th ed. London, Churchill Livingstone, 1983, p. 223.
22. Turley K, Tarnoff H, Snider R, Ebert P: Repair of combined total anomalous pulmonary venous connection and anomalous systemic venous connection. Ann Thorac Surg 31:70, 1981.
23. Ando F, Shirotani H, Kawai J, et al: Successful total repair of complicated cardiac anomalies with asplenia syndrome. J Thorac Cardiovasc Surg 72:33, 1976.
24. Kawashima Y, Kitamura S, Matsuda H, et al: Total cavopulmonary shunt operation in complex cardiac anomalies. J Thorac Cardiovasc Surg 87:74, 1984.
25. Pillai R, Lima R, Anderson RH, et al: Surgical correction in mirror-image atrial arrangement or left atrial isomerism with systemic venous return to the left-sided atrium. J Thorac Cardiovasc Surg 86:288, 1983.
26. De Leon SY, Gidding SS, Ilbawi MN, et al: Surgical management of infants with complex cardiac anomalies associated with reduced pulmonary blood flow and total anomalous pulmonary venous drainage. Ann Thorac Surg 43:207, 1987.

DAVID N. CAMPBELL, MD
DAVID R. CLARKE, MD

AORTIC AND PULMONARY ALLOGRAFTS

A Realistic Appraisal of Their Role in the Surgical Management of Congenital Heart Disease in 1989

From the Department of Surgery
Section of Cardiovascular Surgery
University of Colorado Health
Sciences Center
Denver, Colorado

Reprint requests to:
David N. Campbell, MD
Section of Cardiovascular Surgery
University of Colorado Health
Sciences Center
4200 East Ninth Avenue
Denver, CO 80262

In theory, allografts come very close to fulfilling all the qualities one would like to see in the ideal native valve replacement. Clearly, the allograft is virtually free from thromboembolism, has essentially no transvalvular gradient, resists infection better than mechanical valves, and has a low incidence of valve regurgitation. Unfortunately, availability and durability remain a problem. Small sizes are quite difficult to obtain. These allografts degenerate over time, and in the pediatric population, the rate of degeneration leading to valve failure or conduit dysfunction may be quite rapid. Advocates of the allograft point to the latest evolution in the preservation of human valves, cryopreservation, as the second coming. The question of lasting tissue viability remains at the heart of the matter, and, although reports from O'Brien[1] and Angell[2] suggest better long-term function with cryopreserved valves and valve conduits, cautious optimism is warranted at this time.

HISTORICAL PERSPECTIVE

Early laboratory work with allograft valves began in Detroit in 1952 when Lam[3] placed allograft aortic valves in the descending aorta of dogs. The results were poor because the leaflets became fibrotic. In 1953, Ross at Guy's Hospital in London repeated these studies and demonstrated that the reason Lam's research failed probably had to do with the fact that the valve leaflets were nonfunctional. In Ross' studies, the cusps remained intact but only when the valve had to function with a pulsatile workload (i.e., the native aortic valve was destroyed).[4]

The first successful clinical application of this technique came in 1956 when Murray[5] in Toronto inserted fresh aortic allografts into the descending aortas of three patients with aortic insufficiency. However, it was not until 1962, when Ross[6] and Barratt-Boyes[7] simultaneously in different parts of the world successfully implanted free-sewn aortic allografts in the subcoronary position, that the modern era of orthotopic allograft use in cardiac surgery began in earnest. Ross and colleagues used the single suture layer technique described by Gunning and Duran,[8] whereas Barratt-Boyes used the now-standard double suture line technique.

In 1966, Ross and Somerville[9] introduced the use of aortic valved allograft conduits for reconstruction of the right ventricular outflow tract. This pioneering effort led to extensive use of aortic allograft conduits in the complete repair of many complex congenital cardiac lesions over the next few years. However, by 1972 the enthusiasm for the allograft valved conduit began to lessen when Moodie at the Mayo Clinic[10] reported the intermediate results of 128 patients undergoing aortic allograft reconstruction of the right ventricular outflow tract. Among hospital survivors, the incidence of reoperation for conduit obstruction was 28% at 5 years and 59% at 10 years as indicated by later follow-up.[11] The Mayo Clinic and other centers in the United States[12] switched to the Dacron conduit with a porcine xenograft at that time. Reasons for the abandonment of allografts included long-term degenerative changes leading to wall calcification and valve stenosis, difficulty with graft procurement, sterilization and storage, and primary lack of allograft uniformity. While the major centers in the United States switched to the Dacron conduit, the Europeans mostly out of necessity continued to use the aortic allografts with somewhat variable but reasonably good results.

In 1972, Ross[13-15] began using aortic root replacement with reimplantation of the coronary arteries for infected aortic roots and associated annular abscesses. From there the procedure was adapted to its use in enlargement of congenital tunnel subvalvar and small annulus aortic stenosis. Clarke et al.[16] further modified the technique in combination with the ideas of Rastan and Konno,[17-19] and, in 1985, introduced the concept of extended aortic root replacement for the correction of complex left ventricular outflow obstruction.

The rekindling of interest in homograft conduits for use in right ventricular outflow tract reconstruction began in 1983 when Ross inserted the first pulmonary allograft for reconstruction of the right ventricular outflow tract. The results with this have been excellent,[20-22] and the number of grafts available for correction of congenital defects (either left- or right-sided) has essentially doubled. Pulmonary valved allografts are now the conduit of choice for right ventricular outflow tract reconstruction in congenital heart surgery.

PROCUREMENT AND PRESERVATION

Why have the results of these various reports been so different? The answer initially appears quite simple—variable cell viability. Angell[2,23,24] suggested early on that leaflet viability, i.e., cell viability, was the principal determinant of long-term allograft durability. Barratt-Boyes[25] took a slightly different point of view and presented evidence to suggest that the ground substance (i.e., matrix of the leaflet), including the acid mucopolysaccharides, collagen, and elastin, was more important.

If this material was destroyed, ingrowth of host tissue to form a new matrix could not occur, and the valve would become insufficient. Regardless of which view is more correct, and likely both are contributory, the idea became well established that anything that decreased cell or ground substance viability was detrimental to long-term function of the allograft.

The early experience with homografts clinically in cardiac surgery involved use of "fresh" allografts harvested post mortem often under nonsterile conditions, so that the amount of warm ischemia time was somewhat variable. The grafts were stored at 4° C in tissue culture (nutrient) medium, and the length of storage varied but attempts were made to utilize the valves before 31 days. Early attempts at sterilization included chemical means such as formalin, ethylene oxide, or beta propiolactone. Gamma irradiation was also used as well as freeze drying in the mid-1960s. However, all of these methods led to donor fibroblast and endothelial cell death and disruption of the ground substance. Leaflet thinning, perforation, and/or calcification occurred, and the valve failure rate was higher than that seen with the "fresh" viable allografts used initially without mechanical sterilization.[25]

In 1968, Barratt-Boyes introduced the concept of antibiotic immersion.[25] He continued to collect the allografts unsterilely at autopsy but abandoned chemical sterilization methods for antibiotic sterilization. Initially, the valves were maintained in Hanks solution with PSKA (penicillin 50 mg/ml, streptomycin 1000 mg/ml, kanamycin 1000 mg/ml, and amphotericin 25 mg/ml) at 4° C for eight days. Over the next few years, it became apparent from various studies carried out at Green Lane Hospital that the concentration of antibiotic solution was too strong and damaged the cells and ground substance, so that ingrowth of tissue from the host or possibly maintenance of donor tissue could not occur. Therefore, the concentration, time in contact with the solution, and the solution composition itself were changed in 1983[26,27] to a less toxic mix. CLPVA (cefoxitin 240 mg/ml, lincomycin 120 mg/ml, polymyxin B 100 mg/ml, vancomycin 50 mg/ml, amphotericin B 25 mg/ml) is now the standard antibiotic solution used by most groups, and the solution contact time has been cut to under 48 hours.

As mentioned earlier, the method of procurement of these grafts is also quite important. The longer the warm ischemic time, the less the cell viability. Yankah et al.[28,29] showed rapid dropout of cell viability after 2 hours at room temperature. If the grafts were placed at 4° C, less than 30% of the fibroblasts are viable after 2 weeks of storage and endothelial cells were nonexistent by one week. Age of the donor was also important in that donors over the age of 45–50 had much higher incidence of cusp deterioration; therefore, valves should not be used from donors over this age.[30]

These data suggest that the best method for harvesting the allografts is either from a living, brain-dead donor or from the recipient heart after it is removed for orthotopic cardiac transplantation. With the increasing popularity of orthotopic cardiac transplantation, it is increasingly more difficult to obtain living, brain-dead, donor explants except in smaller children. Obviously, warm ischemia time is minimized by either of these means of procurement, but if only these are utilized, then a significant source of valved allografts will be lost. Autopsy allografts are acceptable, but they should be harvested less than 6–12 hours after death if at all possible. Conditions of retrieval should be as sterile as possible, but it is understood that absolute sterility will be nearly impossible. Given that 95% of these allografts can still be sterilized with antibiotic immersion for 24–48 hours, breaks in sterile technique are not irreversible.

Though procurement continues to be a problem, the more significant problem is long-term availability of a wide range of allografts. Angell[24] in 1973 and O'Brien[1] in 1975 clinically began to address this problem with the use of cryopreservation. The techniques of these two groups are similar for cryopreservation, and although several other centers around the world maintain their own cryopreservation units along with storage banks, the majority of centers now rely on Cryolife, Inc. in Marietta, Georgia for the services of removing the allografts from the hearts, processing the allografts, sterilization, and controlled-rate freezing in pouches that can be sent back to those centers that have their own storage units or kept in storage in Cryolife's central bank.

The technique of cryopreservation is similar to that utilized by Karp et al. previously at the University of Alabama at Birmingham. After antibiotic immersion for 8–24 hours with CLPVA, the tissue is placed in nutrient media (calf serum) with 10% dimethyl sulfoxide (DMSO) and frozen at a regulated rate (1° per minute) to a final liquid nitrogen storage temperature of −196° C. This markedly increases the shelf availability of all types and sizes of allografts.

IMMUNE RESPONSE

Little is known at the present time about the antigenicity of the human valve allograft. Early researchers[31,32] working with freeze-dried allograft valves noted the virtual absence of rejection. Mohri's ingenious canine study in 1967[33] suggested that the aortic valve itself has low antigenicity, particularly in the subcoronary position, a site which he felt was "privileged," i.e., protected from the immune response. McKenzie[34] and Hirsch and Hanke,[35] working with canine allografts as well, reported leaflet thickening, cellular infiltration, development of granulation tissue, fibrin deposition, and eventual fibrosis. Korns[36] in 1971, using a canine aortic valve model, confirmed the earlier work in calves of Baue et al.[37] and suggested that immunologic rejection does occur and that the leaflet thickening and fibrosis were in fact evidence of chronic rejection and not structural injury due to the procedure.

Buck and Angell[38] in the same year presented an elegant study in which a trileaflet valve was constructed and placed long term in 12 dogs in the mitral position. These dogs were sacrificed at various intervals up to 1 year. Each valve had one leaflet as an autograft (from the native mitral valve). The second leaflet was an allograft aortic leaflet from another dog, and the third leaflet was an aortic xenograft (porcine). Buck and Angell found that all leaflets exhibited leaflet thickening in the first few days. They attributed this reactive hyperplasia to the effects of abnormal forces on the connective tissue in the leaflets in the mitral position. However, degenerative changes with endothelial destruction occurred later in the allograft and xenograft and were not seen in the autograft. They believed this to be the result of chronic rejection, and they therefore cautioned against the use of ABO-incompatible allografts.

Karp[39] in 1975 tried to define the exact immune response, if in fact it did exist, that was responsible for immunologic valve failure. He looked for a direct relationship between ABO incompatibility and unsuccessful aortic valve allotransplantation in a selected group of patients undergoing this procedure at UAB between 1968 and 1973. No relationship was found. Karp surmised that ABO compatibility was not necessary for avoidance of the immune response and a successful outcome. In his long-term follow-up of over 300 aortic valve replacement procedures, O'Brien[1] reconfirmed this when he noted that blood mismatch and rhesus mismatch were not associated with increased risk of valve degeneration.

For this reason, some workers in the field believed that the technique of cryopreservation in some way altered the immune response. New information recently presented at the Association for Academic Surgery in Salt Lake City in 1988 would suggest that this is not true. Cochran[40] used a rat model to show that cryopreservation does not alter allograft value antigenicity and recommended that ABO compatibility be honored whenever possible. The reasons for the difference between the laboratory response and the clinical data are unknown.

Perhaps the fate of the endothelial cell during procurement, sterilization, and storage either with cryopreservation or in nutrient medium at 4°C becomes increasingly important. Fibroblasts survive but endothelial cells rapidly become nonviable. Would less degeneration occur to the allograft if the endothelial cells could be better preserved? This is unknown. More likely a greater immunologic response would be mounted to the endothelial cell, a cell that is significantly more active in expression of histocompatibility antigen on the cell membrane.[41] Yacoub[42] in London and Clarke in Denver[43] have raised the question of immunosuppression because recent work indicates that Class I antigens *are* localized to the endothelial cells and *are* targets for the immune response.[44] However, in Yacoub's study[42] of limited immunosuppression using 3 months of steroids and azathioprine after implant of a valve allograft, no difference in intermediate results was noted. He felt that current knowledge did not support the additional risk of immunosuppression to these patients at this time.

PATIENT POPULATION AND SURGICAL TECHNIQUES

Free-sewn Aortic Valve Graft. The technique for free-sewn aortic allograft placement has been previously described in *Cardiac Surgery: State of the Art Reviews* by Sugimoto and Karp[45] and shall not be covered in this chapter. Instead, the technique of extended aortic root replacement and pulmonary allograft reconstruction of the right ventricular outflow tract will be illustrated.

Extended Aortic Root Replacement. In Denver, 21 patients (almost all children) have undergone extended aortic root replacement in the last 3 years. All have had complex left ventricular outflow tract obstruction with various combinations of obstruction including subvalvar, valvar, and supravalvar. In all instances, either severe subvalvar obstruction (tunnel type) or small native annulus was present, making the use of aortic root replacement alone unacceptable. Aortic valve allografts are selected prior to surgery using a weight–internal diameter table. Most patients over 12 kg have an adult-sized aortic conduit placed. (Average internal diameter is around 19 mm.) The patient is prepared for cannulation in standard fashion with two venous right-angled cannulae. After bypass is initiated, the aorta is cross-clamped high on the ascending aorta, and blood cardioplegia is used to protect the myocardium.

Preparation of the allograft is quite important. It is thawed in the transport and storage pouch in a 37°C water bath for 20–25 minutes. After thawing it is carefully rinsed in three successive sterile basins of fetal calf serum with decreasing amounts of DMSO. At the same time the allograft is inspected carefully for evidence of damage to the tissue, including tears or breaks in the aorta itself or leaflet disruption of the aortic valve.

The heart is prepared in a similar fashion to the Konno aortoventriculoplasty previously described.[46] A vertical incision is carried in an oblique fashion from the ascending aorta just above the right coronary artery to the left of the right coronary orifice, and the aortic annulus is transected as the right ventricular outflow tract

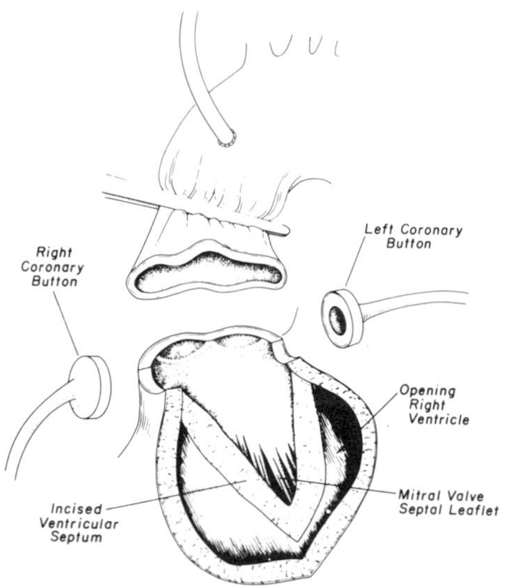

FIGURE 1. The heart is prepared in similar fashion to the aortoventriculoplasty except that the aorta is transected above the aortic valve annulus and coronary buttons are created to sew into the allograft.

is incised just below the pulmonary valve, again in an oblique fashion. The septum is incised vertically to relieve the usually-present tunnel-type muscular obstruction. Preparation is then completed by transecting the ascending aorta, fashioning coronary artery buttons for reimplantation, and removing the aortic leaflets (Fig. 1).

The aortic root is reconstructed by anastomosing the base of the aortic allograft below the valve to the native aortic annulus. The mitral valve leaflet is anchored anteriorly into the septal groove in order to leave the left ventricular outflow tract widely patent (Fig. 2). The coronary artery buttons are sewn into place, first the left then the right. The distal anastomosis is completed after the distal end of the allograft is fashioned to join the ascending aorta. The aortic cross-clamp is removed, and as rewarming is carried out, air is cleared out of the left ventricle and the right ventricular outflow tract is reconstructed with a triangular patch of available remaining allograft (Fig. 3). Caution is suggested: the corners between the right ventricular myocardium and triangular patch allograft should be anchored with care to avoid bleeding. Usually separate, horizontal, mattressed sutures are placed there for this reason. A second word of caution: stab wounds placed in

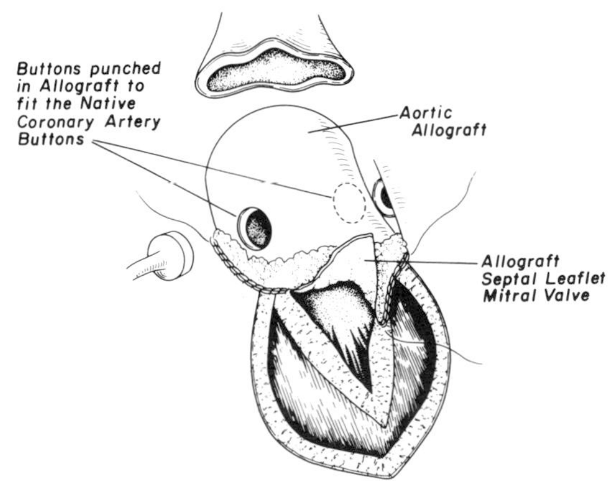

FIGURE 2. The mitral leaflet of the homograft is used to close the incision into the septum, creating a generous outflow tract.

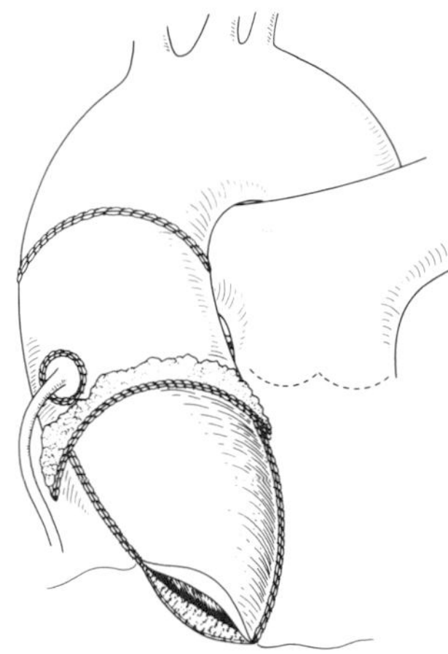

FIGURE 3. The right ventricle is closed with a triangular patch of either remaining allograft or Gor-Tex.

the root to remove air should be avoided since the homograft is initially quite friable and can tear easily when suture closure of the blow hole is attempted.

Pulmonary Allograft RVOT Reconstruction. Pulmonary allografts have been used in 82 patients since 1985 for the reconstruction of the right ventricular outflow tract in complex congenital heart disease. The mean age of these patients was 5 years. In children over 8 kg in weight, adult-sized allografts can be placed routinely. Preparation of the allograft is similar to the aortic allograft previously described. After bypass is initiated, the right ventricle is incised vertically (the aorta may or may not be cross-clamped, depending on the anatomy). The main pulmonary artery, if present, is transected to separate it from the heart. The distal main pulmonary artery as well as the left and right pulmonary arteries are inspected for areas of stenosis. Depending on the situation present, one of three variations for the distal anastomosis can be utilized. A standard circular anastomosis to the opened main pulmonary artery is used if the distal main pulmonary artery and left and right pulmonary arteries are normal. If one side has a stenosis, then the incision in the pulmonary artery can be carried down that side and the distal pulmonary artery allograft can be shaped so that a lip of either one or the other branch pulmonary artery is fitted into the opened distal pulmonary artery and anastomosed (Fig. 4). If both distal pulmonary arteries are narrowed, then the allograft is opened distally through both left and right

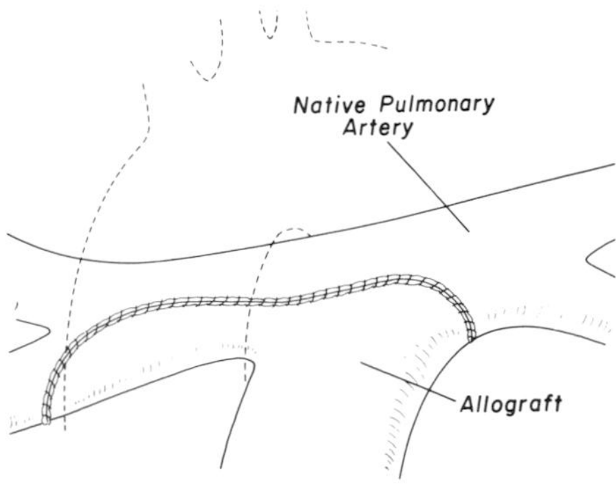

FIGURE 4. If the stenosis of the recipient pulmonary artery is unilateral, an incision is made into that branch, and the distal end of the allograft is sewn into place.

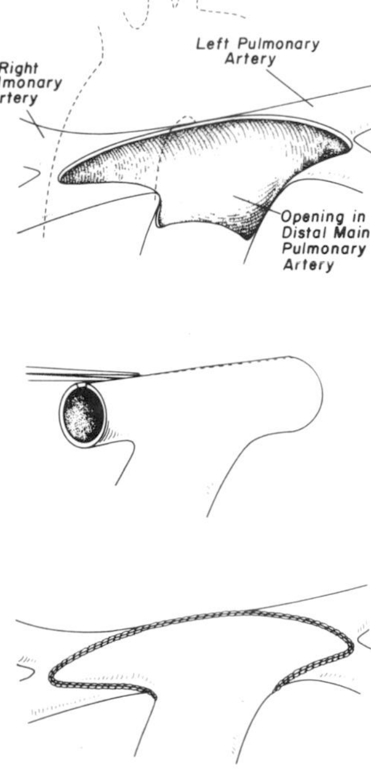

FIGURE 5. If bilateral stenosis of the branch pulmonary arteries exists, incisions are carried down both pulmonary arteries, the allograft is opened through the branches, and the anastomosis is completed.

pulmonary artery, fashioned so that it seats correctly onto the opened native vessel and then is sewn into place (Fig. 5). In situations in which no main pulmonary artery exists, the distal pulmonary homograft can be anastomosed to both hila separately (Fig. 6).

Once the distal end is completed in whatever fashion is necessary, the posterior one-third to one-half of the allograft is anchored to the right ventricle at the superior edge of the incision or at the pulmonary valve annulus if one is present. A triangular hood is fashioned from either Gor-Tex or the remaining allograft tissue, the aortic cross-clamp is released, if one had been used, and rewarming is begun as the hood is sewn into position (Fig. 7). The hood should be triangular and not circumferential so that intimal peel formation (pseudointima) does not occur.

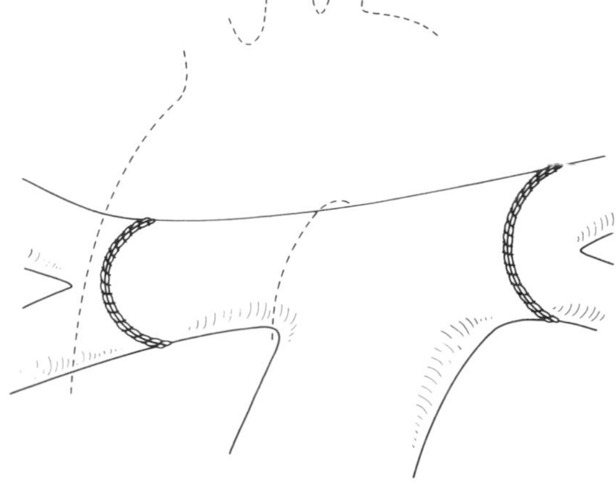

FIGURE 6. If no main pulmonary artery exists, circular anastomosis between the allograft branch pulmonary arteries and the recipient pulmonary arteries is completed.

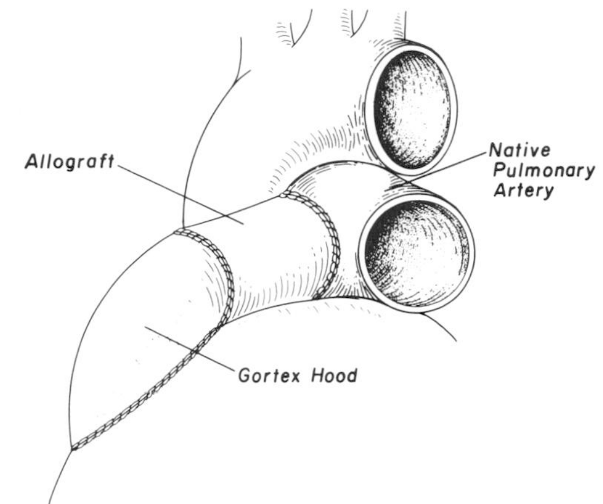

FIGURE 7. The hood used to complete the right ventricular outflow tract should not be circumferential no matter what material is used. Otherwise, the incidence of intimal peel formation and obstruction will be much higher.

RESULTS

Free-sewn Aortic Allografts (Fresh Antibiotic-sterilized). Early morbidity and mortality are similar to other series using mechanical valves and bioprosthesis for comparable time periods. Barratt-Boyes[47] reported a 6% overall 30-day mortality in a total of 393 isolated aortic valve replacements placed in Green Lane Hospital between 1968 and 1974. From this series 248 patients were followed from 9–16.5 years. By actuarial analysis risk of significant incompetence was 5% at 5 years, 22% at 10 years, and 58% at 14 years. However, there were 111 late deaths (47% of the study group). Of interest, the three factors identified as increasing the risk of incompetence included large aortic root size greater than 30 mm, increasing donor valve age greater than 55 years, and recipient age less than 15 years. However, the small number of children in this category[5] made this a tentative conclusion, and he still recommends their use in children.

Free-sewn Aortic Allografts (Cryopreserved). O'Brien[1] reviewed his experience with 124 fresh allografts stored at 4°C and 192 cryopreserved allografts placed at the Prince Charles Hospital between 1969 and 1986 (aortic valve replacement). Interestingly, his early (30-day) mortality was exactly the same as that of Barratt-Boyes, 6%. Overall survival at 15 years was 60% (nearly the same as that of Barratt-Boyes). The risk of significant valve degeneration at 10 years requiring reoperation was 11% in the fresh 4°C storage valves and 0% in the cryopreserved group. At 15 years the risk of valve degeneration requiring reoperation was 41% for the fresh 4°C valves. Fifteen year follow-up unfortunately is not available for the cryopreserved valves since implantation did not begin until 1975. The data are exceptional for both groups. In the subgroup of children undergoing operation, the risk of early valve degeneration was significantly higher in the fresh antibiotic group. Therefore, this must be taken as soft evidence that cryopreserved allografts can be used more safely in children than the fresh valves or other bioprostheses.

Angell,[2] in his review of 23 patients who had cryopreserved valves placed in the aortic position between 1973 and 1975 by the free-sewn technique, found the risk of valve degeneration to be 20% at 10 years. Obviously, this is different from the 0% degeneration that O'Brien found but still is quite good, and probably the true degree of degeneration for cryopreserved valves lies somewhere between the two very different reports.

Ross recently presented data on late results in 108 patients aged 5 to 73 years who underwent aortic root replacement between 1972 and 1986.[48] Indications for this procedure included tunnel subaortic obstruction, para-aortic annular abscesses, homograft valve dysfunction requiring reoperation, and aortic stenosis with hypoplastic aortic annulus. Early (30-day) mortality was 14%, late follow-up indicated a 79% freedom from valve-related death at 8 years and 60% freedom from valve-related complications at 8 years. Ross cautioned against the use of this procedure for Marfan's syndrome, nonspecific aortitis, and ascending aortic aneurysm, because the aortic annulus has a tendency to dilate postoperatively in these disease processes. Finally, he felt that this method of valve replacement in children was "ideal" and that durability was excellent long term in the children in whom he carried out this procedure.

The Denver data on extended aortic root replacement are similar, although a much shorter follow-up period is available. The early (30-day) operative mortality has been 5% and the incidence of valve-related failure at 3 years has been 15%. Two of these children were infants. The significance of this is unknown, but severe rejection of these valves is strongly suspected.

Long-term results of pulmonary valve allograft reconstruction of the right ventricular outflow tract are unknown, but the experiences of Ross, Clarke, and Gonzalez-Lavin indicate a very low incidence of valve failure (less than 2%) at a mean follow-up, however, of less than 5 years. It is hoped that these results will continue to remain excellent with time, in contrast to the Great Ormond Street, London experience. In this group of children, 108 antibiotic-sterilized allografts were placed for right heart, extracardiac conduits. The early mortality was 30%. Late follow-up indicated that these valve conduits were similar to the Dacron conduits in terms of late deaths and conduit obstruction. By 10 years few of the conduits were free from obstruction and/or associated death (25% ± 11.3%). These results are quite disappointing. However, it should be pointed out that the unknown is the degree to which conduit obstruction was involved in the late deaths. It is also likely that much of the obstruction was at the conduit tube and not at the valve, and was related to intimal peel formed in the often-placed circumferential Dacron tube. It is hoped that technical changes today will prevent this cause of late conduit obstruction.

In the Denver experience, trivial pulmonary valve insufficiency was common, but this has not generally progressed with time. The functional results have been excellent. At present a detailed mid-term analysis, including recatheterization of these pulmonary-valved conduits, is under way and the results will be available soon.

Finally, in reviewing his complex congenital experience from 1968 to 1983 with extracardiac conduits in which a free-sewn aortic allograft, a Dacron composite conduit with aortic allograft, or an aortic valved allograft conduit was placed, Fontan[49] reported excellent results with minimal gradients that were not progressive at an average of 5 years' follow-up.

CONCLUSIONS

Over the 30 years that allografts have been used clinically, many changes have occurred. In the beginning allografts appeared to be the perfect answer for the pediatric patient, but the early results with fresh antibiotic-treated allografts stored at 4° C were unfavorable in the young age group.

With the technique of cryopreservation, with better understanding of the immune response, with technical advances such as abandonment of circumferential

Dacron tubes so that intimal peel prevention is markedly lessened, and with use of free-sewn allografts rather than stented valves, the results of allografts placed in younger patients appear comparable to those in older patients. Complex left ventricular outflow tract obstruction is usually best managed by either aortic root replacement or extended aortic root replacement using cryopreserved aortic allografts. Right-sided reconstruction is best managed with the use of a pulmonary allograft. Mitral and tricuspid valve problems are still best managed by plastic procedures. If valve replacement becomes necessary, mechanical valves should be placed in the mitral position. A xenograft or stented allograft can be used in the tricuspid position.

REFERENCES

1. O'Brien MF, Stafford GE, Gardner MAH, et al: A comparison of aortic valve replacement with viable cryopreserved and fresh allograft valves with a note on chromosomal studies. J Thorac Cardiovasc Surg 94:812, 1987.
2. Angell WW, Angell JD, Oury JH, et al: Long-term follow-up of viable frozen aortic homografts: A viable homograft valve bank. J Thorac Cardiovasc Surg 93:815, 1987.
3. Lam CR, Aram HA, Munnell ER: An experimental study of aortic valve homografts. Surg Gynecol Obstet 94:129, 1952.
4. Ross DN: Evolution of the biological concept in cardiac surgery: A Pilgrim's Progress. In Cardiac Valve Allografts 1962–1987. New York, Springer-Verlag, 1988, p 1.
5. Murry G: Homologous aortic valve segment transplant as surgical treatment for aortic and mitral insufficiency. Angiology 7:466, 1956.
6. Ross DN: Homograft replacement of the aortic valve. Lancet 2:487, 1962.
7. Barratt-Boyes BG: Homograft aortic valve replacement in aortic incompetence and stenosis. Thorax 19:131, 1964.
8. Gunning AJ, Duran CG: A method for placing a total homologous aortic valve in the subcoronary position. Lancet 2:488, 1962.
9. Ross DN, Somerville J: Correction of pulmonary atresia with a homograft aortic valve. Lancet 2:1446, 1966.
10. Moodie DS, Mair DD, Fulton RE, et al: Aortic homograft obstruction. J Thorac Cardiovasc Surg 72:553, 1976.
11. McGoon DC, Danielson GK, Puga FJ, et al: Late results after extracardiac conduit repair for congenital cardiac defects. Am J Cardiol 49:1741, 1982.
12. Bowman FO, Hancock WD, Malm JR: A valve-containing dacron prosthesis. Arch Surg 107:724, 1973.
13. Donaldson RM, Ross DN: Homograft aortic root replacement for complicated prosthetic valve endocarditis. Circulation 70(Suppl I):178, 1982.
14. Lau JKH, Robles A, Cherian A, Ross RN: Surgical treatment of prosthetic endocarditis. Aortic root replacement using a homograft. J Thorac Cardiovasc Surg 87:712, 1984.
15. Somerville J, Ross DN: Homograft replacement of aortic root with reimplantation of coronary arteries. Br Heart J 47:473, 1982.
16. McKowen RL, Campbell DN, Woelfel GF, et al: Extended aortic root replacement with aortic allografts. J Thorac Cardiovasc Surg 93:366, 1987.
17. Kono S, Imai Y, Lida Y, et al: A new method for prosthetic valve replacement in congenital aortic stenosis associated with hypoplasia of the aortic valve ring. J Thorac Cardiovasc Surg 70:709, 1975.
18. Rastan H, Abu-Aishah N, Rastan D, et al: Results of aortoventriculoplasty in 21 consecutive patients with left ventricular outflow tract obstruction. J Thorac Cardiovasc Surg 75:659, 1978.
19. Rastan W, Koncz J: A new technique for the treatment of left ventricular outflow tract obstruction. J Thorac Cardiovasc Surg 71:920, 1976.
20. Kay PH, Livi U, Parker R, Ross DN: The pulmonary allograft for right ventricular outflow tract reconstruction. In Cardiac Valve Allografts 1962–1987. New York, Springer-Verlag, 1988, p 189.
21. McGrath LB, Gonzalez-Lavin L, Graf D: Pulmonary valve homograft implantation for ventricular outflow tract reconstruction: Early phase results. Ann Thorac Surg 45:273, 1988.
22. Clarke DR: Pulmonary valve allograft reconstruction of the right ventricular outflow tract. In Cardiac Valve Allografts 1962–1987. New York, Springer-Verlag, 1988, p 195.

23. Mermet B, Buch WS, Angell WW: Viable heart graft: Preservation in the frozen state. Surg Forum 21:157, 1970.
24. Angell JD, Christopher BS, Hawtrey O, Angell WM: A fresh viable human heart valve bank: Sterilization, sterility testing, and cryogenic preservation. Transplant Proc 8(Suppl I):139, 1976.
25. Barratt-Boyes B, Roche A: A review of aortic valve homografts over a six and one half year period. Ann Surg 170:483, 1969.
26. Strickett MG, Barratt-Boyes BG, MacCullough D: Disinfection of human heart valve allografts with antibiotics in low concentration. Pathology 15:457, 1983.
27. Armiger LC, Gavin JB, Barratt-Boyes BG: Histologic assessment of orthotopic aortic valve leaflet allografts: Its role in selecting graft pretreatment. Pathology 15:67, 1983.
28. Yankah AC, Hetzer R: Procurement and viability of cardiac valve allografts. In Cardiac Valve Allografts 1962–1987. New York, Springer-Verlag, 1988, p 23.
29. Yankah AC, Wottge HU, Muller-Hermelink HK, et al: Transplantation of aortic and pulmonary allografts, enhanced viability of endothelial cells by cryopreservation, importance of histocompatibility. J Cardiac Surg 1(Suppl 3):209, 1987.
30. Khanna SK, Ross JK, Monro JL: Homograft aortic valve replacement: 7 years' experience with antibiotic treated valves. Thorax 36:330, 1981.
31. Davies H, Lessof MH, Roberts GI, Ross DN: Homograft replacement of the aortic valve. Follow-up studies in 12 patients. Lancet 1:926, 1965.
32. Hudson REB: Pathology of the human aortic valve homograft. Br Heart J 28:291, 1966.
33. Mohri H, Reichenbach DD, Barnes RW, et al: Studies of antigenicity of the homologous aortic valve. J Thorac Cardiovasc Surg 54:564, 1967.
34. McKenzie MB, Titus JL, Ellis FW Jr, Pappas G: Experimental semilunar valve homografts: Morphological features. J Thorac Cardiovasc Surg 50:410, 1965.
35. Hirsch HH, Hanke H: The cause of transplanted heart valve homograft persistence. Am Heart J 75:568, 1968.
36. Tector AJ, Boyd WC, Korns ME: Aortic valve allograft rejection. J Thorac Cardiovasc Surg 62:592, 1971.
37. Baue AE, Donawicil WJ, Blakemore WS: The immune response to heterotopic allovital aortic valve. Transplants in presensitized and nonsensitized recipients. J Thorac Cardiovasc Surg 56:775, 1968.
38. Buch WS, Kosek JC, Angell WW: The role of rejection and mechanical trauma on graft viability. J Thorac Cardiovasc Surg 62:696, 1971.
39. Balch CM, Karp RB: Blood group compatibility and aortic valve allotransplantation in man. J Thorac Cardiovasc Surg 70:256, 1975.
40. Cochran RP, Kunzelman KS: Cryopreservation does not alter antigenic expression of aortic allografts (in press).
41. Yankah AC, Wottge HU, Muller-Ruchholtz W: Antigenicity and fate of cellular components of heart valve allografts. In Cardiac Valve Allografts 1962–1987. New York, Springer-Verlag, 1988, p. 77.
42. Yacoub MH, Festenstein P, Doyle M, Martin D, et al: The influence of HLA matching in cardiac allograft recipients receiving cyclosporin and azathioprine. Transplant Proc 19:2487, 1987.
43. Campbell DN, Clarke DR: Unpublished data.
44. Yacoub M, Suitters A, Khagani A, Rose M: Localization of major histocompatibility complex (HLA ABC + DR) antigens in aortic homografts. In Bondnar E, Yacoub M (eds): Biologic and Bioprosthetic Valves. New York Yorke Medical Books, 1986, p. 65.
45. Sugimoto JT, Karp RB: Homograft and cryopreserved valves. In Crawford FA Jr (ed): Current Heart Valve Prostheses. Cardiac Surgery: State of the Art Reviews. Philadelphia, Hanley & Belfus, 1987, p. 295.
46. Schaeffer MS, Wiggins JW, Wolfe RR, et al: Aortoventriculoplasty in children. J Thorac Cardiovasc Surg 92:391, 1986.
47. Barratt-Boyes BG, Roche AHG, Subramarman R, Pemberton JR: Long-term followup of patients with the antibiotic-sterilized aortic homograft valve inserted freehand in the aortic position. Circulation 75:768, 1987.
48. Okita Y, Franciosi G, Matsuki O, et al: Early and late results of aortic root replacement with antibiotic-sterilized aortic homograft. J Thorac Cardiovasc Surg 95:696, 1988.
49. Fontan F, Choussat A., Deville C, et al: Aortic valve homografts in the surgical treatment of complex cardiac malformations. J Thorac Cardiovasc Surg 87:649, 1984.

INDEX

Entries in **boldface** type indicate complete chapters